Nutrition Interventions for Healthy Ageing

Nutrition Interventions for Healthy Ageing

Guest Editors

Moustapha Dramé
Lidvine Godaert

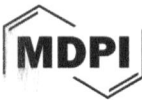

Basel • Beijing • Wuhan • Barcelona • Belgrade • Novi Sad • Cluj • Manchester

Guest Editors

Moustapha Dramé
Department of Clinical
Research and Innovation
University Hospitals
of Martinique
Martinique
France

Lidvine Godaert
Department of Geriatrics
General Hospital
of Valenciennes
Valenciennes
France

Editorial Office
MDPI AG
Grosspeteranlage 5
4052 Basel, Switzerland

This is a reprint of the Special Issue, published open access by the journal *Nutrients* (ISSN 2072-6643), freely accessible at: https://www.mdpi.com/journal/nutrients/special_issues/76M853WU19.

For citation purposes, cite each article independently as indicated on the article page online and as indicated below:

Lastname, A.A.; Lastname, B.B. Article Title. *Journal Name* **Year**, *Volume Number*, Page Range.

ISBN 978-3-7258-2715-2 (Hbk)
ISBN 978-3-7258-2716-9 (PDF)
https://doi.org/10.3390/books978-3-7258-2716-9

© 2025 by the authors. Articles in this book are Open Access and distributed under the Creative Commons Attribution (CC BY) license. The book as a whole is distributed by MDPI under the terms and conditions of the Creative Commons Attribution-NonCommercial-NoDerivs (CC BY-NC-ND) license (https://creativecommons.org/licenses/by-nc-nd/4.0/).

Contents

Valérie Dormal, Barbara Pachikian, Elena Debock, Marine Buchet, Sylvie Copine and Louise Deldicque
Evaluation of a Dietary Supplementation Combining Protein and a Pomegranate Extract in Older People: A Safety Study
Reprinted from: *Nutrients* **2022**, *14*, 5182, https://doi.org/10.3390/nu14235182 1

Charlotte Mortensen, Inge Tetens, Michael Kristensen and Anne Marie Beck
Vitamin D and Calcium Supplementation in Nursing Homes—A Quality Improvement Study
Reprinted from: *Nutrients* **2022**, *14*, 5360, https://doi.org/10.3390/nu14245360 10

Miho Kanazashi, Tadayuki Iida, Ryosuke Nakanishi, Masayuki Tanaka, Hiromi Ikeda, Naomi Takamiya, et al.
Brazilian Propolis Intake Decreases Body Fat Mass and Oxidative Stress in Community-Dwelling Elderly Females: A Randomized Placebo-Controlled Trial
Reprinted from: *Nutrients* **2023**, *15*, 364, https://doi.org/10.3390/nu15020364 20

Moustapha Dramé and Lidvine Godaert
The Obesity Paradox and Mortality in Older Adults: A Systematic Review
Reprinted from: *Nutrients* **2023**, *15*, 1780, https://doi.org/10.3390/nu15071780 32

Muhammed Tunc, Pinar Soysal, Ozge Pasin, Lee Smith, Masoud Rahmati, Veliye Yigitalp, et al.
Hypomagnesemia Is Associated with Excessive Daytime Sleepiness, but Not Insomnia, in Older Adults
Reprinted from: *Nutrients* **2023**, *15*, 2467, https://doi.org/10.3390/nu15112467 47

Nadine Simo-Tabue, Denis Boucaud-Maitre, Laurys Letchimy, Jeff Guilhem-Decleon, Jeannie Helene-Pelage, Guillaume T. Duval and Maturin Tabue-Teguo
Correlates of Undernutrition in Older People in Guadeloupe (French West Indies): Results from the KASADS Study
Reprinted from: *Nutrients* **2023**, *15*, 2950, https://doi.org/10.3390/nu15132950 59

Theng Choon Ooi, Azizan Ahmad, Nor Fadilah Rajab and Razinah Sharif
The Effects of 12 Weeks Colostrum Milk Supplementation on the Expression Levels of Pro-Inflammatory Mediators and Metabolic Changes among Older Adults: Findings from the Biomarkers and Untargeted Metabolomic Analysis
Reprinted from: *Nutrients* **2023**, *15*, 3184, https://doi.org/10.3390/nu15143184 68

Lei An, Qiu Lu, Ke Wang and Yousheng Wang
Urolithins: A Prospective Alternative against Brain Aging
Reprinted from: *Nutrients* **2023**, *15*, 3884, https://doi.org/10.3390/nu15183884 83

Sapna Virdi, Abbey M. McKee, Manogna Nuthi and Nafisa M. Jadavji
The Role of One-Carbon Metabolism in Healthy Brain Aging
Reprinted from: *Nutrients* **2023**, *15*, 3891, https://doi.org/10.3390/nu15183891 108

Nadja-R. Baer, Noemi Vanessa Grissmer, Liane Schenk, Hanna R. Wortmann, Petra Warschburger and Ulrike A. Gisch
Practicing Interoceptive Sensitivity as a Couple: A Mixed-Methods Acceptance Analysis of a Dyadic vs. Single Pilot Randomized Controlled Trial
Reprinted from: *Nutrients* **2024**, *16*, 1949, https://doi.org/10.3390/nu16121949 119

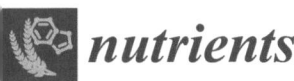

Article

Evaluation of a Dietary Supplementation Combining Protein and a Pomegranate Extract in Older People: A Safety Study

Valérie Dormal [1,2], Barbara Pachikian [1], Elena Debock [1], Marine Buchet [1], Sylvie Copine [1] and Louise Deldicque [1,2,*]

1. Center of Investigation in Clinical Nutrition, Université Catholique de Louvain, 1348 Louvain-la-Neuve, Belgium
2. Institute of Neuroscience, Université Catholique de Louvain, 1348 Louvain-la-Neuve, Belgium
* Correspondence: louise.deldicque@uclouvain.be

Abstract: Malnutrition is a highly prevalent condition in older adults. It is associated with low muscle mass and function and increased occurrence of health problems. Maintaining an adequate nutritional status as well as a sufficient nutrient intake in older people is therefore essential to address this public health problem. For this purpose, protein supplementation is known to prevent the loss of muscle mass during aging, and the consumption of various pomegranate extracts induces numerous health benefits, mainly through their antioxidant properties. However, to our knowledge, no study has to date investigated the impact of their combination on the level of malnutrition in older people. The objective of this preliminary study was thus to evaluate the safety of a combination of protein and a pomegranate extract in healthy subjects aged 65 years or more during a 21-day supplementation period. Thirty older participants were randomly assigned to receive protein and a pomegranate extract (Test group) or protein and maltodextrin (Control group) during a 21-day intervention period. The primary outcomes were the safety and tolerability of the supplementation defined as the occurrence of adverse events, and additional secondary outcomes included physical examination and hematological and biochemical parameters. No serious adverse events were reported in any group. Changes in physical, hematological, and biochemical parameters between the initial screening and the end of the study were equivalent in both groups, except for glutamate-pyruvate transaminase (GPT) and prealbumin, for which a decrease was observed only in the Test group. Our initial findings support the safety of the combination of protein and a pomegranate extract in healthy elderly people. Future clinical trials on a larger sample and a longer period are needed to determine the efficacy of this combination.

Keywords: protein; pomegranate extract; older people; safety; clinical trial

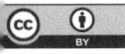

1. Introduction

Malnutrition in older adults has been recently identified as a challenging public health problem associated not only with a high mortality and morbidity rate but also with physical, psychological, and functional decline [1,2]. In particular, protein–energy malnutrition (PEM), resulting from a decrease in protein and energy intake, has been associated with a number of health problems such as sarcopenia [3,4]. Sarcopenia is characterized by a gradual loss of muscle mass leading to a decrease in muscle strength and physical performance. This condition can have functional consequences, such as falls and fractures, and worsens the health and the quality of life of the elderly [5].

The treatment of malnutrition requires early identification and efficient intervention, both in hospitalized patients and community-dwelling older adults. Higher protein intake recommendations are made to older adults suffering from malnutrition. Beyond its role in the accretion of muscle mass, protein has been identified as a key nutrient for elderly people. Slightly higher protein intake than usually recommended may improve muscle health and help maintain energy balance, weight management, and cardiovascular function [6], all of which may contribute to an improved quality of life. Compared to the typical recommended protein intake of 0.83 g·kg^{-1}·d^{-1} in healthy adults, the recommended intake rises to 1 g·kg^{-1}·d^{-1} in older malnourished persons with a body mass index (BMI) under 21 kg/m^2 [7]. Currently, the most common method to reach that recommendation is consuming oral nutritional supplements (ONS). Several clinical studies in elderly people have shown that protein- and vitamin-D-rich ONS improve protein synthesis, muscle mass, and performance but also functional parameters, evaluated, for example, by the chair rise test [8–10]. However, evidence investigating ONS compliance and effectiveness is conflicting [11]. In addition, those supplements are rarely effectively consumed by the elderly because of their taste, their satietogenic texture, and/or their high cost [12].

More tolerable and appropriate alternatives that meet the needs of malnourished older people are therefore required. Besides integrating protein directly into the food consumed, the combination with other substances beneficial to the elderly may constitute another strategy. In this study, protein of high biological value was combined with a pomegranate extract, a rich source of various phytochemicals, including anthocyanins, ellagitannins, gallotannins, proanthocyanidins, flavonols, and lignans, which are known to induce beneficial effects on human health [13]. The pomegranate extract used here was particularly rich in ellagitannins, more specifically in punicalagins, as well as in ellagic acid. Thanks to its antioxidant and anti-inflammatory mechanisms, pomegranate is known to improve muscle function [14] and performance [15] in resistance-trained men. In addition to the positive effects of pomegranate on muscles, pomegranate also has other very interesting properties, including protection against metabolic and cardiovascular diseases [16,17]. Pomegranate polyphenols are able to inhibit low-density lipoprotein (LDL) oxidation and to increase the activity of serum paraoxonase, an esterase that protects lipids against peroxidation in humans [18]. Here, we chose to test whey protein, a protein source of high biological value due to its high content of essential amino acids, particularly leucine. This amino acid is particularly effective at stimulating protein synthesis in the skeletal muscle [19]. Whey protein has proven to be a very efficient protein source to stimulate protein synthesis and the accretion of muscle mass in diverse populations, including older people [20,21].

Altogether, these data show that protein and pomegranate extract supplementation are effective nutritional strategies to improve health status, at least when taken separately. Whether there is an added value in combining them and whether pomegranate extracts provide health benefits in older persons is unknown. Combining protein and a pomegranate extract would be innovative but safety issues may arise as their combination has never been tested in an older population. The aim of this study was therefore to evaluate the safety of a 21-day supplementation combining protein and a pomegranate extract in healthy subjects aged 65 years or more compared to protein alone.

2. Materials and Methods

2.1. Participants

A total of 39 participants were assessed for eligibility, and 30 participants were randomized between December 2021 and February 2022 into the Test (n = 15) or the Control (n = 15) groups (Figure 1). One participant from the Test group dropped out of the study for personal reasons. Participants were recruited by posters, mail, social networks, and local newspapers. To be included, the participants had to meet the following criteria: woman or man aged over 65 years; presenting a BMI from 20 to 30; and in good general health as evidenced by medical history and physical examination. The participants were excluded if they presented one of the following exclusion criteria: severe psychiatric disorder or disease within 6 months before inclusion (such as depression, bipolar disorder, severe anxiety, psychosis, schizophrenic disorders, or dementia) or a severe neurologic trouble (such as Alzheimer's, autism, or Parkinson's disease); cancer within less than 3 years before the screening visit (except basal cell skin cancer or squamous cell skin cancer); a severe gastro-intestinal, hepatic, respiratory, kidney, or cardiovascular disorder or severe infection (such as HIV or hepatitis); uncontrolled hormonal disorders (such as thyroid problems or Cushing's syndrome); uncontrolled type 1 or 2 diabetes; known allergy or intolerance to one of the components of the administered products; and participants consuming ONS or protein supplements up to one month before the screening.

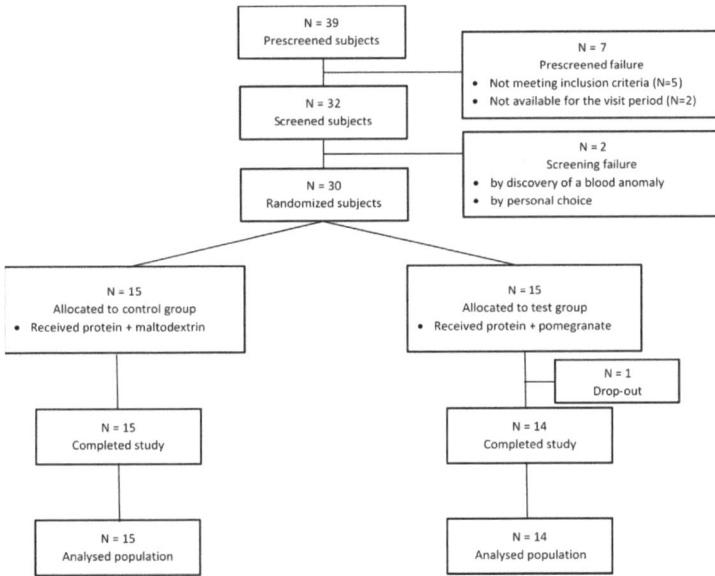

Figure 1. Flow chart of the study samples, including the number of participants who were screened, underwent randomization, completed the study treatment, and were analyzed for the primary and secondary outcomes.

All selected participants provided written informed consent. The trial was approved by the local ethical committee and was carried out in accordance with the Declaration of Helsinki and the Good Clinical Practice guidelines as required by the following regulations: the Belgian law of 7 May 2004 regarding experiments on human beings and the EU Directive 2001/20/EC on Clinical Trials (registration at clinicaltrials.gov accessed on 6 November 2022 as NCT05527249).

2.2. Study Design and Randomization

This was a randomized double-blind placebo-controlled interventional study. A prescreening was proposed with an online questionnaire sent by email. Then, the screening visit, comprising a physical examination (including measurement of body weight, height, heart rate, and blood pressure) and a blood sampling, was organized within 4 weeks before subject inclusion. The participants who met all the criteria were randomly assigned to the Test or the Control groups. Both groups were instructed (1) to consume 20 g protein mixed into vegetable milk, orange juice, or soup and (2) to ingest one capsule with a glass of water every day before lunch for 3 weeks. The participants of both groups received the same protein powder (Fresubin®) with a neutral taste and containing 100% whey protein. The capsule contained 650 mg pomegranate extract (Oxylent GR) in the Test group and 650 mg maltodextrin (Delical, BS Nutrition) in the Control group. Each capsule of pomegranate extract contained at least 65 mg punicalagins (>10%), 260 mg polyphenols (>40%), and more than 13 mg ellagic acid (>2%). The dose of 650 mg was chosen based on the efficacy of this dose to improve muscle strength recovery after eccentric exercise [22]. The capsules containing maltodextrin or pomegranate extract were prepared by a pharmacist. The appearance, i.e., white color, did not distinguish the 2 capsules. All products were stored in a closed room at a controlled temperature between 18 and 25 °C and protected from light. Study outcomes were assessed at baseline (V1), in the middle of the intervention (day 10; V2), and at the end of the intervention (day 21; V3). Protocol deviations and subjects' withdrawals were monitored regularly during the study. The database was locked, and the blinding was broken after completion of the whole quality control of the data.

2.3. Safety Measurements

The primary outcomes were safety and tolerability of the protein/pomegranate combination defined as occurrence of adverse events. All these events were recorded from the signature of the informed consent to the end of the study.

The secondary outcomes were changes in physical examination, including weight, heart rate, and systolic and diastolic blood pressure; changes in hematological parameters, including hemoglobin and hematocrit levels and white blood cell, red blood cell, and platelet counts; and changes in biochemical parameters (Lims Mbnext group), including uric acid, creatinine, total bilirubin, glutamate oxaloacetic transaminase (GOT), glutamate pyruvate transaminase (GPT), total cholesterol, triglyceride, sodium, potassium, total protein, prealbumin, urea, blood glucose, alkaline phosphatase, gamma-glutamytranspeptidase (GGT), lactate dehydrogenase (LDH), and C-reactive protein (CRP). Compliance to protein and pomegranate/maltodextrin ingestion was assessed at the end of the study by weighing the remaining quantity of powder and capsules and comparing to the quantity given at the beginning of the study.

2.4. Statistical Analyses

Given the pilot nature of this study, a sample size of 30 participants was determined based on feasibility considerations. All the continuous variables are presented as mean ± SD. Statistical analyses were performed using the software systems SAS 9.4 (SAS Institute Inc., Cary, NC, USA). Baseline differences in demographic characteristics between the groups were examined using χ^2 tests and independent t tests. Differences in physical, hematological, and biochemical parameters between groups (Control and Test) at each visit (V1, V2, and V3) were analyzed using a linear mixed model for repeated measurements with subjects as the random variable, and groups, visits, and their interaction as fixed independent variables. As variables were not normally distributed, a logarithmic transformation was applied, and when appropriate, post hoc comparison was performed using the Wilcoxon matched-pairs signed-rank test for analyses of within-group differences and the Wilcoxon Mann–Whitney two-sample test for analyses of differences between groups. All analyses were conducted at an alpha level of 0.05.

3. Results

3.1. Participants' Characteristics

The Test group was composed of 5 men and 9 women, and the mean age was 68.4 ± 2.4 years, while the Control group was composed of 9 men and 6 women, and the mean age was 68.7 ± 2.8 years. There were no significant differences in age, gender ratio, weight, BMI, or blood pressure between the two groups at baseline.

3.2. Primary Outcomes

The protein/pomegranate combination was well tolerated, with no serious adverse event reported and no difference in the mild and moderate adverse events reported by the Test (n = 5) and the Control (n = 6) groups. None of these mild or moderate adverse effects, including lung infection, COVID-19, and painful tooth extraction, were deemed to be related to the supplementation (Table 1).

Table 1. Description of mild and moderate adverse events observed in the Test and Control groups.

		Description of the Adverse Event	Intensity of the Event	Causal Relation of the Event to the Study Product
Test		COVID	Moderate	Not related
		Intestinal problems	Moderate	Maybe related
		Intestinal problems	Moderate	Unlikely related
		Headache	Mild	Not related
		Tendinitis	Moderate	Not related
Control		Lung infection	Moderate	Not related
		COVID	Mild	Not related
		COVID	Moderate	Not related
		Eczema	Moderate	Unlikely related
		Sciatic nerve inflammation	Moderate	Not related
		Painful tooth extraction	Moderate	Not related

3.3. Secondary Outcomes

Data related to physical, hematological, and biochemical parameters are presented in Table 2 and Figures 2 and 3.

Table 2. Physical, hematological, and biochemical parameters.

	Test (n = 14)			Control (n = 15)		
	V1	V2	V3	V1	V2	V3
Physical parameters						
Weight (kg)	70.9 ± 14.7	72.8 ± 16.7	72.1 ± 16.0	72.3 ± 10.6	70.2 ± 10.4	72.3 ± 11.6
Heart rate (bpm)	64.9 ± 6.9	66.6 ± 11.4	71.1 ± 12.0	65.3 ± 11.0	67.4 ± 17.7	65.9 ± 12.3
Body Mass Index (kg/m^2)	25.7 ± 3.2	26.8 ± 3.5	26.5 ± 3.3	24.7 ± 2.2	24.3 ± 2.5	25.0 ± 3.1
Hematological parameters						
White blood cells (10^3/μL)	5.89 ± 1.38	5.82 ± 1.24	5.83 ± 1.13	5.57 ± 1.01	5.83 ± 1.37	5.50 ± 1.21
Red blood cells (10^6/μL)	4.62 ± 0.30	4.59 ± 0.29	4.53 ± 0.26	4.68 ± 0.42	4.69 ± 0.35	4.64 ± 0.35
Hemoglobin (g/dL)	13.9 ± 1.2	13.7 ± 0.9	13.6 ± 0.9 *	14.1 ± 1.1	14.0 ± 1.0	14.0 ± 1.0 *
Hematocrit (%)	41.0 ± 2.8	40.6 ± 2.4	40.2 ± 2.4	41.3 ± 3.1	41.4 ± 2.8	41.3 ± 2.7
Platelet count (10^3/μL)	267.6 ± 40.6	265.1 ± 47.7	265.6 ± 36.8	241.8 ± 46.6	248.3 ± 45.3	245.7 ± 42.9
Biochemical parameters						
Uric acid (mg/dL)	5.20 ± 1.26	4.76 ± 1.12 ***	4.59 ± 1.07 ***	5.52 ± 1.33	4.96 ± 1.39 ***	4.99 ± 1.17 ***
Creatinine (mg/dL)	0.80 ± 0.17	0.77 ± 0.12	0.74 ± 0.15	0.81 ± 0.15	0.80 ± 0.16	0.80 ± 0.17
Total bilirubin (mg/dL)	0.77 ± 0.27	0.72 ± 0.24	0.69 ± 0.26	0.84 ± 0.40	0.79 ± 0.39	0.82 ± 0.41
GOT (U/L)	23.4 ± 6.6	22.6 ± 5.5	21.4 ± 4.0	22.6 ± 4.2	23.6 ± 9.7	23.7 ± 5.8
Triglycerides (mg/dL)	121.9 ± 72.5	109.2 ± 45.9	106.8 ± 59.9	98.2 ± 43.6	99.1 ± 48.9	94.5 ± 44.2
Sodium (mmol/L)	139.6 ± 2.3	139.7 ± 2.5	140.1 ± 2.1	139.5 ± 2.0	139.5 ± 2.8	139.5 ± 2.2
Potassium (mmol/L)	4.32 ± 0.30	4.68 ± 0.37 ***	4.59 ± 0.37 ***	4.37 ± 0.21	4.78 ± 0.36 ***	4.53 ± 0.40 ***
Total protein (g/L)	68.4 ± 3.7	68.0 ± 3.1	66.5 ± 3.7	66.9 ± 3.0	67.2 ± 2.7	66.8 ± 3.3
Urea (mg/dL)	37.1 ± 10.4	42.1 ± 10.0 *	40.1 ± 6.1	35.7 ± 10.2	39.7 ± 9.4 *	37.7 ± 7.8
Blood glucose (mg/dL)	89.3 ± 9.2	87.6 ± 8.1	90.1 ± 11.5	89.1 ± 8.6	88.1 ± 7.3	89.9 ± 9.6
Alkaline phosphatase (U/L)	69.1 ± 22.9	68.4 ± 21.4	68.5 ± 20.8	68.8 ± 15.4	68.0 ± 13.8	68.3 ± 12.6
GGT (U/L)	27.4 ± 19.2	25.2 ± 16.8	24.6 ± 15.2	23.3 ± 8.5	24.2 ± 11.7	24.7 ± 14.4
LDH (U/L)	168.1 ± 21.1	168.9 ± 21.8	166.5 ± 26.6	175.2 ± 29.6	169.5 ± 24.2	174.2 ± 23.3
CRP (mg/L)	2.26 ± 1.75	2.71 ± 1.43	3.88 ± 6.86	1.79 ± 1.12	1.55 ± 0.85	1.65 ± 1.21

Values are means ± SD. n: number of subjects; bpm: beats per minute; GOT: glutamate oxaloacetic transaminase; GGT: gamma-glutamyltranspeptidase; LDH: lactate dehydrogenase; CRP: C-reactive protein. * $p < 0.05$ vs. V1, *** $p < 0.001$ vs. V1.

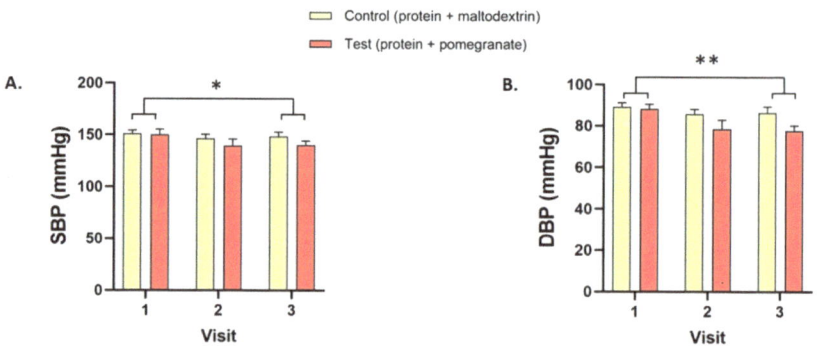

Figure 2. Systolic and diastolic blood pressures. (**A**) Systolic (SBP) and (**B**) diastolic (DBP) blood pressures in the Test and Control groups at V1, V2, and V3. * $p < 0.05$, ** $p < 0.01$.

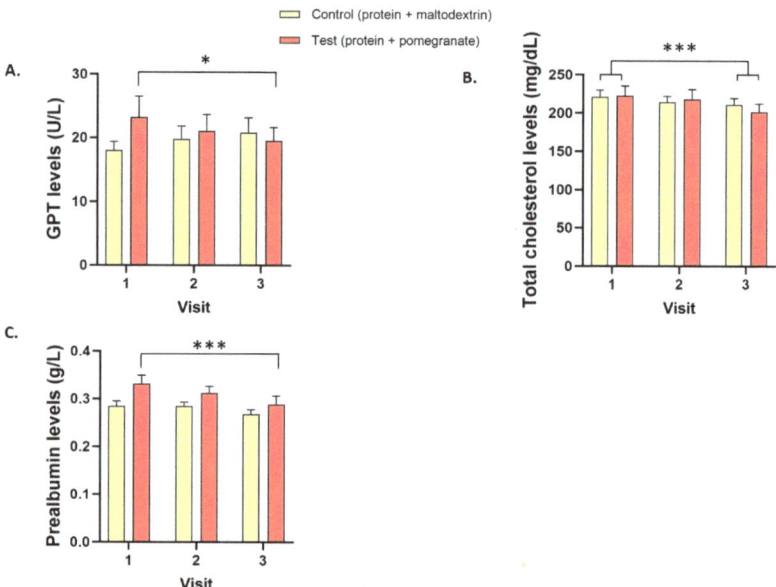

Figure 3. Glutamate pyruvate transaminase, total cholesterol, and prealbumin levels. Plasma (**A**) glutamate pyruvate transaminase (GPT), (**B**) total cholesterol, and (**C**) prealbumin levels in the Test and Control groups at V1, V2, and V3. * $p < 0.05$, *** $p < 0.001$.

3.3.1. Physical Parameters

The systolic (-4.2%, $p = 0.046$, Figure 2A) and diastolic (-7.5%, $p = 0.003$, Figure 2B) blood pressures decreased between V1 and V3 in both the Control and Test groups, with no difference between the two groups. No difference between conditions was observed in the weight, the BMI, or the heart rate (Table 2).

3.3.2. Hematological Parameters

Plasma hemoglobin levels decreased between V1 and V3 in both groups (-1.8%, $p = 0.038$), with no difference between groups (Table 2). No difference between conditions was observed in the hematocrit levels or the white blood cell, red blood cell, or platelet counts.

3.3.3. Biochemical Parameters

Plasma GPT levels decreased between V1 and V3 only in the Test group (-15.7%, $p = 0.039$, Figure 3A). Total plasma cholesterol levels decreased between V1 and V3 in both groups (-6.9%, $p < 0.001$), with no difference between groups (Figure 3B). Plasma prealbumin levels decreased between V1 and V3 in the Test group (-12.1%, $p < 0.001$) and tended to decrease in the Control group (-3.6%, $p = 0.071$, Figure 3C). In both groups, the levels of plasma uric acid decreased between V1 and V2 (-9.3%, $p < 0.001$) and V1 and V3 (-10.6%, $p < 0.0001$) while the levels of urea increased at the same time between V1 and V2 ($+12.5\%$, $p = 0.011$), with no difference between groups (Table 1). Plasma potassium levels increased similarly in both groups between V1 and V2 ($+8.9\%$, $p < 0.001$) and between V1 and V3 ($+4.9\%$, $p < 0.001$). Finally, plasma creatinine, total bilirubin, GOT, triglyceride, sodium, protein, blood glucose, alkaline phosphatase, GGT, LDH, and CRP levels were stable throughout the study and did not differ among groups (Table 2).

3.3.4. Compliance

A high compliance percentage in both groups was found, with an intake of $100.0 \pm 5.7\%$ in the Test group and $100.0 \pm 6.8\%$ in the Control group, with no difference between the two groups (Table S1).

4. Discussion

Malnutrition is a highly prevalent condition in older adults. It is associated with low muscle mass and function and increased occurrence of health problems [1–4]. Maintaining an adequate nutritional status as well as a sufficient nutrient intake in older people is therefore essential to address this public health problem. For this purpose, protein supplementation is known to prevent the loss of muscle mass during aging [8–10], and the consumption of various pomegranate extracts induces numerous health benefits, mainly through their antioxidant properties [13]. Combining protein and a pomegranate extract would be innovative but safety issues may arise as this combination has never been tested in an older population. The aim of this study was therefore to evaluate the safety of a 21-day supplementation combining protein and a pomegranate extract in healthy subjects aged 65 years or more compared to protein alone.

Our results showed that the daily combination of 20 g protein and 650 mg pomegranate extract for 21 days was safe and well tolerated. No serious adverse events were observed, and all mild or moderate adverse events were not related to the dietary supplement consumption. These results reinforce previous studies showing the safety of pomegranate extract supplementation at similar or higher doses in different adult populations, e.g., 1050 mg in hemodialysis patients [23] or 710 and 1420 mg in overweight individuals [24]. In addition, there were no differences between the Test and Control groups in physical and hematological parameters. In line with previous results dealing with protein or pomegranate supplementation [25,26], a decrease in systolic and diastolic blood pressure was observed between the start and the end of the study in both groups. While beyond the primary scope of the present study, these results suggest beneficial actions of protein and protein/pomegranate supplementation on blood pressure. To confirm these preliminary observations, a proper control group with neither protein nor pomegranate supplementation needs to be included in our follow-up study investigating the efficacy of those compounds on physical and hematological parameters in malnourished older people.

Most of the differences in the biochemical parameters observed between baseline screening and the end of the study were present in both groups. Plasma potassium and urea levels increased while uric acid and total cholesterol decreased similarly in both groups, which is consistent with previous reports following protein intake in healthy and pathological populations [27–29]. Here, we did not find any additional effect of combined protein/pomegranate supplementation compared to protein alone on the different biochemical parameters studied, possibly excepting GPT, a marker of liver function [30]. The latter decreased in the Test group only. In addition to its already known effects on metabolic risk factors [16], pomegranate could have a potential beneficial effect on parameters related to liver function. Here as well, a proper control group with neither protein nor pomegranate supplementation will be necessary when investigating the efficacy of those compounds on biochemical parameters in malnourished older people. Globally, given the preliminary nature of this safety study, the small number of participants resulted in limited statistical power to demonstrate specific benefits of protein and pomegranate on health-related parameters. That said, the primary aim of the present study was fulfilled, namely, the investigation of the safety and tolerance of combined protein/pomegranate supplementation in a limited sample of older people. Despite some statistical changes, all parameters studied here remained within healthy thresholds. Therefore, our supplementation can be considered safe and well tolerated.

In conclusion, we found that a combined protein/pomegranate supplementation for 21 days was safe and well tolerated in older participants. This first study was required before investigating the efficacy of this combination in a larger sample of older malnourished people for a longer duration to detect changes in muscle mass, and in a more appropriate form such as directly integrated into food to increase ONS compliance.

Supplementary Materials: The following supporting information can be downloaded at: https://www.mdpi.com/article/10.3390/nu14235182/s1. Table S1: Individual compliance (%) in the Control and Test groups.

Author Contributions: Conceptualization, B.P., S.C. and L.D.; methodology, B.P., E.D. and S.C.; data analysis, V.D., B.P. and E.D.; investigation, B.P., E.D., M.B. and S.C.; writing—original draft preparation, V.D. and B.P.; writing—review and editing, B.P., E.D., M.B., S.C. and L.D.; project administration, V.D., B.P., E.D. and S.C. All authors have read and agreed to the published version of the manuscript.

Funding: This work was supported by the Region Wallonne (Delicen's).

Institutional Review Board Statement: The study was conducted according to the guidelines of the Declaration of Helsinki and approved by the Institutional Review Board (or Ethics Committee) of Comité d'Ethique Hospitalo-Facultaire de Saint-Luc (protocol code 2021/21SEP/387).

Informed Consent Statement: Informed consent was obtained from all subjects involved in the study.

Data Availability Statement: Data are available upon request by sending an e-mail to cicn@uclouvain.be

Acknowledgments: We thank Céline Bugli (SMCS, UCLouvain) for the helpful statistical analysis of the data.

Conflicts of Interest: The authors have no conflict of interest to disclose.

References

1. Correia, M.I.; Waitzberg, D.L. The impact of malnutrition on morbidity, mortality, length of hospital stay and costs evaluated through a multivariate model analysis. *Clin. Nutr.* **2003**, *22*, 235–239. [CrossRef]
2. Norman, K.; Hass, U.; Pirlich, M. Malnutrition in Older Adults-Recent Advances and Remaining Challenges. *Nutrients* **2021**, *13*, 2764. [CrossRef]
3. Corish, C.A.; Kennedy, N.P. Protein-energy undernutrition in hospital in-patients. *Br. J. Nutr.* **2000**, *83*, 575–591. [CrossRef]
4. Sieber, C.C. Malnutrition and sarcopenia. *Aging Clin. Exp. Res.* **2019**, *31*, 793–798. [CrossRef]
5. Beaudart, C.; Reginster, J.Y.; Petermans, J.; Bruyere, O. [Quality of life of sarcopenic patients: Contribution of the SarcoPhAge study]. *Geriatr. Psychol. Neuropsychiatr. Vieil.* **2015**, *13*, 391–395. [CrossRef]
6. Baum, J.I.; Kim, I.Y.; Wolfe, R.R. Protein Consumption and the Elderly: What Is the Optimal Level of Intake? *Nutrients* **2016**, *8*, 359. [CrossRef]
7. Volkert, D.; Beck, A.M.; Cederholm, T.; Cruz-Jentoft, A.; Goisser, S.; Hooper, L.; Kiesswetter, E.; Maggio, M.; Raynaud-Simon, A.; Sieber, C.C.; et al. ESPEN guideline on clinical nutrition and hydration in geriatrics. *Clin. Nutr.* **2019**, *38*, 10–47. [CrossRef]
8. Chanet, A.; Verlaan, S.; Salles, J.; Giraudet, C.; Patrac, V.; Pidou, V.; Pouyet, C.; Hafnaoui, N.; Blot, A.; Cano, N.; et al. Supplementing Breakfast with a Vitamin D and Leucine-Enriched Whey Protein Medical Nutrition Drink Enhances Postprandial Muscle Protein Synthesis and Muscle Mass in Healthy Older Men. *J. Nutr.* **2017**, *147*, 2262–2271. [CrossRef]

9. Houston, D.K.; Nicklas, B.J.; Ding, J.; Harris, T.B.; Tylavsky, F.A.; Newman, A.B.; Lee, J.S.; Sahyoun, N.R.; Visser, M.; Kritchevsky, S.B.; et al. Dietary protein intake is associated with lean mass change in older, community-dwelling adults: The Health, Aging, and Body Composition (Health ABC) Study. *Am. J. Clin. Nutr.* **2008**, *87*, 150–155. [CrossRef]
10. Volkert, D.; Hubsch, S.; Oster, P.; Schlierf, G. Nutritional support and functional status in undernourished geriatric patients during hospitalization and 6-month follow-up. *Aging* **1996**, *8*, 386–395. [CrossRef]
11. Mathewson, S.L.; Azevedo, P.S.; Gordon, A.L.; Phillips, B.E.; Greig, C.A. Overcoming protein-energy malnutrition in older adults in the residential care setting: A narrative review of causes and interventions. *Ageing Res. Rev.* **2021**, *70*, 101401. [CrossRef]
12. Clegg, M.E.; Williams, E.A. Optimizing nutrition in older people. *Maturitas* **2018**, *112*, 34–38. [CrossRef]
13. Jauhar, S.; Ismail-Fitry, M.R.; Chong, G.H.; NorKhaizura, M.A.R.; Ibadullah, W.Z.W. Polyphenol Compounds from Pomegranate (Punica Granatum) Extracted via Various Methods and its Application on Meat and Meat Products: A Review. *J. Adv. Res. Appl. Sci. Eng. Technol.* **2018**, *12*, 1–12.
14. Trombold, J.R.; Reinfeld, A.S.; Casler, J.R.; Coyle, E.F. The effect of pomegranate juice supplementation on strength and soreness after eccentric exercise. *J. Strength Cond. Res.* **2011**, *25*, 1782–1788. [CrossRef]
15. Torregrosa-Garcia, A.; Avila-Gandia, V.; Luque-Rubia, A.J.; Abellan-Ruiz, M.S.; Querol-Calderon, M.; Lopez-Roman, F.J. Pomegranate Extract Improves Maximal Performance of Trained Cyclists after an Exhausting Endurance Trial: A Randomised Controlled Trial. *Nutrients* **2019**, *11*, 721. [CrossRef]
16. Laurindo, L.F.; Barbalho, S.M.; Marquess, A.R.; Grecco, A.I.S.; Goulart, R.A.; Tofano, R.J.; Bishayee, A. Pomegranate (*Punica granatum* L.) and Metabolic Syndrome Risk Factors and Outcomes: A Systematic Review of Clinical Studies. *Nutrients* **2022**, *14*, 1665. [CrossRef]
17. Vucic, V.; Grabez, M.; Trchounian, A.; Arsic, A. Composition and Potential Health Benefits of Pomegranate: A Review. *Curr. Pharm. Des.* **2019**, *25*, 1817–1827. [CrossRef]
18. Aviram, M.; Dornfeld, L.; Kaplan, M.; Coleman, R.; Gaitini, D.; Nitecki, S.; Hofman, A.; Rosenblat, M.; Volkova, N.; Presser, D.; et al. Pomegranate juice flavonoids inhibit low-density lipoprotein oxidation and cardiovascular diseases: Studies in atherosclerotic mice and in humans. *Drugs Exp. Clin. Res.* **2002**, *28*, 49–62.
19. Koopman, R.; Wagenmakers, A.J.; Manders, R.J.; Zorenc, A.H.; Senden, J.M.; Gorselink, M.; Keizer, H.A.; van Loon, L.J. Combined ingestion of protein and free leucine with carbohydrate increases postexercise muscle protein synthesis in vivo in male subjects. *Am. J. Physiol. Endocrinol. Metab.* **2005**, *288*, E645–E653. [CrossRef]
20. Colonetti, T.; Grande, A.J.; Milton, K.; Foster, C.; Alexandre, M.C.; Uggioni, M.L.; Rosa, M.I. Effects of whey protein supplement in the elderly submitted to resistance training: Systematic review and meta-analysis. *Int. J. Food Sci. Nutr.* **2017**, *68*, 257–264. [CrossRef]
21. Kuo, Y.Y.; Chang, H.Y.; Huang, Y.C.; Liu, C.W. Effect of Whey Protein Supplementation in Postmenopausal Women: A Systematic Review and Meta-Analysis. *Nutrients* **2022**, *14*, 4210. [CrossRef]
22. Machin, D.R.; Christmas, K.M.; Chou, T.H.; Hill, S.C.; Van Pelt, D.W.; Trombold, J.R.; Coyle, E.F. Effects of Differing Dosages of Pomegranate Juice Supplementation after Eccentric Exercise. *Physiol. J.* **2014**, *2014*, 271959. [CrossRef]
23. Rivara, M.B.; Mehrotra, R.; Linke, L.; Ruzinski, J.; Ikizler, T.A.; Himmelfarb, J. A pilot randomized crossover trial assessing the safety and short-term effects of pomegranate supplementation in hemodialysis patients. *J. Ren. Nutr.* **2015**, *25*, 40–49. [CrossRef]
24. Heber, D.; Seeram, N.P.; Wyatt, H.; Henning, S.M.; Zhang, Y.; Ogden, L.G.; Dreher, M.; Hill, J.O. Safety and antioxidant activity of a pomegranate ellagitannin-enriched polyphenol dietary supplement in overweight individuals with increased waist size. *J. Agric. Food Chem.* **2007**, *55*, 10050–10054. [CrossRef]
25. Goodarzi, R.; Jafarirad, S.; Mohammadtaghvaei, N.; Dastoorpoor, M.; Alavinejad, P. The effect of pomegranate extract on anthropometric indices, serum lipids, glycemic indicators, and blood pressure in patients with nonalcoholic fatty liver disease: A randomized double-blind clinical trial. *Phytother. Res.* **2021**, *35*, 5871–5882. [CrossRef]
26. Wolfe, R.R.; Miller, S.L.; Miller, K.B. Optimal protein intake in the elderly. *Clin. Nutr.* **2008**, *27*, 675–684. [CrossRef]
27. Kesteloot, H.E.; Joossens, J.V. Relationship between dietary protein intake and serum urea, uric acid and creatinine, and 24-hour urinary creatinine excretion: The BIRNH Study. *J. Am. Coll. Nutr.* **1993**, *12*, 42–46. [CrossRef]
28. Nuttall, F.Q.; Gannon, M.C.; Saeed, A.; Jordan, K.; Hoover, H. The metabolic response of subjects with type 2 diabetes to a high-protein, weight-maintenance diet. *J. Clin. Endocrinol. Metab.* **2003**, *88*, 3577–3583. [CrossRef]
29. Oh, C.; No, J.K. Appropriate protein intake is one strategy in the management of metabolic syndrome in Korean elderly to mitigate changes in body composition. *Nutr. Res.* **2018**, *51*, 21–28. [CrossRef]
30. Huang, X.J.; Choi, Y.K.; Im, H.S.; Yarimaga, O.; Yoon, E.; Kim, H.S. Aspartate aminotransferase (AST/GOT) and alanine aminotransferase (ALT/GPT) detection techniques. *Sensors* **2006**, *6*, 756–782. [CrossRef]

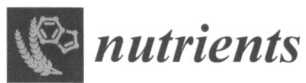

Article

Vitamin D and Calcium Supplementation in Nursing Homes—A Quality Improvement Study

Charlotte Mortensen [1,*], Inge Tetens [2], Michael Kristensen [1] and Anne Marie Beck [3]

[1] Department of Nursing and Nutrition, Faculty of Health, University College Copenhagen, 2200 Copenhagen, Denmark
[2] Department of Nutrition, Exercise and Sports, Faculty of Science, University of Copenhagen, 1958 Frederiksberg, Denmark
[3] Dietetic and Nutritional Research Unit, Herlev Gentofte Hospital, 2730 Herlev, Denmark
* Correspondence: cpet@kp.dk; Tel.: +45-51380364

Abstract: Even though dietary supplements with vitamin D and calcium are recommended to nursing home residents, we recently reported a low adherence to this recommendation. The objective of this 20-week quality improvement study was to use the Model for Improvement and Plan-Do-Study-Act (PDSA) cycles to improve adherence in Danish nursing homes. We included two nursing homes with 109 residents at baseline. An information sheet including the rationale for the recommendation was developed for the nurses to urge residents to take the supplements and seek approval by the general practitioner afterwards (PDSA cycle 1). Moreover, it was included in admission meetings with new residents to address supplementation (PDSA cycle 2). A nurse reviewed patient records for number of residents prescribed adequate doses of vitamin D ($\geq$20 µg) and calcium ($\geq$800 mg) before, during and after the intervention. At baseline, 32% (n = 35) of the residents had adequate doses of vitamin D and calcium. After implementation of the information sheet and adjustment to admission meetings, this increased to 65% (n = 71) at endpoint (p < 0.001). In conclusion, in this quality improvement study, we improved the number of prescriptions of adequate doses of vitamin D and calcium over 20 weeks using the Model for Improvement and PDSA experiments.

Keywords: vitamin D; calcium; supplements; nursing homes; adherence; Model for Improvement

1. Introduction

Despite recommendations of supplementation with vitamin D or vitamin D and calcium to older adults and nursing home residents in a variety of countries, vitamin D deficiency (serum 25-hydroxyvitamin D < 30 nmol/L [1–3]) is continuously reported to be widespread among this vulnerable group [4–8]. This can have negative consequences for, physical functioning and bone health, as well as increased risk of falling and mortality [8–13]. Recently, our online survey among randomly selected nursing homes in Denmark (n = 41) showed that only 8% of nursing homes have a high adherence to the recommendation of giving residents 20 µg vitamin D and 800–1000 mg calcium [14]. A poor adherence was also reported for similar vitamin D and calcium supplement recommendations among nursing home residents in the USA [15,16], Canada [17], Australia [18] and England [19]. Our online survey also showed that the health care professionals' (HCPs) main reason for not providing the recommended supplements to the residents was that the general practitioners (GPs) did not prescribe vitamin D and calcium to the residents [14]. As the HCPs can only administer the supplements after either a prescription or written consent from the GPs [20], the result is a poor adherence. This is despite the recommendation being a preventive recommendation and not only for treatment [21]. Our data are in accordance with a Belgian survey where 45% of the GPs did not systematically prescribe vitamin D, and, of these, one third only prescribe vitamin D when they remember to [22]. This highlights

Citation: Mortensen, C.; Tetens, I.; Kristensen, M.; Beck, A.M. Vitamin D and Calcium Supplementation in Nursing Homes—A Quality Improvement Study. *Nutrients* 2022, 14, 5360. https://doi.org/10.3390/nu14245360

Academic Editors: Moustapha Dramé and Bruce W. Hollis

Received: 4 November 2022
Accepted: 13 December 2022
Published: 16 December 2022

Publisher's Note: MDPI stays neutral with regard to jurisdictional claims in published maps and institutional affiliations.

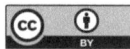

Copyright: © 2022 by the authors. Licensee MDPI, Basel, Switzerland. This article is an open access article distributed under the terms and conditions of the Creative Commons Attribution (CC BY) license (https://creativecommons.org/licenses/by/4.0/).

the need to find strategies to target this underutilization of recommended supplements in long-term care.

The lack of incorporation of a recommendation into routine clinical practice is well-known. Studies report that it may take on average 17 years for evidence-based practice within healthcare to be incorporated into routine clinical practice [23,24]. Thus, there is a need for implementation science, which targets the experienced barriers with strategies considered feasible by the involved HCPs. A widely used method of quality improvement in health care is the Model for Improvement including the Plan-Do-Study-Act (PDSA) cycle, in which small-scale experiments are conducted together with the HCPs to accelerate improvements [25–27]. This model has previously been used in two studies targeting low adherence to vitamin D supplementation among nursing home residents. In both studies, adherence improved after 6 [16] and 12 months [17], respectively. However, it has previously been stated that resources are often underestimated when it comes to using the PDSA cycle in quality improvement [28] and that health care studies using the Model for Improvement do often not comply with the key principals of the method [25]. In addition, it has been reported that HCPs find it difficult and time-consuming to follow the method parallel to their primary health care tasks [29]. It could be a barrier for using the Model for Improvement, that it is resource-demanding and leaves less time for primary health care tasks. The objective of this study was to investigate whether using the Model for Improvement in a realistic setting could increase adherence to the vitamin D and calcium supplement recommendation in Danish nursing homes.

2. Materials and Methods

2.1. Study Design

This was a quality improvement study designed to measure effectiveness, i.e., measure the degree of effect through an intervention conducted under real-world settings. The purpose of the intervention was to increase adherence to the supplement recommendation for nursing home residents. Effectiveness was calculated as the number of prescriptions of vitamin D and calcium to the residents before and after the intervention. The intervention was conducted simultaneously at two Danish nursing homes during 20 weeks from October 2021 to March 2022. No control nursing homes were included.

2.2. Recruitment of Nursing Homes

Two nursing homes in the Region of Zealand, Denmark, were included: nursing home 1 (NH1) and nursing home 2 (NH2). NH1 was recruited based on their participation in our online survey on adherence and barriers to supplementation [14]. NH2 was recruited through use of professional contacts. The inclusion criterion for the nursing homes was an estimated adherence of <40% to the recommendation of residents receiving both supplements, as previously suggested as the definition of low adherence [14].

2.3. Baseline Data

Baseline data included number of residents per nursing home, whether a GP was affiliated at the nursing home, and number of residents prescribed adequate doses of vitamin D and calcium (≥ 20 µg of vitamin D and ≥ 800 mg calcium, respectively).

2.4. Steps in the Model for Improvement

The three initial steps in the Model for Improvement are shown in Figure 1 [26]. The goal was set for both nursing homes in accordance with the SMART criteria (Figure 1, step 1) [26], as at least 80% of the residents should have both vitamin D and calcium prescribed in at least the recommended doses after a 20-week intervention period. To determine if adherence improved during the intervention, patient journals were reviewed approximately every third week to see if and from when additional residents were prescribed the recommended supplements (Figure 1, step 2). As input before selecting the strategy most suitable to reach the goal (Figure 1, step 3), an interview was performed with each of the involved nurses, and a driver diagram with factors affecting the goal was correspondingly made (Supplementary Figure S1) [26].

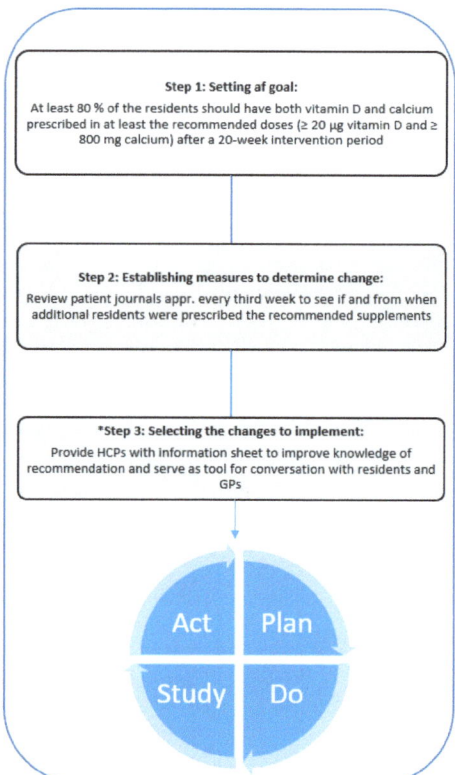

Figure 1. The Model for Improvement. Visual overview of the three initial steps followed by the PDSA cycle. * Input to step three from driver diagram (see Supplementary Figure S1). Abbreviations: GPs; General practitioner, HCPs; Health care professionals. Figure inspired by [25].

2.5. The Plan-Do-Study-Act Cycles

The project's supervisor and the nurses involved in the project planned the first PDSA cycle. The nurses expressed a need for information about the specific recommendation, e.g., the doses recommended and the health reasons to follow it in order to talk with both residents and their GP about supplementation. Therefore, the project's supervisor created an information sheet on laminated paper easy for the nurses to bring around to the residents and advise them to have the supplements. Thus, the purpose of this information sheet was to contribute to increased knowledge on the reasoning behind the recommendation of vitamin D and calcium supplements, as this was a prerequisite for the HCPs to be able to argue for supplementation and thereby work for improved adherence. As the recommendation is a general preventive recommendation for all, regardless of vitamin D status and bone health, all residents were targeted this intervention. If a resident agreed to have vitamin D and calcium, the nurse contacted the GP to ensure that supplementation would not interact with any disease conditions or medicine, and the GP correspondingly prescribed the supplements, if appropriate. During PDSA cycle 1, all residents were asked about supplementation (Figure 2). However, to address the turnover of residents, we conducted a PDSA cycle 2 to ensure that new residents were asked to initiate supplementation as early as possible. Therefore, the nurses made a note that all future admission meetings should include urging new residents and their relatives to consider the supplements (PDSA cycle 2).

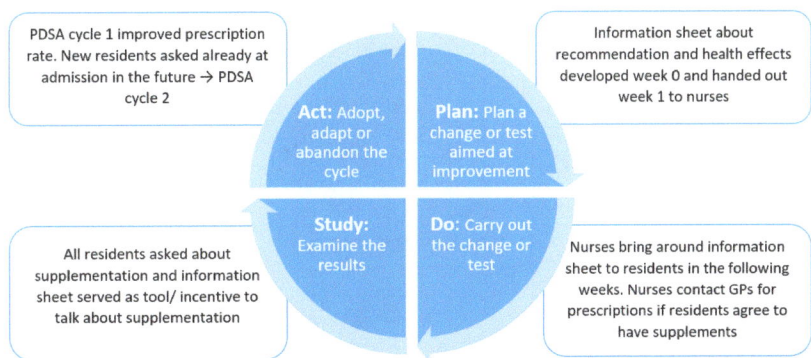

Figure 2. Illustration of the four phases Plan-Do-Study-Act of the PDSA cycle 1 in the project.

2.6. Effect Evaluation

Approximately every third week, the project's supervisor contacted the nurse by telephone or attended a meeting (due to the COVID-19 pandemic, most meetings were conducted via telephone). Here, the nurse checked resident journals to see if additional residents had been prescribed vitamin D and calcium supplements, and number of residents and week number were noted by the project's supervisor. Only residents having ≥20 µg vitamin D and ≥800 mg calcium were noted. Although a written agreement from the GP is sufficient, as vitamin D and calcium are not medicine but dietary supplements [20], the HCPs at both nursing homes only wished to provide supplements if a prescription from the GP was made, and thus the number of prescriptions was chosen as effect evaluation.

2.7. Process Evaluation

Process evaluation was planned to include number of residents presented to the information sheet in each week (PDSA cycle 1), as well as numbers of meetings held with new residents and relatives where vitamin D and calcium supplementation was a topic (PDSA cycle 2).

2.8. Statistics

Data were analyzed using the statistical software IBM SPSS Statistics 28.0. Descriptive statistics are presented as numbers and frequencies. McNemar's test was used to determine if proportions of residents prescribed adequate doses of vitamin D and calcium changed during the intervention from week 1 to 20. A *p*-value of 0.05 determined significance.

2.9. Ethics

The study was conducted in accordance with the Declaration of Helsinki and approved by the Scientific Ethics Committees of The Capital Region of Denmark (H-20031971, 2 December 2020). We anonymized and handled data from the two nursing homes in accordance with the General Data Protection Regulation and the Data protection act. As per the data protection law of 2018, the study was not to be reported to the Danish Data Protection Agency [30]. Data in this paper constitutes a part of data collected at the two nursing homes. Additional data, which will be reported elsewhere, include vitamin D status, muscle strength and physical function in a subgroup of 40 residents. The project is registered at ClinicalTrials.gov as NCT04956705.

3. Results

3.1. Baseline Data

Characteristics of the two nursing homes at baseline are shown in Table 1. Initial reviews of patient records by the involved nurses revealed that adherence was below 40% and 30% at NH1 and NH2, respectively. All residents at NH1 had the same GP, as this nursing home had their own GP affiliated. Contrary, no GP was affiliated at NH2, so residents at NH2 had different GPs in the municipality.

Table 1. Table of characteristics of the two nursing homes at baseline.

	Nursing Home 1	Nursing Home 2
Number of residents (n)	45	64
Adherence to the recommendation n (%)	17 (37.8)	18 (28.1)
General practitioner affiliated	Yes	No

Adherence was defined as the number of residents prescribed ≥ 20 μg vitamin D and ≥ 800 mg calcium after review of resident's journals.

3.2. Effect of the Intervention

During the intervention period, four residents (two at each NH) passed away and three new residents moved in (one at NH1 and two at NH2). The primary intervention was the use of the information sheet by the nurses. Collectively, for both nursing homes, adherence increased from around 32% at baseline to 65% at endpoint in week 20 (Table 2), which was a 102.8% improvement ($p < 0.001$).

Table 2. Adherence to the recommendation at the nursing homes at baseline and at endpoint after the 20-week intervention period.

	Baseline Week 1 n (%)	Endpoint Week 20 n (%)	Week 1–20 [1] p-Values
NH1 (n = 45)	17 (37.8%)	33 (73.3%)	<0.001
NH2 (n = 64)	18 (28.1%)	38 (59.4%)	<0.001
NH1 + NH2 (n = 109)	35 (32.1%)	71 (65.1%)	<0.001

[1] Calculated using the McNemar test, statistical significance $p < 0.05$. Adherence was defined as the number of residents prescribed ≥ 20 μg vitamin D and ≥ 800 mg calcium after review of resident's journals. Abbreviations: NH; Nursing home.

In Figure 3, the vitamin D and calcium adherence rate (percentage, %) is shown for each of the 20 intervention weeks at the two nursing homes separately.

3.3. Process Evaluation

It was not compatible with a busy day for the nurses to quantify the number of residents who were presented with the information sheet (PDSA cycle 1) on a weekly basis during the intervention. Moreover, in some cases, the information sheet served more as a background-knowledge tool for the nurses in their correspondence with residents rather than a visual tool used in the conversation. When it comes to process evaluation of incorporating the admission meetings to bring up supplementation (PDSA cycle 2), NH1 had one and NH2 had two meetings during the intervention period, at which the residents were encouraged to begin supplementation. This was agreed at all three meetings and supplements correspondingly prescribed by the GPs. Thus, 100% of the meetings with new residents resulted in commencement of supplementation.

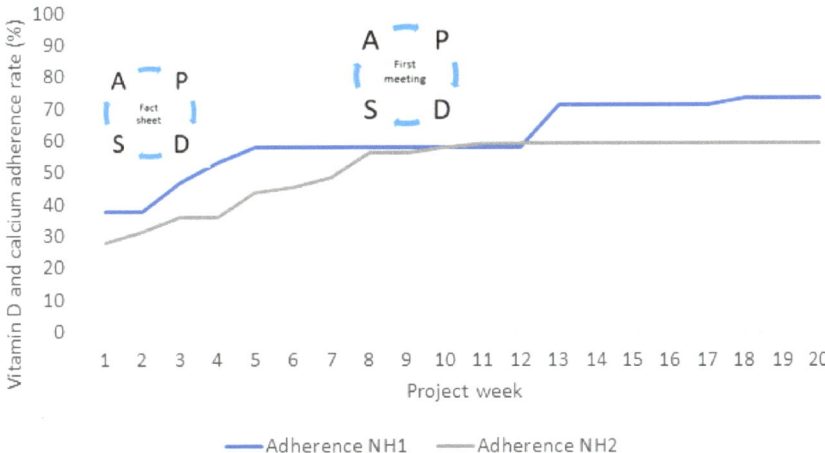

Figure 3. Development of adherence to the recommendation of vitamin D and calcium supplementation (≥20 μg vitamin D and ≥800 mg calcium) at two Danish nursing homes during the 20-week intervention period. "Fact sheet" refers to the information sheet used by the nurses to urge residents to have the supplements, and "first meeting" refers to the adjustment of admission meetings to include supplementation as a topic. Abbreviations: NH; Nursing home, PDSA; Plan-Do-Study-Act.

4. Discussion

This quality improvement study showed that it is possible to improve adherence to a recommendation of vitamin D and calcium supplementation at nursing homes using the Model for Improvement as a quality improvement method. By use of a simple information sheet about the recommendation and a small adjustment to the admission meetings, adherence at the two included nursing homes increased from baseline values of 38% and 28% of residents having the supplements prescribed to 73% and 59%, respectively. As previously stated, using the Model for Improvement has been reported to be resource-demanding and time-consuming and problematic for the HCPs to follow [25,28,29]. However, we have found that a simple and cheap strategy primarily involving one HCP at each site, who mainly conducted the data collection, and one project supervisor, who created the tool for a simple intervention and assisted with the data collection, can lead to changes in health care.

Although not based on the Model for Improvement, Munir et al. used a similarly simple approach in an American quality improvement study among 83 long-term care residents. In that study, the medical director at the facility created an educational letter to the GPs with the rationale for calcium and vitamin D supplementation, including the recommended doses. This increased calcium supplementation from 45% to 80% and vitamin D supplementation from 35% to 78% [15]. Thus, the GPs were informed about the benefits of the supplements directly by letter whereas the present study focused on educating the nurses and urged them to contact the GPs (by e-mail or at personal meetings) and argue for an increased adherence to the recommendation. It could be hypothesized that these different communication pathways may explain why adherence was higher in the study by Munir et al. The authors noted, however, making these orders on supplementation a routine on admission for new residents should be considered, which agrees with our strategy on adjustments to admission meetings (PDSA cycle 2). Another American study did use the PDSA cycle approach to improve adherence to vitamin D prescription rates at nursing homes by primarily educating HCPs at a nursing home with a similar sample size (101 residents) and during a similar time frame (five months) as in the present study. In that study, Yanamadala et al., found that vitamin D prescription rate increased from 35% to 86% [16]. The study had a considerably larger project staff compared to the simpler approach with one project supervisor and one involved nurse at each nursing home in our study. Moreover, while the present study only noted prescriptions of both vitamin D and calcium in at least the recommended doses, the study by Yanamadala et al., also counted prescriptions of only vitamin D and vitamin D in multivitamins, which may give higher adherence rates. Tablets containing both micronutrients are larger and may not be prescribed if the resident has chewing-swallowing difficulties. Moreover, some GPs may omit calcium tablets to some residents as they may cause constipation, kidney stones and increased risk of myocardial infarction [9]. However, as the aim of the present study was to evaluate adherence to the national recommendation, only prescriptions in accordance with this were included.

Other international studies have targeted vitamin D adherence-improvement in larger samples and longer periods. For instance, a Canadian study found that 12 months of knowledge translation strategies based on PDSA cycles in 19 long-term care settings increased vitamin D prescriptions by 22% from a baseline of 36% of residents [17]. Contrary, an Australian study did not find improved vitamin D supplement use after six months of knowledge translation at 17 residential aged care facilities. The authors stated, however, that most of the interventions were not implemented after six months, which could explain the lack of effect [18]. Moreover, one explanation of the different outcomes in the studies could be different baseline prevalence, i.e., 36% had vitamin D prescribed initially in the Canadian intervention homes compared to 57% in the Australian intervention homes. Thus, ours and other studies indicate, that with an initially low adherence of <40%, it is possible to improve prescription rate by targeting the experienced barriers. As we have recently showed that 35% of a representative sample of Danish nursing homes have a low adherence [14], there is a large potential for adherence-improvement in Denmark.

Despite improved adherence, neither of the nursing homes involved in our study had a high adherence (>80% [16]) at endpoint. NH1 had the highest endpoint adherence of 73%, which could indicate that having a nursing home-affiliated GP is preferable, since it is easier to make several requests for prescriptions at the time. An explanation for why higher adherence was not achieved could be that the residents at the two nursing homes were included in the decision of having the supplements prescribed or not, which was not the case in the studies by Munir et al., and Yanamadala et al. [15,16]. Therefore, even though presented with the positive effects of vitamin D and calcium, some residents refused to have the supplements prescribed. A contributing factor to not reaching a high adherence in the present study could be the general health condition of Danish nursing home residents. The average age of becoming a resident in Danish nursing homes is 84 years old [31] and around one third only live less than one year [32], so most nursing home residents are very vulnerable when moving in. Moreover, approximately 50% of Danish nursing home residents have one or more chronic diseases and approximately 40% are diagnosed with dementia [31]. It could be considered whether strategies other than daily tablets are appropriate for the most vulnerable residents, such as administering higher doses of vitamin D less frequently [33].

This study has some limitations. A major limitation was that we did not include any control nursing homes. Therefore, we cannot know if our intervention caused improved adherence, or if the nursing homes would have increased prescription rates during winter in general. For the Danish adult population in general, vitamin D supplements are recommended from October to March [21] due to lack of cutaneous vitamin D synthesis at this latitude [34], which results in many being vitamin D-deficient during spring [35]. Even though the recommendation for nursing home residents is a general preventive recommendation all year round, it is possible that HCPs and GPs have increased awareness of the recommended supplements during winter and that some improvement in adherence would take place irrespective of an intervention. Based on this, our results may be overestimated and should be interpreted with caution. Another limitation is that the primary outcome was the number of prescriptions of adequate doses of vitamin D and calcium and not the actual consumption of the supplements. As most residents consumed their tablets in their own room after dosage by the HCPs, it was not possible for them to supervise every resident as they consumed the supplements. However, according to the HCPs, prescribed tablets were also dosed, and actual consumption checked regularly by inspection of the dosage boxes. Another limitation is the lack of information on numbers of rejections and reasoning behind rejection of supplementation by either the resident or the GP. This information would be valuable when discussing further strategies to improve adherence. In this regard, it should be mentioned that the present study did not include a third PDSA cycle, as HCPs stated that all residents had already been asked to take a stand, which should be accepted as their final decision from an ethical perspective. The relatively short intervention period of 20 weeks was chosen, as this constitutes the months where no cutaneous vitamin D synthesis occurs at this northern latitude, and since other data collected as part of this study (as vitamin D status measured in a subgroup of residents as presented in Section 2.9) were dependent on lack of cutaneous vitamin D synthesis. Moreover, as previously mentioned, others have found significant improvements with the same study duration as in the present study [16]. However, we cannot rule out that duration of the study or number of PDSA cycles could influence endpoint adherence.

Strengths of the present study include the simple and cheap intervention with limited demands on resources, e.g., documentation. Even though the two involved nurses invested time in the project and its purpose, their participation in the study did not seem to interfere much with routine care tasks, as the chosen intervention could be fitted in. Another strength is the involvement of the relevant HCPs, which ensured that the most relevant barriers were targeted during the intervention. Moreover, as the initial interviews with the nurses confirmed some of the same barriers identified in our previous online survey [14], we find that the targeted barriers are transferable to other nursing homes.

Another important group to consider is the community-dwelling older adults at 70+ years, as the recommendation of year-round vitamin D and calcium supplementation in Denmark is also targeted at this group and considering that a previous Danish study showed that only 32% of 70+ year-olds still living in own home take the recommended supplements [36]. A higher adherence in this group could automatically improve adherence among the older adults in long-term care, as it will be part of their daily routine before admission. In addition, older adults could stay self-reliant for a longer period as prolonged vitamin D insufficiency reduces bone mineral density and type 2 muscle fibers, leading to increased fragility [37]. Moreover, supplementation with calcium and vitamin D can already reduce bone loss rate and fracture risk in 50+ year-olds [38].

5. Conclusions

In conclusion, we have demonstrated that an initially low adherence to the vitamin D and calcium supplement recommendation among Danish nursing home residents can improve within a relatively short period when the nurses are provided with information about the recommendation and make small adjustments to their admission meetings. Our results should, however, be interpreted with caution due to a lack of control nursing homes. Further implementation research projects, preferably including control groups, are needed to evaluate and target experienced barriers among the HCPs. This is not only relevant when it comes to vitamin D and calcium supplementation, but also considering other relevant topics within health care.

Supplementary Materials: The following supporting information can be downloaded at: https://www.mdpi.com/article/10.3390/nu14245360/s1, Figure S1: driver diagram.

Author Contributions: Conceptualization, C.M., I.T., M.K. and A.M.B.; methodology, C.M., I.T., M.K. and A.M.B.; software, C.M.; validation, C.M., I.T., M.K. and A.M.B.; formal analysis, C.M.; investigation, M.K. and C.M.; resources, C.M., I.T., M.K. and A.M.B.; data curation, C.M., I.T., M.K. and A.M.B.; writing—original draft preparation, C.M.; writing—review and editing, I.T., M.K. and A.M.B.; visualization, C.M.; supervision, I.T., M.K. and A.M.B.; project administration, C.M.; funding acquisition, C.M., I.T., M.K. and A.M.B. All authors have read and agreed to the published version of the manuscript.

Funding: This research was funded by the Innovation Fund in Denmark, grant number 9164-000001B.

Institutional Review Board Statement: The study was conducted in accordance with the Declaration of Helsinki, and approved by the Scientific Ethics Committees of The Capital Region of Denmark (H-20031971, 02.12.2020).

Informed Consent Statement: Patient consent was waived as data collection was limited to review of prescriptions in patient records.

Data Availability Statement: The data presented in this study are available on request from the corresponding author.

Acknowledgments: We would like to acknowledge and thank all the health care professionals at the two nursing homes for being open-minded and positive about the study. A special thanks to the involved nurses at the two participating nursing homes for their valuable time, contribution, and dedication to the study, especially in the difficult time of the COVID-19 pandemic. We also thank all the residents and their relatives for their involvement and openness to the study and its purpose.

Conflicts of Interest: The authors declare no conflict of interest. The funders had no role in the design of the study, in the collection, analyses, or interpretation of data, in the writing of the manuscript, or in the decision to publish the results.

References

1. Nordic Council of Ministers. *Nordic Nutrition Recommendations 2012: Integrating Nutrition and Physical Activity*, 1st ed.; Norden: Copenhagen, Denmark, 2014; Volume 5, ISBN 978-92-893-2670-4.
2. EFSA NDA Panel (EFSA Panel on Dietetic Products, Nutrition and Allergies). Scientific Opinion on Dietary Reference Values for Vitamin D. *Eur. Food Saf. Authority J.* **2016**, *14*, 4547. [CrossRef]
3. Byers, A.W.; Connolly, G.; Campbell, W.W. Vitamin D Status and Supplementation Impacts on Skeletal Muscle Function: Comparisons between Young Athletes and Older Adults. *Curr. Opin. Clin. Nutr. Metab. Care* **2020**, *23*, 421–427. [CrossRef] [PubMed]
4. Rolland, Y.; de Souto Barreto, P.; van Kan, G.A.; Annweiler, C.; Beauchet, O.; Bischoff-Ferrari, H.; Berrut, G.; Blain, H.; Bonnefoy, M.; Cesari, M.; et al. Vitamin D Supplementation in Older Adults: Searching for Specific Guidelines in Nursing Homes. *J. Nutr. Health Aging* **2013**, *17*, 402–412. [CrossRef] [PubMed]
5. Itkonen, S.T.; Andersen, R.; Björk, A.K.; Brugård Konde, Å.; Eneroth, H.; Erkkola, M.; Holvik, K.; Madar, A.A.; Meyer, H.E.; Tetens, I.; et al. Vitamin D Status and Current Policies to Achieve Adequate Vitamin D Intake in the Nordic Countries. *Scand. J. Public Health* **2020**, *49*, 616–627. [CrossRef]
6. Pludowski, P.; Holick, M.F.; Grant, W.B.; Konstantynowicz, J.; Mascarenhas, M.R.; Haq, A.; Povoroznyuk, V.; Balatska, N.; Barbosa, A.P.; Karonova, T.; et al. Vitamin D Supplementation Guidelines. *J. Steroid Biochem. Mol. Biol.* **2018**, *175*, 125–135. [CrossRef]
7. Amrein, K.; Scherkl, M.; Hoffmann, M.; Neuwersch-Sommeregger, S.; Köstenberger, M.; Tmava Berisha, A.; Martucci, G.; Pilz, S.; Malle, O. Vitamin D Deficiency 2.0: An Update on the Current Status Worldwide. *Eur. J. Clin. Nutr.* **2020**, *74*, 1498–1513. [CrossRef]
8. Samefors, M.; Östgren, C.J.; Mölstad, S.; Lannering, C.; Midlöv, P.; Tengblad, A. Vitamin D Deficiency in Elderly People in Swedish Nursing Homes Is Associated with Increased Mortality. *Eur. J. Endocrinol.* **2014**, *170*, 667–675. [CrossRef]
9. Reid, I.R.; Bolland, M.J. Controversies in Medicine: The Role of Calcium and Vitamin D Supplements in Adults. *Med. J. Aust.* **2019**, *211*, 468–473. [CrossRef]
10. Houston, D.K.; Cesari, M.; Ferrucci, L.; Cherubini, A.; Maggio, D.; Bartali, B.; Johnson, M.A.; Schwartz, G.G.; Kritchevsky, S.B. Association between Vitamin D Status and Physical Performance: The InCHIANTI Study. *J. Gerontol. A Biol. Sci. Med. Sci.* **2007**, *62*, 440–446. [CrossRef]
11. Cameron, I.D.; Dyer, S.M.; Panagoda, C.E.; Murray, G.R.; Hill, K.D.; Cumming, R.G.; Kerse, N. Interventions for Preventing Falls in Older People in Care Facilities and Hospitals. *Cochrane Database Syst. Rev.* **2018**, *2018*, CD005465. [CrossRef]
12. Kojima, G.; Tanabe, M. Frailty Is Highly Prevalent and Associated with Vitamin D Deficiency in Male Nursing Home Residents. *J. Am. Geriatr. Soc.* **2016**, *64*, e33–e35. [CrossRef] [PubMed]
13. Pilz, S.; Dobnig, H.; Tomaschitz, A.; Kienreich, K.; Meinitzer, A.; Friedl, C.; Wagner, D.; Piswanger-Sölkner, C.; März, W.; Fahrleitner-Pammer, A. Low 25-Hydroxyvitamin D Is Associated with Increased Mortality in Female Nursing Home Residents. *J. Clin. Endocrinol. Metab.* **2012**, *97*, E653–E657. [CrossRef] [PubMed]
14. Mortensen, C.; Tetens, I.; Kristensen, M.; Snitkjaer, P.; Beck, A.M. Adherence and Barriers to the Vitamin D and Calcium Supplement Recommendation at Danish Nursing Homes: A Cross-Sectional Study. *BMC Geriatr.* **2022**, *22*, 27. [CrossRef] [PubMed]
15. Munir, J.; Wright, R.J.; Carr, D.B. A Quality Improvement Study on Calcium and Vitamin D Supplementation in Long-Term Care. *J. Am. Med. Dir. Assoc.* **2006**, *7*, 305–309. [CrossRef]

16. Yanamadala, M.; Heflin, M.T.; White, H.K.; Buhr, G.T. Ensuring Vitamin D Supplementation in Nursing Home Patients—A Quality Improvement Project. *J. Nutr. Gerontol. Geriatr.* **2012**, *31*, 158–171. [CrossRef]
17. Kennedy, C.C.; Ioannidis, G.; Thabane, L.; Adachi, J.D.; Marr, S.; Giangregorio, L.M.; Morin, S.N.; Crilly, R.G.; Josse, R.G.; Lohfeld, L.; et al. Successful Knowledge Translation Intervention in Long-Term Care: Final Results from the Vitamin D and Osteoporosis Study (ViDOS) Pilot Cluster Randomized Controlled Trial. *Trials* **2015**, *16*, 214. [CrossRef]
18. Walker, P.; Kifley, A.; Kurrle, S.; Cameron, I.D. Increasing the Uptake of Vitamin D Supplement Use in Australian Residential Aged Care Facilities: Results from the Vitamin D Implementation (ViDAus) Study. *BMC Geriatr.* **2020**, *20*, 383. [CrossRef]
19. Williams, J.; Williams, C. Responsibility for Vitamin D Supplementation of Elderly Care Home Residents in England: Falling through the Gap between Medicine and Food. *BMJ Nutr. Prev. Health* **2020**, *3*, 256–262. [CrossRef]
20. Danish Patient Safety Authority. Proper handling of medication. A tool for care centers, home care etc. Responsibility, safety and tasks [Korrekt håndtering af medicin. Et værktøj for plejecentre, hjemmepleje, hjemmesyge, bosteder m.v. Ansvar, sikkerhed og opgaver]. 2019, Volume 2; pp. 1–20. Available online: https://stps.dk/da/udgivelser/2019/korrekt-medicinhaandtering/~{}/media/0E30EDB960FA47DBA41FDA577A0AB979 (accessed on 15 September 2022). (In Danish)
21. Danish Health Authority. Recommendations on Vitamin D [Anbefalinger om D-vitamin]. Available online: https://www.sst.dk/da/viden/ernaering/anbefalinger-om-d-vitamin (accessed on 15 March 2021). (In Danish)
22. Buckinx, F.; Reginster, J.Y.; Cavalier, E.; Petermans, J.; Ricour, C.; Dardenne, C.; Bruyère, O. Determinants of Vitamin D Supplementation Prescription in Nursing Homes: A Survey among General Practitioners. *Osteoporos. Int.* **2016**, *27*, 881–886. [CrossRef]
23. Bauer, M.S.; Damschroder, L.; Hagedorn, H.; Smith, J.; Kilbourne, A.M. An Introduction to Implementation Science for the Non-Specialist. *BMC Psychol.* **2015**, *3*, 32. [CrossRef]
24. Morris, Z.S.; Wooding, S.; Grant, J. The Answer Is 17 Years, What Is the Question: Understanding Time Lags in Translational Research. *J. R. Soc. Med.* **2011**, *104*, 510–520. [CrossRef] [PubMed]
25. Taylor, M.J.; McNicholas, C.; Nicolay, C.; Darzi, A.; Bell, D.; Reed, J.E. Systematic Review of the Application of the Plan–do–study–act Method to Improve Quality in Healthcare. *BMJ Qual. Saf.* **2014**, *23*, 290–298. [CrossRef] [PubMed]
26. Crowl, A.; Sharma, A.; Sorge, L.; Sorensen, T. Accelerating Quality Improvement within Your Organization: Applying the Model for Improvement. *J. Am. Pharm. Assoc.* **2015**, *55*, e364–e376. [CrossRef] [PubMed]
27. Knudsen, S.V.; Laursen, H.V.B.; Johnsen, S.P.; Bartels, P.D.; Ehlers, L.H.; Mainz, J. Can Quality Improvement Improve the Quality of Care? A Systematic Review of Reported Effects and Methodological Rigor in Plan-Do-Study-Act Projects. *BMC Health Serv. Res.* **2019**, *19*, 683. [CrossRef] [PubMed]
28. Reed, J.E.; Card, A.J. The Problem with Plan-Do-Study-Act Cycles. *BMJ Qual. Saf.* **2016**, *25*, 147–152. [CrossRef]
29. Kring Schjørring, M.; Tjørnhøj-Thomsen, T.; Hulvej Rod, M. Evaluation of "in Safe Hands" [Evaluering Af I Sikre Hænder]. *Natl. Inst. Public Health Dan. Statens Inst. Folk.* **2017**, *2017*, 1–45. (In Danish)
30. The Danish Data Protection Agency. The General Notification System Ends [Den Generelle Anmeldelsesordning Ophører]. Available online: https://www.datatilsynet.dk/presse-og-nyheder/nyhedsarkiv/2018/maj/den-generelle-anmeldelsesordning-ophoerer (accessed on 22 February 2022). (In Danish)
31. Ministry of Health and the Elderly. National Examination of Conditions in Nursing [National Undersøgelse Af Forholdende På Plejecentre]. Available online: https://dsr.dk/sites/default/files/192/undersoegelse-af-forholdene-paa-plejecentreashx_.pdf (accessed on 22 February 2022). (In Danish)
32. The Danish Health Data Authority [Sundhedsdatastyrelsen]. Many Have a Long Stay in Nursing Home [Mange Bor Længe På Plejehjem]. Available online: https://sundhedsdatastyrelsen.dk/da/nyheder/2020/plejehjemsbeboere_161220 (accessed on 22 February 2022). (In Danish)
33. Mol, R.; Kansu, A.D.; Cebe, T.; Yildiz, S.; Butun, V.K.; Simsek, B.; Cakatay, U. High versus Moderate Dosage of Daily and Weekly Administration of Vitamin D Supplements in the Form of Oil Drop in Nursing Home Residents. *J. Coll. Physicians Surg. Pak.* **2018**, *28*, 618–622. [CrossRef]
34. O'Neill, C.M.; Kazantzidis, A.; Ryan, M.J.; Barber, N.; Sempos, C.T.; Durazo-Arvizu, R.A.; Jorde, R.; Grimnes, G.; Eiriksdottir, G.; Gudnason, V.; et al. Seasonal Changes in Vitamin D-Effective UVB Availability in Europe and Associations with Population Serum 25-Hydroxyvitamin D. *Nutrients* **2016**, *8*, 533. [CrossRef]
35. Hansen, L.; Tjønneland, A.; Køster, B.; Brot, C.; Andersen, R.; Cohen, A.S.; Frederiksen, K.; Olsen, A. Vitamin D Status and Seasonal Variation among Danish Children and Adults: A Descriptive Study. *Nutrients* **2018**, *10*, 1801. [CrossRef]
36. Frantzen, C.; Videbæk, P.N.; Andersen, B.V.; Kidmose, U.; Lähteenmäki, L.; Grønhøj, A. Anbefalinger Om Tilskud Af D-Vitamin Og Calcium-Viden, Accept Og Efterlevelse Blandt de 55+ Årige. *Aarhus Univ.* **2019**, *157*, 59.
37. Sanders, K.M.; Scott, D.; Ebeling, P.R. Vitamin D Deficiency and Its Role in Muscle-Bone Interactions in the Elderly. *Curr. Osteoporos. Rep.* **2014**, *12*, 74–81. [CrossRef] [PubMed]
38. Tang, B.M.; Eslick, G.D.; Nowson, C.; Smith, C.; Bensoussan, A. Use of Calcium or Calcium in Combination with Vitamin D Supplementation to Prevent Fractures and Bone Loss in People Aged 50 Years and Older: A Meta-Analysis. *Lancet* **2007**, *370*, 657–666. [CrossRef] [PubMed]

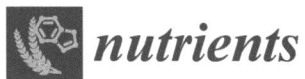 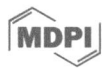

Article

Brazilian Propolis Intake Decreases Body Fat Mass and Oxidative Stress in Community-Dwelling Elderly Females: A Randomized Placebo-Controlled Trial

Miho Kanazashi [1], Tadayuki Iida [1], Ryosuke Nakanishi [2], Masayuki Tanaka [3], Hiromi Ikeda [1], Naomi Takamiya [1], Noriaki Maeshige [4], Hiroyo Kondo [5], Tomohiko Nishigami [1], Toshihide Harada [1] and Hidemi Fujino [4,*]

1. Department of Physical Therapy, Faculty of Health and Welfare, Prefectural University of Hiroshima, Mihara 723-0053, Japan
2. Department of Physical Therapy, Faculty of Rehabilitation, Kobe International University, Kobe 658-0032, Japan
3. Department of Physical Therapy, Faculty of Health Sciences, Okayama Healthcare Professional University, Okayama 700-0913, Japan
4. Department of Rehabilitation Science, Kobe University Graduate School of Health Sciences, Kobe 654-0142, Japan
5. Department of Food Science and Nutrition, Nagoya Women's University, Nagoya 467-8611, Japan
* Correspondence: fujino@phoenix.kobe-u.ac.jp; Tel.: +81-78-796-4542

Abstract: This study aimed to investigate the effects of Brazilian propolis on body fat mass and levels of adiponectin and reactive oxygen species among community-dwelling elderly females. This was a double-blind randomized placebo-controlled trial. Altogether, 78 females aged 66–84 years were randomly assigned to the propolis (PRO; $n = 39$) or placebo (PLA; $n = 39$) group. For 12 weeks, the PRO group were given three capsules containing 227 mg of propolis twice a day. Meanwhile, the PLA group were given daily placebo capsules. Of 78 participants, 53 (PLA group: $n = 28$, PRO group: $n = 25$) completed the study. Although no changes were observed in absolute or relative fat mass in the PLA group, they showed a significant decline in the PRO group. The level of serum adiponectin in the PLA group did not change, although that of the PRO group significantly increased. The level of d-ROMs in the PLA group significantly increased, whereas that of the PRO group significantly decreased. The serum SOD activity in the PLA group significantly decreased, whereas that of the PRO group tended to increase. These results suggest that propolis supplementation may decrease body fat mass and oxidative stress among community-dwelling elderly females.

Keywords: supplementation; body composition; adiponectin; oxidative stress; antioxidant

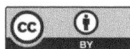

1. Introduction

Females undergoing the menopause experience a considerable change in metabolic activity [1]. Postmenopausal females present with a remarkably higher incidence of visceral obesity than that presented by premenopausal females [2]. In elderly females, fat accumulation is accelerated by not only age-related declines in muscle mass and physical activity, but also by changes in carbohydrate and lipid metabolism patterns associated with lower levels of sex steroid hormones caused by the menopause [1]. Fat accumulation can result in obesity. This, in turn, causes different metabolic complications, such as type 2 diabetes and cardiovascular diseases [1], consequently resulting in severe limitations to daily activities and higher mortality rates. Therefore, decreasing fat accumulation is important for maintaining health among elderly postmenopausal females.

Body fat mass shows a positive correlation with systemic oxidative stress in clinically healthy middle-aged females [3]. Oxidative stress is enhanced by increased adipose tissues associated with the menopause [1]. Therefore, postmenopausal females are at a high risk of oxidative stress caused by increased adipose tissues. Different cytokines are secreted from adipose tissues [4], which are involved in the increase or decrease in oxidative stress. The level of circulating adiponectin, which is a favorable adipokine, unlike others, decreases with increased adipose tissues [5,6]. Moreover, it enhances the antioxidant capacity via mitochondrial biogenesis and leads to a higher expression of antioxidant enzymes [7,8]. Therefore, the effects of changes in fat mass on oxidative stress can be partially explained by adiponectin levels.

Exercise and dietary restrictions are effective in controlling fat accumulation. However, since these countermeasures can be difficult to continue, alternative methods should be considered. Daily nutritional supplementation has been found to be effective against obesity and metabolic complications [9,10]. Recently, the effects of polyphenols have been comprehensively assessed in clinical trials in humans [11]. Propolis, a substance produced by bees from the resin collected from trees and shrubs, has long been used as a nonpharmacologic agent [12]. In particular, a growing body of evidence has shown that Brazilian green propolis is beneficial to health because it has different bioactive activities [13]. Previous studies have revealed that Brazilian propolis decreases visceral fat accumulation in ob/ob mice with high fat diet-induced obesity [14] and type 2 diabetes [15]. Therefore, further studies must be conducted to verify the effects of Brazilian propolis on fat mass among humans. To date, numerous studies have examined the therapeutic effects of propolis of various origins among patients with diabetes and other diseases [16–19]. However, the effect of propolis intake on body fat mass among community-dwelling healthy females remains unknown.

Based on previous reports, we hypothesized that Brazilian propolis supplementation would reduce fat mass and promote adiponectin secretion among females, thereby optimizing an integrated balance between reactive oxygen species (ROS) and antioxidants. This randomized, double-blind, placebo-controlled trial aimed to investigate the effects of ethanol extracts of Brazilian green propolis on fat mass, adiponectin secretion, and oxidative stress among community-dwelling elderly females. This study could contribute to the development of novel therapeutic strategies for preventing obesity and its associated metabolic disorders, such as vascular disease and Alzheimer's disease, among elderly females.

2. Materials and Methods

2.1. Participants

Healthy postmenopausal elderly females were recruited as trial volunteers for this study via the use of a public relations magazine in Mihara City, Japan. The inclusion criteria were healthy, postmenopausal females aged 65 years or older who were independent in their daily lives. Meanwhile, the exclusion criteria were females with orthopedic diseases, psychiatric disorders, and dementia; those on medication; those taking other supplements; and those who missed at least 3 days of supplementation during the 12-week intervention period. The participants received a detailed explanation regarding the contents and methods of this study before the trial began. Written informed consent was obtained from 82 volunteers. Among them, 78 attended the baseline examination session and were randomly assigned to either the propolis or the placebo group. The participants were provided with individual identification numbers to ensure anonymity. After matching according to age (± 3 years) and body mass index (BMI; ± 3 kg/m2), the participants were divided into the group receiving propolis capsules (PRO; $n = 39$) and the group receiving placebo capsules (PLA; $n = 39$). The authors were blinded to the information regarding the groups to which the participants were assigned. Eleven participants (PRO group, $n = 6$; PLA group, $n = 5$) dropped out of the study because they missed taking the supplementation more than three times during the 12-week intervention period. In addition, 14 participants (PRO group, $n = 8$; PLA group, $n = 6$) who did not participate in the measurement after the 12-week intervention or declined some measurements were excluded from the analysis. Finally, we analyzed 25 and 28 participants in the PRO and PLA groups, respectively. Figure 1 shows the sampling scheme of this study.

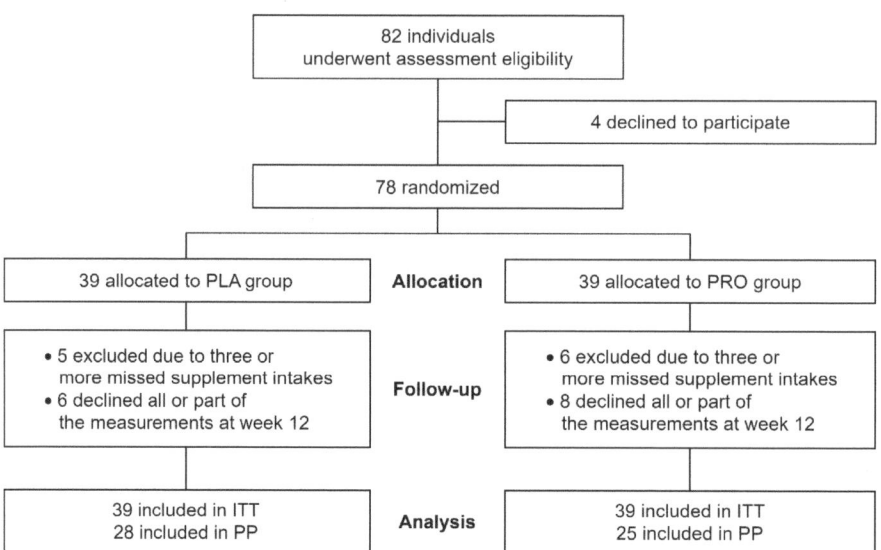

Figure 1. CONSORT flowchart. PLA, placebo; PRO, propolis; ITT, intention-to-treat; PP, per-protocol. Obtained from honeybee hives and extracted using ethanol. Wheat germ oil is extracted by pressing the wheat germ and is used as a solvent for propolis supplements. Therefore, it was selected as a placebo in this study. The supplements used in the present study are commercially available as health foods. As for the dosage of propolis, an animal toxicity study has shown that the non-observed effect level is 1400 mg/kg/day [20]. In reports on human subjects, 400–900 mg/day of propolis has been applied to patients with rheumatoid arthritis [21], type 2 diabetes mellitus [22], or COVID-19 [23] and elderly people (average 72.8 years) [24]. In the present study, 454 mg/day of propolis was administered to the subjects and none of them complained of side effects. This suggests that propolis and its dosage used in the present study are likely to be safe.

2.2. Study Design

This was a randomized, double-blind, and placebo-controlled trial. The PRO group were given three soft capsules containing 227 mg/3 capsules of propolis twice per day, i.e. after breakfast and dinner (total intake: 454 mg/6 capsules/day) for 12 weeks. Meanwhile, the PLA group were given placebo capsules at the same dosage and frequency for 12 weeks. The participants were instructed to take the capsules with water or tea. Furthermore, all participants were required to not alter their lifestyle habits, such as diet and exercise, during the study period. To assess compliance, the participants were instructed to record changes in their lifestyle and health status and daily capsule intake.

The study was conducted in accordance with the Declaration of Helsinki and approved by the Institutional Review Board (or Ethics Committee) of the Prefectural University of Hiroshima (15MH064) and Kobe University Graduate School of Health Sciences (277-2). Furthermore, the trial was registered at the University Hospital Medical Information Network (UMIN) Center (ID: UMIN000020459). Informed consent was obtained from all subjects involved in the study.

2.3. Brazilian Propolis Supplementation

We prepared 227 mg/3 capsules of propolis supplement using Propolis 300® (Yamada Bee Farm, Okayama, Japan), which is a commercial product, and the placebo supplement by replacing propolis with wheat germ oil. The raw materials for propolis supplementation include gelatin, propolis extract, glycerin fatty acid ester, glycerin, arginine, pectin, and cocoa color. The propolis extract was mainly composed of flavonoids

2.4. Assessment Procedures

All assessments were performed by a physician, radiologist, nurse, dietitian, and ten physical therapists. The assessments before and after the intervention lasted for approximately 60 min. They were conducted at the Mihara Campus of Prefectural University of Hiroshima using a standardized protocol by the same researcher.

All assessments were conducted between 09:00 and 15:00 in the same laboratories. The participants were instructed to fast for 2 h before the assessments. The consumption of Japanese tea was allowed before and during the assessments to prevent dehydration. Upon arrival, the participants were instructed to sit. Next, their blood pressure and heart rate were evaluated and their health was examined by the physician. Their body mass was measured at increments of 0.1 kg using a calibrated digital scale and their height was evaluated at increments of 0.1 cm using a wall-mounted height meter. Body mass index (BMI) was calculated as weight (kg) divided by squared height (m^2). With reference to the participant's lifestyle and other records, dietitians and physical therapists interviewed the participants about their lifestyle habits, including diet and exercise, during the intervention period.

While in the sitting position, the nurse collected blood samples from a superficial vein in the forearm of all patients via venipuncture. Approximately 4 mL blood was collected and placed into prechilled silicone-coated and lithium heparin-coated tubes. A portion of the blood sample was used to measure the level of diacron-reactive oxygen metabolites (d-ROMs), which is an indicator of blood oxidative stress, using the FREE Carrio Duo (WISMERLL Co., Tokyo, Japan) as per the manufacturer's instructions. The level of d-ROMs was expressed in Carratelli units (U.CARR) [25] (normal range: 250–300 U.CARR), where 1 U.CARR corresponds to 0.08 mg/dL of H_2O_2. To collect serum, the remaining blood sample was centrifuged at $3000 \times g$ for 15 min at 4 °C. The collected serum was stored in a deep freezer at -80 °C until subsequent biochemical analysis. Antioxidative superoxide dismutase (SOD) activity and adiponectin concentration were evaluated using the serum sample. SOD activity was assessed using the SOD Assay Kit-WST (S311, Dojindo, Kumamoto, Japan) by employing the colorimetric quantification method as per the manufacturer's instructions. The adiponectin concentration was evaluated using the commercial ELISA kit (Human Total Adiponectin/Acrp30 Quantikine ELISA Kit/514-96041, DRP300, R&D Systems, Minneapolis, MN, the USA) as per the manufacturer's instructions.

Body composition and bone mineral density (BMD) were assessed by a radiologist using Discovery (Hologic, Inc., Bedford, MA, USA) with dual-energy X-ray absorptiometry (DXA), which is a highly accurate method [26,27]. Absolute and relative fat mass and absolute lean body mass, except that of the head, were evaluated. The BMD of the lumbar spine (L2–L4) and the left femur was evaluated.

To evaluate hand grip and knee extension strength, which are significantly correlated with the total body skeletal muscle mass, skeletal muscle function was assessed by physical therapists. The hand grip strength of the dominant hand was analyzed to the nearest 0.5 kg using a hydraulic hand dynamometer (T.K.K. 5401; Takei Scientific Instruments Co., Ltd., Niigata, Japan) while the participants remained in a standing position and the upper limbs remained in a drooping position. Evaluations were conducted twice at intervals of 1 min, and the best score was recorded as the hand grip strength. The knee extension strength of the dominant leg was evaluated using a seated measuring device (Isoforce GT-330, OG Giken, Okayama, Japan). The measurements were conducted while the participants were sitting in a chair with the backrest tilted back at 12° from upright position, with two belts on the thighs and one on the waist, and with the knee joint flexed at 90°. Measurements were conducted at intervals of 2 min, and the best score was recorded as the knee extension strength. During the measurements of hand grip and knee extension, the participants were instructed not to stop breathing to prevent the occurrence of the Valsalva effect.

2.5. Statistical Analysis

All continuous data were presented as mean standard error of the mean or median (interquartile range) for parametric or nonparametric continuous variables, respectively.

The baseline characteristics between the two groups were compared using a Student's unpaired t-test or a Mann–Whitney U-test for parametric or nonparametric continuous variables, respectively. All 78 subjects were analyzed using mixed-effects models for repeated measures with intervention, study time point, and their interaction according to intention-to-treat (ITT). As per-protocol (PP) analysis, 53 subjects were using a two-factor repeated-measures analysis of variance with time as the within-participant factor and group as the between-participant factor. If there was a significant time × group interaction, post hoc analyses with Bonferroni correction were performed to identify significant within-group effects. Intragroup changes in the levels of blood markers before and after the intervention were compared using the Wilcoxon rank-sum test. For all statistical analyses, a p value of <0.05 was considered statistically significant. All statistical analyses and graphical data representations were performed using IBM SPSS Statistics 27 (IBM Japan Ltd., Tokyo, Japan) and Prism version 7 (GraphPad Software Inc, San Diego, CA, USA).

The sample size calculation and power analysis were performed as follows: First, we estimated a treatment effect of 1 kg and standard deviation of 5 kg on fat mass and calculated effect size before study. Next, we calculated the sample size using the G*Power 3.1 software (Heinrich-Heine-Universität Düsseldorf) for MAC. A two-way repeated measures ANOVA indicated that a total sample size of 52 was needed to reach 80% power, in order to detect the interaction effect size of 0.20 at a significance level of 0.05.

3. Results

Table 1 shows the baseline characteristics of elderly females in each group. No significant differences were noted in any measurement between the two groups. Based on lifestyle and health records during the experimental period, no change was observed in the participant's lifestyle habits, such as exercise and diet.

Table 1. Baseline characteristics of the participants in each group.

	PLA (n = 28)	Propolis (n = 25)	p Value
Physical characteristics			
Age (years)	75 (69–78)	75 (72–78)	0.447 [a]
Height (cm)	149.7 ± 1.0	151.2 ± 1.1	0.287 [b]
Body mass (kg)	53.0 ± 1.6	55.1 ± 1.6	0.368 [b]
BMI (kg/m^2)	23.7 ± 0.7	24.0 ± 0.6	0.716 [b]
Body composition			
Fat mass (kg)	16.2 ± 1.1	17.0 ± 0.9	0.576 [b]
Fat mass (%)	32.4 ± 1.2	33.0 ± 1.0	0.675 [b]
Lean body mass (kg)	32.8 ± 0.7	33.8 ± 0.7	0.368 [b]
Bone mineral density			
Lumbar spine (g/cm^2)	0.80 ± 0.02	0.80 ± 0.03	0.955 [b]
Proximal femur (g/cm^2)	0.70 ± 0.02	0.69 ± 0.02	0.556 [b]
Muscle function			
Hand grip strength (kg)	25.1 ± 0.6	25.0 ± 0.6	0.841 [b]
Knee extension strength (Nm)	94.0 ± 3.5	92.7 ± 4.1	0.809 [b]
Blood markers			
Adiponectin (µg/mL)	7.8 (3.1–11.0)	5.3 (2.8–10.0)	0.675 [a]
d-ROMs (U. CARR)	374.5 ± 9.1	385.6 ± 11.8	0.451 [b]
SOD activity (U/mL)	134 (122–162)	136 (119–152)	0.539 [a]

Data are presented as mean ± standard error of the mean or median (interquartile range). Significant differences were analyzed using the Student's unpaired t-test. A p value of <0.05 was considered statistically significant. There was no significant difference between the two groups in any measurements at baseline. BMI, body mass index; d-ROMs, diacron-reactive oxygen metabolites; SOD, superoxide dismutase. [a] Derived by Mann–Whitney U-test. [b] Derived by independent samples t-test.

An interaction effect was observed for absolute and relative fat mass (p = 0.005 and p < 0.001, respectively; Figure 2a,b), i.e., the absolute and relative fat mass in the PLA group did not change (pre: 16.2 ± 1.1 kg, post: 16.4 ± 1.1 kg, p = 0.657; pre: 32.4% ± 1.2%, post

32.7% ± 1.2%; p = 0.255, respectively). Meanwhile, those of the PRO group significantly decreased (pre: 17.0 ± 0.9 kg, post: 16.7 ± 1.0 kg, p = 0.007; pre: 33.1% ± 1.0%, post: 32.3% ± 1.1%, p = 0.002, respectively). An interactive effect was observed for absolute lean body mass (p = 0.005; Figure 2c), i.e., the absolute lean body mass in the PLA group did not change (pre: 32.8 ± 0.7 kg, post: 32.5 ± 0.7 kg, p = 0.114). However, that of the PRO group tended to increase (pre: 33.8 ± 0.7 kg, post: 34.1 ± 0.7 kg, p = 0.058).

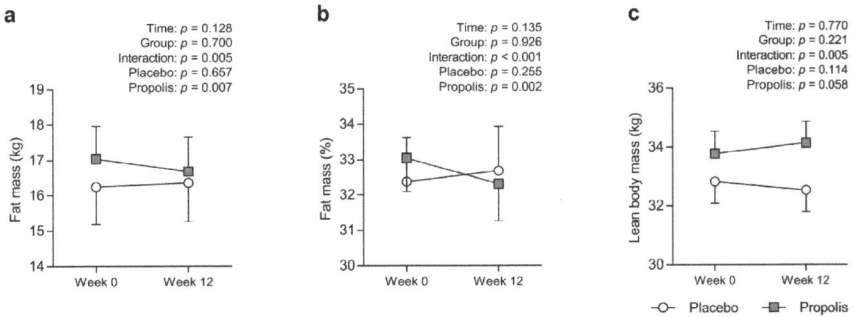

Figure 2. Absolute fat mass (**a**), relative fat mass (**b**), and absolute lean body mass (**c**), with the exception of the head in the placebo (white) and propolis (gray) groups. Values were presented as mean ± standard error of the mean. Variables were analyzed via two-factor repeated-measures analysis of variance, with time (week 0 vs. 12) and group (placebo vs. propolis) as factors. A p value of <0.05 was considered significant. If there was a significant time × group interaction, post hoc analyses with Bonferroni correction were performed to identify significant within-group effects.

There was no significant change between body mass, BMI, lumbar spine, proximal femur BMD, hand grip strength, or knee extension strength before and after the intervention (Table 2).

Table 2. Measurements before and after 12 weeks of supplementation with propolis and placebo Data are presented as mean ± standard error of the mean. Results from both ITT and PP analysis are shown. Variables were analyzed via two-factor repeated-measures analysis of variance, with time (week 0 vs. 12) and group (placebo vs. propolis) as factors. A p value of <0.05 was considered statistically significant. For variables with a significant time × group interaction, post hoc analyses with Bonferroni correction were conducted to identify significant within-group effects. * Significantly different from before the intervention. PP, per-protocol; ITT, intention-to-treat; BMI, body mass index; BMD, bone mineral density.

	Placebo (n = 28)		Propolis (n = 25)		p Value (PP Analysis)			p Value (ITT Analysis)		
	Week 0	Week 12	Week 0	Week 12	Time	Group	Interaction	Time	Group	Interaction
Body mass (kg)	53.0 ± 1.6	52.8 ± 1.7	55.1 ± 1.6	54.9 ± 1.5	0.170	0.361	0.830	0.039	0.497	0.368
BMI (kg/m^2)	23.7 ± 0.7	23.6 ± 0.7	24.0 ± 0.6	24.0 ± 0.6	0.157	0.700	0.755	0.037	0.701	0.328
Fat mass (kg)	16.2 ± 1.1	16.4 ± 1.1	17.0 ± 0.9	16.7 ± 1.0 *	0.128	0.700	0.005	0.384	0.479	0.077
Fat mass (%)	32.4 ± 1.2	32.7 ± 1.3	33.0 ± 1.0	32.3 ± 1.0 *	0.135	0.926	<0.001	0.297	0.440	0.005
Lean body mass (kg)	32.8 ± 0.7	32.5 ± 0.7	33.8 ± 0.7	34.1 ± 0.7	0.770	0.221	0.005	0.941	0.509	0.003
Lumbar spine BMD (g/cm^2)	0.80 ± 0.02	0.79 ± 0.02	0.80 ± 0.03	0.80 ± 0.04	0.855	0.920	0.569	0.663	0.563	0.496
Proximal femur BMD (g/cm^2)	0.70 ± 0.02	0.70 ± 0.02	0.69 ± 0.02	0.68 ± 0.02	0.522	0.556	0.989	0.267	0.284	0.664
Hand grip strength (kg)	25.1 ± 0.6	24.6 ± 0.6	25.0 ± 0.6	25.1 ± 0.7	0.491	0.860	0.265	0.203	0.550	0.294
Knee extension strength (Nm)	94.0 ± 3.5	97.1 ± 4.4	92.7 ± 4.1	97.2 ± 4.9	0.043	0.921	0.684	<0.001	0.813	0.498

The level of serum adiponectin in the PLA group did not change after the intervention (pre: 7.9 (3.3–11.1) µg/mL, post: 5.8 (2.5–9.9) µg/mL; p = 0.145), but significantly increased in the PRO group (pre: 5.3 (2.8–10.0) µg/mL, post: 9.0 (3.8–10.6) µg/mL; p = 0.007; Figure 3a). The blood level of d-ROMs in the PLA group significantly increased (pre: 374.5 ± 8.9 U.CARR, post: 402.4 ± 12.5 U.CARR; p < 0.001), but significantly decreased in the PRO group (pre: 385.6 ± 111.8 U.CARR, post: 365.7 ± 10.5 U.CARR; p = 0.013;

Figure 3b). The serum SOD activity in the PLA group significantly decreased (pre: 132 (122–162) U/mL, post: 127 (115–143) U/mL; $p = 0.015$), but tended to increase in the PRO group (pre: 136 (119–152) U/mL, post: 143 and (124–168) U/mL; $p = 0.070$; Figure 3c). None of the participants presented with life-threatening side effects following supplementation with propolis and placebo during the experimental period.

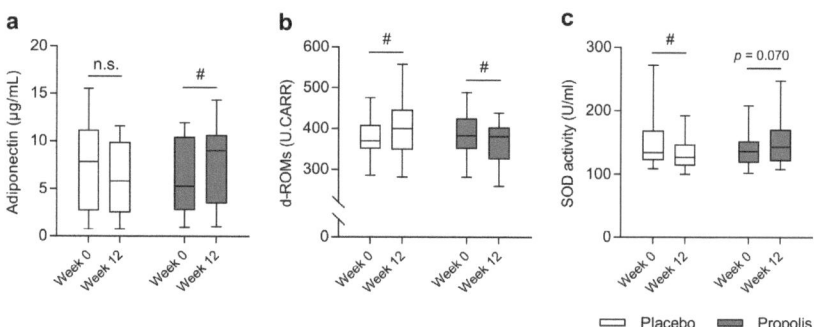

Figure 3. Boxplots showing values of serum levels of adiponectin (**a**), blood levels of d-ROMs (**b**), and serum SOD activity (**c**) before and after the intervention in the placebo (white) and propolis (gray) groups. Boxplots show the median, upper and lower quartiles, and maximum and minimum values. The differences between before and after the intervention in each group were compared using a Mann–Whitney U-test. A p value of <0.05 was considered significant. # Significantly different between before and after the intervention. d-ROMs, diacron-reactive oxygen metabolites; SOD, superoxide dismutase.

4. Discussion

Our prospective interventional study showed that propolis had a positive effect on absolute and relative fat mass, relative lean body mass, and levels of adiponectin and ROS among community-dwelling elderly females. Therefore, propolis supplementation may be an effective strategy for preventing disorders caused by body fat accumulation among elderly females. In previous studies, the anti-obesity and antioxidant properties of propolis have been found to be effective against diseases such as type 2 diabetes [13,14,16–19,22]. To the best of our knowledge, this is the first study that has shown the efficacy of propolis supplementation among community-dwelling healthy elderly females.

Propolis supplementation caused the absolute and relative fat mass to decrease among elderly females. The DXA method, which is the gold standard for body composition measurements, was used to assess fat mass, and the results of this study were highly reliable. Propolis has been shown to reduce fat mass in obese animal models [14]. The mechanism was correlated with the fact that propolis induces the activation of peroxisome proliferator-activated receptor γ (PPARγ) [13], which causes browning of white adipocytes. Artepillin C, an ingredient derived from propolis, can induce brown-like adipocytes' formation [28], which increase energy expenditure and promote fat loss. Moreover, decreased fat mass may be associated with the positive effects of propolis on AMP-activated protein kinase (AMPK) in the skeletal muscle [29]. AMPK is a key factor for metabolic activity, including lipid metabolism [30]. Therefore, propolis supplementation may increase skeletal muscle lipid metabolism via AMPK activation, which may also promote fat loss. Taken together, a lower fat mass, as observed in this study, may be accounted for by a higher lipolytic capacity in adipocytes and skeletal muscles. In addition, another possible explanation for reduced fat mass may be attributed to the positive effect of propolis on skeletal muscle mass, resulting in increased energy expenditure through the basal metabolic rate. A previous study that has reported on propolis indicated that propolis has a protective effect on aged skeletal muscle via various biological activities such as anti-inflammatory and antioxidative actions [31]. Indeed, among the elderly females in this study, lean body mass tended to increase following supplementation with propolis. In contrast, hand grip and knee extension strength did not change with or without propolis supplementation. Increased lean body mass is not always accompanied by changes in limb muscle strength [32,33]. In addition, licorice flavonoid oil supplementation consisting of another type of polyphenol increased the trunk muscle mass but not limb muscle mass, with no improvement observed in limb muscle strength in older adults [34]. Therefore, propolis supplementation may have increased lean body mass mainly in the trunk region in this study as well, resulting in higher energy expenditure. Taken together, these results indicate that propolis supplementation is an effective strategy for reducing fat mass, which may prevent obesity-related metabolic complications among elderly females.

Propolis supplementation increased the levels of adiponectin among elderly females. To the best of our knowledge, this is the first study to show that propolis increases the level of adiponectin in humans. Brazilian propolis-derived components have molecular mechanisms that act on adiponectin expression. Previous research has shown that Brazilian propolis is associated with adiponectin expression via the activation of PPARγ in adipocytes [35]. This report supports the results of the present study, i.e., the circulating level of adipokines, including adiponectin, is a good indicator of fat mass and other body properties. Age-related changes in body fat distribution include loss of subcutaneous fat, accumulation of visceral fat, and deposition of ectopic fat [36]. Furthermore, the changes in sex hormones associated with the menopause cause visceral adiposity among elderly females [1]. Visceral fat accumulation shows a negative correlation with the circulating levels of adiponectin [37–39]. From these reports, the increased adiponectin level with propolis intake could be also attributed to a possible decrease in visceral fat mass. Therefore, propolis supplementation may have a positive effect on visceral fat accumulation among elderly postmenopausal females.

Oxidative stress, as assessed using blood levels of d-ROMs, decreased with propolis supplementation among elderly females. Brazilian propolis contains different bioactive components, such as artepillin C and baccharin, and has antioxidant effects [40–43]. Therefore, decreased ROS accumulation in the blood samples of propolis-treated elderly females may be partially attributed to the antioxidant activity of Brazilian propolis per se. However, the activation of PPARγ enhances antioxidative capacity by increasing antioxidant expression, including that of SOD [44,45]. In addition, adiponectin stimulates antioxidant enzyme expression [7]. Therefore, propolis supplementation may enhance antioxidant expression, including that of SOD, as evidenced in the PRO group that showed a tendency of increase in SOD activity. This might have reduced the level of ROS in the blood of the propolis-treated group. Oxidative stress is associated with the pathology of various age-related conditions [46]. Furthermore, postmenopausal females are highly exposed to the effects of ROS owing to a decreased antioxidant capacity and low levels of estrogen [47]. Therefore, the effect of propolis on reducing the risk of oxidative stress may partially prevent oxidative stress-related diseases in postmenopausal aging females.

However, propolis did not affect BMD. Nevertheless, it is premature to conclude that it did not have a protective effect on human bones based on this 12-week intervention study. The estrogenic effects of propolis, which can reduce the development of postmenopausal symptoms, were observed in an ovariectomized animal model [48]. Changes in the levels of estrogen and other sex hormones associated with the menopause can contribute to osteoporosis [49] among elderly females. Therefore, propolis may be effective against osteoporosis among elderly females who have gone through the menopause. However, further research must be conducted to evaluate the appropriate dosage and duration of propolis treatment.

As medical care costs continually rise with the increase in the elderly population, elderly individuals must manage their own health. Fat accumulation can be prevented or decreased to a certain degree via self-management. To reduce body fat mass, regular exercise and dietary restriction are required. However, the lifestyle habits of elderly individuals are difficult to modify. In association with this, the intake of functional foods, including propolis, can be considered without making any major alterations to lifestyle habits and can be a practical and sustainable method.

This study had several limitations. First, we failed to report the food consumption and the levels of physical activity of participants during the study period. We confirmed through interviews that there were no changes in the eating or exercise habits of the participants. However, because the specific quantification of these factors was not performed, their effects cannot be taken into account in this study. Second, we only included elderly females. Therefore, the effects of propolis supplementation on reducing body fat and blood levels of ROS cannot be generalized to males and younger individuals. Third, although body fat was evaluated accurately using the DXA method, the distribution of adipose tissues was not assessed. In particular, visceral and ectopic fats are involved in the development of insulin resistance and vascular disorders [50,51]. Therefore, future studies must be conducted to evaluate the distribution of body fat. Fourth, general blood properties, such as the levels of triglyceride and low-density lipoprotein, were not investigated. These indices are commonly used as indicators of metabolic function, including lipid metabolism. Therefore, they should be evaluated in future studies. Fifth, the data at week 12 should have been obtained for subjects (placebo, $n = 5$; propolis, $n = 6$) who were excluded from the experiment due to missed supplement intakes during the experiment. Since there was no discrepancy between the ITT and PP analyses in fat mass for the primary outcome, the results of the PP analysis were used in this study.

5. Conclusions

Propolis supplementation reduced body fat accumulation, increased blood levels of adipokine, and decreased blood levels of ROS among elderly females, which are all beneficial to health. Therefore, propolis may be effective in preventing various disorders, especially those associated with fat accumulation among elderly females.

Author Contributions: Conceptualization, M.K. and H.F.; methodology, M.K., R.N. and H.F.; software, T.I., N.T., M.T. and T.N.; validation, T.H. and H.F.; formal analysis, M.K., T.I., R.N., M.T. and T.N.; investigation, M.K., T.I., R.N., M.T., H.I., N.T., N.M., H.K. and T.H.; resources, M.K., T.I., H.K., T.H. and H.F.; data curation, R.N., N.T., N.M. and T.N.; writing—original draft preparation, M.K., R.N and M.T; writing—review and editing, T.I., T.N. and H.F.; visualization, M.K. and M.T.; supervision, T.H. and H.F.; project administration, M.K. and H.F.; funding acquisition, M.K., M.T. and H.F. All authors have read and agreed to the published version of the manuscript.

Funding: This study was supported by Grants-in-Aid for Scientific Research (No. 15K16516, No. 16H07361) from the Japanese Ministry of Education, Culture, Sports, Science and Technology and Yamada Research Grant. The funder had no role in the study design, data collection, and analysis; decision to publish; or preparation of the manuscript.

Institutional Review Board Statement: The study was conducted in accordance with the Declaration of Helsinki and approved by the Institutional Review Board (or Ethics Committee) of the Prefectural University of Hiroshima (15MH064) and Kobe University Graduate School of Health Sciences (277-2). Furthermore, the trial was registered at the University Hospital Medical Information Network (UMIN) Center (ID: UMIN000020459).

Informed Consent Statement: Informed consent was obtained from all subjects involved in the study.

Data Availability Statement: The data that support the findings of this study are available from the corresponding author upon reasonable request.

Conflicts of Interest: The authors declare no conflict of interest.

References

1. Kozakowski, J.; Gietka-Czernel, M.; Leszczynska, D.; Majos, A. Obesity in menopause—Our negligence or an unfortunate inevitability? *Przegląd Menopauzalny* **2017**, *16*, 61–65. [CrossRef]
2. Donato, G.B.; Fuchs, S.C.; Oppermann, K.; Bastos, C.; Spritzer, P.M. Association between menopause status and central adiposity measured at different cutoffs of waist circumference and waist-to-hip ratio. *Menopause* **2006**, *13*, 280–285. [CrossRef] [PubMed]

3. Wu, B.; Fukuo, K.; Suzuki, K.; Yoshino, G.; Kazumi, T. Relationships of systemic oxidative stress to body fat distribution, adipokines and inflammatory markers in healthy middle-aged women. *Endocr. J.* **2009**, *56*, 773–782. [CrossRef] [PubMed]
4. Fantuzzi, G. Adipose tissue, adipokines, and inflammation. *J. Allergy Clin. Immunol.* **2005**, *115*, 911–919. [CrossRef]
5. Weyer, C.; Funahashi, T.; Tanaka, S.; Hotta, K.; Matsuzawa, Y.; Pratley, R.E.; Tataranni, P.A. Hypoadiponectinemia in obesity and type 2 diabetes: Close association with insulin resistance and hyperinsulinemia. *J. Clin. Endocrinol. Metab.* **2001**, *86*, 1930–1935. [CrossRef]
6. Ryan, A.S.; Berman, D.M.; Nicklas, B.J.; Sinha, M.; Gingerich, R.L.; Meneilly, G.S.; Egan, J.M.; Elahi, D. Plasma adiponectin and leptin levels, body composition, and glucose utilization in adult women with wide ranges of age and obesity. *Diabetes Care* **2003**, *26*, 2383–2388. [CrossRef]
7. Kim, Y.; Park, C.W. Mechanisms of Adiponectin Action: Implication of Adiponectin Receptor Agonism in Diabetic Kidney Disease. *Int. J. Mol. Sci.* **2019**, *20*, 1782. [CrossRef] [PubMed]
8. Iwabu, M.; Yamauchi, T.; Okada-Iwabu, M.; Sato, K.; Nakagawa, T.; Funata, M.; Yamaguchi, M.; Namiki, S.; Nakayama, R.; Tabata, M.; et al. Adiponectin and AdipoR1 regulate PGC-1alpha and mitochondria by Ca^{2+} and AMPK/SIRT1. *Nature* **2010**, *464*, 1313–1319. [CrossRef]
9. Martínez-Fernández, L.; Laiglesia, L.M.; Huerta, A.E.; Martínez, J.A.; Moreno-Aliaga, M.J. Omega-3 fatty acids and adipose tissue function in obesity and metabolic syndrome. *Prostaglandins Other Lipid Mediat.* **2015**, *121*, 24–41. [CrossRef]
10. Meydani, M.; Hasan, S.T. Dietary polyphenols and obesity. *Nutrients* **2010**, *2*, 737–751. [CrossRef]
11. Mongioi, L.M.; La Vignera, S.; Cannarella, R.; Cimino, L.; Compagnone, M.; Condorelli, R.A.; Calogero, A.E. The Role of Resveratrol Administration in Human Obesity. *Int. J. Mol. Sci.* **2021**, *22*, 4362. [CrossRef] [PubMed]
12. Pasupuleti, V.R.; Sammugam, L.; Ramesh, N.; Gan, S.H. Honey, Propolis, and Royal Jelly: A Comprehensive Review of Their Biological Actions and Health Benefits. *Oxid Med. Cell Longev.* **2017**, *2017*, 1259510. [CrossRef] [PubMed]
13. Kitamura, H. Effects of Propolis Extract and Propolis-Derived Compounds on Obesity and Diabetes: Knowledge from Cellular and Animal Models. *Molecules* **2019**, *24*, 4394. [CrossRef] [PubMed]
14. Sakai, T.; Ohhata, M.; Fujii, M.; Oda, S.; Kusaka, Y.; Matsumoto, M.; Nakamoto, A.; Taki, T.; Nakamoto, M.; Shuto, E. Brazilian Green Propolis Promotes Weight Loss and Reduces Fat Accumulation in C57BL/6 Mice Fed A High-Fat Diet. *Biol. Pharm. Bull.* **2017**, *40*, 391–395. [CrossRef]
15. Kitamura, H.; Naoe, Y.; Kimura, S.; Miyamoto, T.; Okamoto, S.; Toda, C.; Shimamoto, Y.; Iwanaga, T.; Miyoshi, I. Beneficial effects of Brazilian propolis on type 2 diabetes in ob/ob mice: Possible involvement of immune cells in mesenteric adipose tissue. *Adipocyte* **2013**, *2*, 227–236. [CrossRef]
16. Silveira, M.A.D.; Teles, F.; Berretta, A.A.; Sanches, T.R.; Rodrigues, C.E.; Seguro, A.C.; Andrade, L. Effects of Brazilian green propolis on proteinuria and renal function in patients with chronic kidney disease: A randomized, double-blind, placebo-controlled trial. *BMC Nephrol.* **2019**, *20*, 140. [CrossRef] [PubMed]
17. El-Sharkawy, H.M.; Anees, M.M.; Van Dyke, T.E. Propolis Improves Periodontal Status and Glycemic Control in Patients With Type 2 Diabetes Mellitus and Chronic Periodontitis: A Randomized Clinical Trial. *J. Periodontol.* **2016**, *87*, 1418–1426. [CrossRef]
18. Gao, W.; Pu, L.; Wei, J.; Yao, Z.; Wang, Y.; Shi, T.; Zhao, L.; Jiao, C.; Guo, C. Serum Antioxidant Parameters are Significantly Increased in Patients with Type 2 Diabetes Mellitus after Consumption of Chinese Propolis: A Randomized Controlled Trial Based on Fasting Serum Glucose Level. *Diabetes Ther. Res. Treat. Educ. Diabetes Relat. Disord.* **2018**, *9*, 101–111. [CrossRef]
19. Hesami, S.; Hashemipour, S.; Shiri-Shahsavar, M.R.; Koushan, Y.; Khadem Haghighian, H. Administration of Iranian Propolis attenuates oxidative stress and blood glucose in type II diabetic patients: A randomized, double-blind, placebo-controlled, clinical trial. *Casp. J. Intern. Med.* **2019**, *10*, 48–54. [CrossRef]
20. Burdock, G.A. Review of the biological properties and toxicity of bee propolis (propolis). *Food Chem. Toxicol.* **1998**, *36*, 347–363. [CrossRef]
21. Matsumoto, Y.; Takahashi, K.; Sugioka, Y.; Inui, K.; Okano, T.; Mandai, K.; Yamada, Y.; Shintani, A.; Koike, T. Double-blinded randomized controlled trial to reveal the effects of Brazilian propolis intake on rheumatoid arthritis disease activity index; BeeDAI. *PLoS ONE* **2021**, *16*, e0252357. [CrossRef]
22. Zhao, L.; Pu, L.; Wei, J.; Li, J.; Wu, J.; Xin, Z.; Gao, W.; Guo, C. Brazilian Green Propolis Improves Antioxidant Function in Patients with Type 2 Diabetes Mellitus. *Int. J. Environ. Res. Public Health* **2016**, *13*, 498. [CrossRef]
23. Silveira, M.A.D.; de Souza, S.P.; Dos Santos Galvão, E.B.; Teixeira, M.B.; Gomes, M.M.D.; Damiani, L.P.; Bahiense, B.A.; Cabral, J.B.; De Oliveira, C.; Mascarenhas, T.R.; et al. The use of standardized Brazilian green propolis extract (EPP-AF) as an adjunct treatment for hospitalized COVID-19 patients (BeeCovid2): A structured summary of a study protocol for a randomized controlled trial. *Trials* **2022**, *23*, 255. [CrossRef]
24. Zhu, A.; Wu, Z.; Zhong, X.; Ni, J.; Li, Y.; Meng, J.; Du, C.; Zhao, X.; Nakanishi, H.; Wu, S. Brazilian Green Propolis Prevents Cognitive Decline into Mild Cognitive Impairment in Elderly People Living at High Altitude. *J. Alzheimers Dis.* **2018**, *63*, 551–560. [CrossRef]
25. Fukui, T.; Yamauchi, K.; Maruyama, M.; Yasuda, T.; Kohno, M.; Abe, Y. Significance of measuring oxidative stress in lifestyle-related diseases from the viewpoint of correlation between d-ROMs and BAP in Japanese subjects. *Hypertens. Res.* **2011**, *34*, 1041–1045. [CrossRef]
26. Shepherd, J.A.; Ng, B.K.; Sommer, M.J.; Heymsfield, S.B. Body composition by DXA. *Bone* **2017**, *104*, 101–105. [CrossRef]

27. Ponti, F.; Santoro, A.; Mercatelli, D.; Gasperini, C.; Conte, M.; Martucci, M.; Sangiorgi, L.; Franceschi, C.; Bazzocchi, A. Aging and Imaging Assessment of Body Composition: From Fat to Facts. *Front. Endocrinol.* **2019**, *10*, 861. [CrossRef]
28. Nishikawa, S.; Aoyama, H.; Kamiya, M.; Higuchi, J.; Kato, A.; Soga, M.; Kawai, T.; Yoshimura, K.; Kumazawa, S.; Tsuda, T. Artepillin C, a Typical Brazilian Propolis-Derived Component, Induces Brown-Like Adipocyte Formation in C3H10T1/2 Cells, Primary Inguinal White Adipose Tissue-Derived Adipocytes, and Mice. *PLoS ONE* **2016**, *11*, e0162512. [CrossRef]
29. Ueda, M.; Hayashibara, K.; Ashida, H. Propolis extract promotes translocation of glucose transporter 4 and glucose uptake through both PI3K- and AMPK-dependent pathways in skeletal muscle. *Biofactors* **2013**, *39*, 457–466. [CrossRef]
30. Day, E.A.; Ford, R.J.; Steinberg, G.R. AMPK as a Therapeutic Target for Treating Metabolic Diseases. *Trends Endocrinol. Metab.* **2017**, *28*, 545–560. [CrossRef]
31. Ali, A.M.; Kunugi, H. Apitherapy for Age-Related Skeletal Muscle Dysfunction (Sarcopenia): A Review on the Effects of Royal Jelly, Propolis, and Bee Pollen. *Foods* **2020**, *9*, 1362. [CrossRef]
32. Goodpaster, B.H.; Park, S.W.; Harris, T.B.; Kritchevsky, S.B.; Nevitt, M.; Schwartz, A.V.; Simonsick, E.M.; Tylavsky, F.A.; Visser, M.; Newman, A.B. The loss of skeletal muscle strength, mass, and quality in older adults: The health, aging and body composition study. *J. Gerontology. Ser. A Biol. Sci. Med. Sci.* **2006**, *61*, 1059–1064. [CrossRef]
33. Ten Haaf, D.S.M.; Eijsvogels, T.M.H.; Bongers, C.; Horstman, A.M.H.; Timmers, S.; de Groot, L.; Hopman, M.T.E. Protein supplementation improves lean body mass in physically active older adults: A randomized placebo-controlled trial. *J. Cachexia Sarcopenia Muscle* **2019**, *10*, 298–310. [CrossRef]
34. Kinoshita, T.; Matsumoto, A.; Yoshino, K.; Furukawa, S. The effects of licorice flavonoid oil with respect to increasing muscle mass: A randomized, double-blind, placebo-controlled trial. *J. Sci. Food Agric.* **2017**, *97*, 2339–2345. [CrossRef]
35. Ikeda, R.; Yanagisawa, M.; Takahashi, N.; Kawada, T.; Kumazawa, S.; Yamaotsu, N.; Nakagome, I.; Hirono, S.; Tsuda, T. Brazilian propolis-derived components inhibit TNF-α-mediated downregulation of adiponectin expression via different mechanisms in 3T3-L1 adipocytes. *Biochim. Biophys. Acta* **2011**, *1810*, 695–703. [CrossRef]
36. Cartwright, M.J.; Tchkonia, T.; Kirkland, J.L. Aging in adipocytes: Potential impact of inherent, depot-specific mechanisms. *Exp. Gerontol.* **2007**, *42*, 463–471. [CrossRef]
37. Okamoto, Y.; Kihara, S.; Funahashi, T.; Matsuzawa, Y.; Libby, P. Adiponectin: A key adipocytokine in metabolic syndrome. *Clin. Sci.* **2006**, *110*, 267–278. [CrossRef]
38. Matsuzawa, Y. Therapy Insight: Adipocytokines in metabolic syndrome and related cardiovascular disease. *Nat. Clin. Pract. Cardiovasc. Med.* **2006**, *3*, 35–42. [CrossRef]
39. Cho, S.A.; Joo, H.J.; Cho, J.Y.; Lee, S.H.; Park, J.H.; Hong, S.J.; Yu, C.W.; Lim, D.S. Visceral Fat Area and Serum Adiponectin Level Predict the Development of Metabolic Syndrome in a Community-Based Asymptomatic Population. *PLoS ONE* **2017**, *12*, e0169289. [CrossRef]
40. Guimaraes, N.S.; Mello, J.C.; Paiva, J.S.; Bueno, P.C.; Berretta, A.A.; Torquato, R.J.; Nantes, I.L.; Rodrigues, T. Baccharis dracunculifolia, the main source of green propolis, exhibits potent antioxidant activity and prevents oxidative mitochondrial damage. *Food Chem. Toxicol.* **2012**, *50*, 1091–1097. [CrossRef]
41. Veiga, R.S.; De Mendonca, S.; Mendes, P.B.; Paulino, N.; Mimica, M.J.; Lagareiro Netto, A.A.; Lira, I.S.; Lopez, B.G.; Negrao, V.; Marcucci, M.C. Artepillin C and phenolic compounds responsible for antimicrobial and antioxidant activity of green propolis and Baccharis dracunculifolia DC. *J. Appl. Microbiol.* **2017**, *122*, 911–920. [CrossRef]
42. Nakamura, T.; Ohta, Y.; Ohashi, K.; Ikeno, K.; Watanabe, R.; Tokunaga, K.; Harada, N. Protective effect of Brazilian propolis against hepatic oxidative damage in rats with water-immersion restraint stress. *Phytother. Res.* **2012**, *26*, 1482–1489. [CrossRef]
43. Ni, J.; Wu, Z.; Meng, J.; Zhu, A.; Zhong, X.; Wu, S.; Nakanishi, H. The Neuroprotective Effects of Brazilian Green Propolis on Neurodegenerative Damage in Human Neuronal SH-SY5Y Cells. *Oxid Med. Cell Longev.* **2017**, *2017*, 7984327. [CrossRef]
44. Kim, T.; Yang, Q. Peroxisome-proliferator-activated receptors regulate redox signaling in the cardiovascular system. *World J. Cardiol.* **2013**, *5*, 164–174. [CrossRef]
45. Corona, J.C.; Duchen, M.R. PPARγ as a therapeutic target to rescue mitochondrial function in neurological disease. *Free. Radic. Biol. Med.* **2016**, *100*, 153–163. [CrossRef]
46. Liguori, I.; Russo, G.; Curcio, F.; Bulli, G.; Aran, L.; Della-Morte, D.; Gargiulo, G.; Testa, G.; Cacciatore, F.; Bonaduce, D.; et al. Oxidative stress, aging, and diseases. *Clin. Interv. Aging* **2018**, *13*, 757–772. [CrossRef]
47. Doshi, S.B.; Agarwal, A. The role of oxidative stress in menopause. *J. Mid-Life Health* **2013**, *4*, 140–146. [CrossRef]
48. Okamoto, Y.; Tobe, T.; Ueda, K.; Takada, T.; Kojima, N. Oral administration of Brazilian propolis exerts estrogenic effect in ovariectomized rats. *J. Toxicol. Sci.* **2015**, *40*, 235–242. [CrossRef]
49. Stepan, J.J.; Hruskova, H.; Kverka, M. Update on Menopausal Hormone Therapy for Fracture Prevention. *Curr. Osteoporos. Rep.* **2019**, *17*, 465–473. [CrossRef]

50. Mangge, H.; Zelzer, S.; Puerstner, P.; Schnedl, W.J.; Reeves, G.; Postolache, T.T.; Weghuber, D. Uric acid best predicts metabolically unhealthy obesity with increased cardiovascular risk in youth and adults. *Obes. (Silver Spring)* **2013**, *21*, E71–E77. [CrossRef]
51. Lim, S.; Meigs, J.B. Links between ectopic fat and vascular disease in humans. *Arterioscler. Thromb. Vasc. Biol.* **2014**, *34*, 1820–1826. [CrossRef]

Disclaimer/Publisher's Note: The statements, opinions and data contained in all publications are solely those of the individual author(s) and contributor(s) and not of MDPI and/or the editor(s). MDPI and/or the editor(s) disclaim responsibility for any injury to people or property resulting from any ideas, methods, instructions or products referred to in the content.

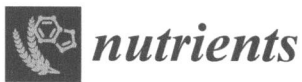 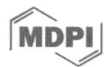

Systematic Review

The Obesity Paradox and Mortality in Older Adults: A Systematic Review

Moustapha Dramé [1,2,*] and Lidvine Godaert [1,3]

1. EpiCliV Research Unit, Faculty of Medicine, University of the French West Indies, 97261 Fort-de-France, France; godaert-l@ch-valenciennes.fr
2. Department of Clinical Research and Innovation, University Hospitals of Martinique, 97261 Fort-de-France, France
3. Department of Geriatrics, General Hospital of Valenciennes, 59300 Valenciennes, France
* Correspondence: moustapha.drame@chu-martinique.fr

Abstract: "Obesity paradox" describes the counterintuitive finding that aged overweight and obese people with a particular disease may have better outcomes than their normal weight or underweight counterparts. This systematic review was performed to summarize the publications related to the obesity paradox in older adults, to gain an in-depth understanding of this phenomenon. PubMed©, Embase©, and Scopus© were used to perform literature search for all publications up to 20 March 2022. Studies were included if they reported data from older adults on the relation between BMI and mortality. The following article types were excluded from the study: reviews, editorials, correspondence, and case reports and case series. Publication year, study setting, medical condition, study design, sample size, age, and outcome(s) were extracted. This review has been registered with PROSPERO (no. CRD42021289015). Overall, 2226 studies were identified, of which 58 were included in this systematic review. In all, 20 of the 58 studies included in this review did not find any evidence of an obesity paradox. Of these 20 studies, 16 involved patients with no specific medical condition, 1 involved patients with chronic diseases, and 2 involved patients with type 2 diabetes mellitus. Seven out of the nine studies that looked at short-term mortality found evidence of the obesity paradox. Of the 28 studies that examined longer-term mortality, 15 found evidence of the obesity paradox. In the studies that were conducted in people with a particular medical condition ($n = 24$), the obesity paradox appeared in 18 cases. Our work supports the existence of an obesity paradox, especially when comorbidities or acute medical problems are present. These findings should help guide strategies for nutritional counselling in older populations.

Keywords: obesity paradox; aged adults; body mass index; mortality

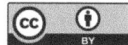

1. Introduction

Obesity, usually defined by the body mass index (BMI), is considered a public health problem, and is associated with many diseases [1–3]. The prevalence of obesity is high in younger adults but also in older people [4], and evidence suggests that prevalence of obesity will continue to increase [5]. The term "obesity paradox" is used to describe the counterintuitive finding that aged overweight and obese people with a particular disease may have better outcomes than their normal weight or underweight counterparts. However, there is wide heterogeneity between studies regarding the association between obesity and mortality in older adults, depending on the diseases concerned, the presence or absence of a particular disease, or the BMI level considered [6–8]. In aged people, body composition tends to change, and body weight tends to decrease, and some authors have suggested that fatness could be healthy [9]. Thus, it is important to confirm whether an "obesity paradox" truly exists, with a view to adapting management policies for overweight or obese old people.

In this context, the objective of the study was to summarize the publications in the literature relating to the obesity paradox in older adults, to enhance our understanding of this phenomenon.

2. Methods

2.1. Literature Search

A preliminary check was made in PubMed©, Scopus©, Embase©, Prospero©, and the Cochrane Library© to ensure that no systematic reviews had previously been conducted on this specific topic.

A literature search was performed using PubMed©, Embase©, and Scopus© to cover all publications up to March 20, 2022. The search terms defined by the two researchers (LG, MD) included the following keywords in the title and/or the abstract: ("obesity paradox" OR "reverse epidemiology" OR "body mass index" OR BMI OR overweight OR obesity) AND (mortality OR death OR survival)). The search included studies in the French or English language and studies on human subjects, and excluded the following publication types: reviews, editorials, correspondence, and case reports and case series. A manual check was performed for potential additional studies. This systematic review was based on the Preferred Reporting Items for Systematic Reviews and Meta-Analyses (PRISMA) guidelines. This study was registered with PROSPERO (an International prospective register of systematic reviews) (number CRD42021289015, available at https://www.crd.york.ac.uk/prospero/display_record.php?ID=CRD42021289015, accessed on 20 March 2023.

2.2. Study Selection

Study eligibility criteria were defined a priori by the two researchers (LG, MD) within the PICOS framework. Studies were eligible if they reported data on "obesity paradox" (using body mass index as a nutritional indicator). The population was restricted to studies that included persons 65 years or older, whatever their sex, ethnicity, or living place. The intervention (exposure) was a presence of overweight or obesity as defined by the baseline BMI value. The control was those who were underweight or a normal weight. The outcome was death, whatever the timepoint. When the study was not specifically conducted in older adults, only data concerning those aged 65 years or over were taken into account (provided that the information was available). Correspondence, editorials, reviews, basic science articles, and case reports and case series were excluded.

2.3. Data Extraction

The Covidence systematic review software© (Veritas Health Innovation, Melbourne, Australia), available at www.covidence.org, was used to perform data analysis. After elimination of duplicates, the two researchers (LG, MD) made a blind review of titles and abstracts of all articles. When there was disagreement about whether or not to include an article, they discussed the case until consensus was reached. Overlap between studies was verified. Data extraction was realised independently by the two researchers (LG, MD), using the same extraction form. The following data were extracted: publication year, study setting, medical condition, study design, sample size, age (mean or median and their statistical dispersion parameters, when available), and outcome(s). To check whether the obesity paradox was present or not, the following information was collected: outcome(s), BMI classes, type of analysis (whether multivariable or not), statistical estimates (Hazard ratio, Odds ratio, Rate ratio, Rates) and their respective 95% confidence intervals (95% CI), and the level of significance (p-values).

2.4. Quality Assessment

The Newcastle–Ottawa Scale (NOS) [10] was used to assess the quality of included studies. This scale is composed of three quality criteria: selection (4 points), comparability (2 points), and outcome assessment (3 points). This gives a total of between 0 and 9 points.

Scores of 7 or more are considered high quality studies, scores of 5–6 as moderate quality, and scores below 5 as low quality. Disagreements in scoring were resolved by a joint review of the manuscript to reach consensus.

Where possible and appropriate, some parameters were calculated from available data (e.g., mean age and/or standard deviation, rate ratio, odds ratio, etc.).

3. Results

As shown in Figure 1, 2226 studies were identified by the literature search. Among these, 1285 duplicates were found and excluded. After checking titles and abstracts of the remaining 942 studies, 273 articles were included for full-text assessment. After full-text examination of these 273 studies, 215 were excluded for at least one of the following reasons: lack of relevant information, overlapping data, or inappropriate age of the study population. Thus, 58 studies were retained in this review.

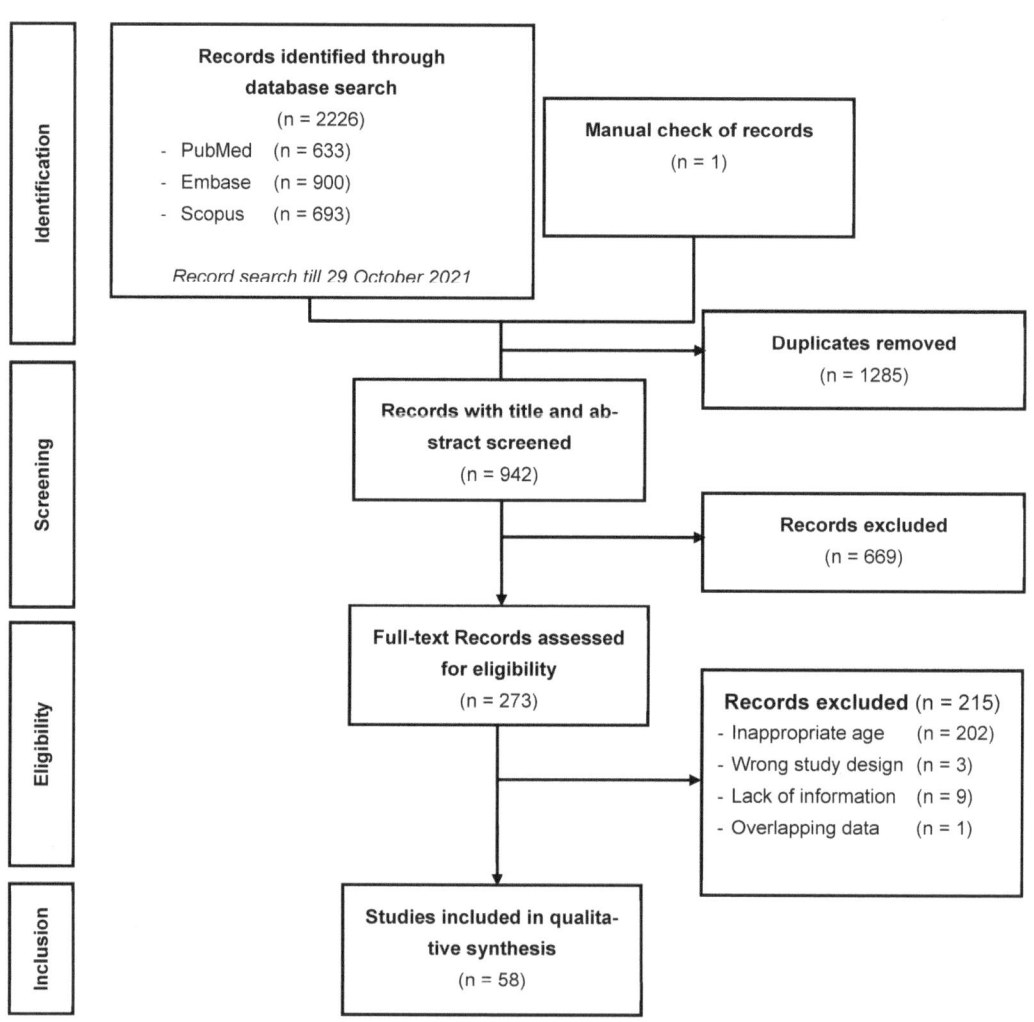

Figure 1. PRISMA flow diagram of the records included in the systematic review.

Table 1 summarizes the characteristics of the studies included in the review. All studies were observational cohorts; 41 were prospective [11–51] and 17 were retrospective [52–68]

Table 1. Description of the studies included in the present systematic review.

Author, Year	Country	Study Design	Study Setting	Medical Condition	Sample Size	Age (Years) Mean ± SD
Kananen, 2022 [68]	Sweden	Retrospective cohort	Hospital, Geriatrics	COVID-19	1409	77 [65–104] ♣
Amin, 2021 [11]	USA	Prospective cohort	Hospital, Surgery	Hip fracture	52,729	x ± x
Danninger, 2021 [52]	USA	Retrospective cohort	Hospital, ICU	Sepsis	8707	x ± x
El Moheb, 2021 [12]	USA	Prospective cohort	Hospital, Surgery	Emergent surgery	78,704	75 ± x
Lin, 2021 [13]	Taiwan	Prospective cohort	Community	None specific	81,221	74 ± 6
Martinez-Tapia, 2021 [14]	France	Prospective cohort	Hospital, Geriatrics	Cancer	2071	81 ± 6
Lai, 2020 [15]	Taiwan	Prospective cohort	LTCF	None specific	182	79 ± 8
Schneider, 2020 [16]	Germany	Prospective cohort	Hospital, Neurosurgery	Glioblastoma	110	72 [65–86] ♣
Seino, 2020 [53]	Japan	Retrospective cohort	Community	None specific	1977	72 ± 6 *
Nishida, 2019 [17]	Japan	Prospective cohort	Community	None specific	1229	74 ± 5
Om, 2019 [18]	Korea	Prospective cohort	Hospital, Cardiology	Aortic stenosis	379	79 ± x *
Tokarek, 2019 [54]	Poland	Retrospective cohort	Hospital, Cardiology	TAVI patients	147	82 [x–x] ♣
Yoshihisa, 2019 [19]	Japan	Prospective cohort	Hospital, Cardiology	Acute heart failure	2410	x ± x
Crotti, 2018 [20]	Italy	Prospective cohort	Community	None specific	4970	72 ± 5
De Palma, 2018 [21]	Sweden	Prospective cohort	Hospital, Cardiology	TAVI patients	492	83 ± 6
Keller, 2018 [55]	Germany	Retrospective cohort	Hospital, Cardiology	AMI	122,607	80 ± x
Kim, 2018 [22]	Korea	Prospective cohort	Community	None specific	170,639	72 ± 5
Lee, 2018 [56]	Korea	Retrospective cohort	Community	None specific	11,844	72 ± 5
Lv, 2018 [23]	China	Prospective cohort	Community	None specific	4361	92 ± 8
de Souto Barreto, 2017 [24]	France	Prospective cohort	Nursing home	Dementia	3741	86 ± 8
Wu, 2017 [25]	China	Prospective cohort	Hospital, ED	Atrial fibrillation	1321	x ± x
Cheng, 2016 [57]	USA	Retrospective cohort	Community	None specific	4565	74 ± 5
Flodin, 2016 [26]	Sweden	Prospective cohort	Hospital	Hip fracture	843	82 ± 7
Calabia, 2015 [58]	Spain	Retrospective cohort	Hospital, Nephrology	Haemodialysis	3978	75 ± 6
Kim, 2015 [59]	Korea	Retrospective cohort	Community	Chronic diseases	x	x ± x
Kubota, 2015 [60]	Japan	Retrospective cohort	Community	T2DM	16,304 #	x ± x
Kuo, 2015 [27]	Taiwan	Prospective cohort	Outpatients	T2DM	x	x ± x
Shil Hong, 2015 [61]	Korea	Retrospective cohort	Community	None specific	1000	76 ± 9
Buys, 2014 [28]	USA	Prospective cohort	Community	None specific	1257	75 ± 7
Clark, 2014 [62]	USA/Nigeria	Retrospective cohort	Community	None specific	2466	77 ± 5 *
Ford, 2014 [29]	USA	Prospective Cohort	Community	None specific	2995	81 ± 4
Lang, 2014 [30]	France	Prospective cohort	Hospital, ED	None specific	1306	85 ± 6

Table 1. Cont.

Author, Year	Country	Study Design	Study Setting	Medical Condition	Sample Size	Age (Years) Mean ± SD
Lee, 2014 [31]	Korea	Prospective cohort	Community	None specific	11,844	73 ± 7
Murphy, 2014 [63]	Iceland	Retrospective cohort	Community	T2DM	637	77 [66–96] ♠
Wu, 2014 [32]	Taiwan	Prospective cohort	Community	None specific	77,541	73 ± 7
Yamauchi, 2014 [64]	Japan	Retrospective cohort	Hospital, Pulmonology	COPD	263,940	78 ± 7
Chen, 2013 [33]	Taiwan	Prospective cohort	Veterans	None specific	1257	83 ± 5
Dahl, 2013 [34]	Sweden	Prospective cohort	Community	None specific	882	80 ± 6
Nakazawa, 2013 [35]	Japan	Prospective cohort	Nursing home	None specific	8510	84 ± 8
Takata, 2013 [36]	Japan	Prospective cohort	Community	None specific	675	80 ± 0
Tseng, 2013 [37]	Taiwan	Prospective cohort	Community	T2DM	34,825	x ± x
Veronese, 2013 [38]	Italy	Prospective cohort	Nursing home	None specific	181	81 ± 8
Woo, 2013 [39]	China	Prospective cohort	Community	None specific	4000	73 ± 5
Yamamoto, 2013 [40]	France	Prospective cohort	Hospital, Cardiology	TAVI patients	3072	83 ± 7
Zekry, 2013 [41]	Switzerland	Prospective cohort	Hospital, Geriatric	None specific	444	85 ± 7
de Hollander, 2012 [42]	Netherlands	Prospective cohort	Community	None specific	1980	73 ± 2
Kvamme, 2012 [43]	Norway	Prospective cohort	Community	None specific	16,711	73 ± 5
Mihel, 2012 [44]	Croatia	Prospective cohort	Community	Hypertension	2507	x ± x
Tsai, 2012 [65]	Taiwan	Retrospective cohort	Community	None specific	2892	x ± x
Cereda, 2011 [45]	Italy	Prospective cohort	LTCF	None specific	533	84 ± 8
Berraho, 2010 [46]	France	Prospective cohort	Community	None specific	3646	75 ± 7
Han, 2010 [47]	Korea	Prospective cohort	Community	None specific	877	75 ± 8
Kitamura, 2010 [48]	Japan	Prospective cohort	Home care	None specific	205	84 ± 8
Lea, 2009 [66]	USA	Retrospective cohort	Hospital, Cardiology	AMI	74,167	77 ± x *
Luchsinger, 2008 [49]	USA	Prospective cohort	Community	None specific	1372	78 ± 6
Locher, 2007 [50]	USA	Prospective cohort	Community	None specific	983	75 ± 7
Takata, 2007 [51]	Japan	Prospective cohort	Community	None specific	697	80 ± 0
Grabowski, 2001 [67]	USA	Retrospective cohort	Community	None specific	7527	77 ± 6

SD: Standard deviation; ICU: Intensive care unit; ED: Emergency department; TAVI: Transcatheter Aortic Valve Implementation; COPD: Chronic Obstructive Pulmonary Disease; AMI: Acute Myocardial Infarction; T2DM: Type 2 Diabetes Mellitus; LTCF: Long-term care facility. x: Missing information; #: Person-years; *: Pooled mean and/or standard deviation have been calculated with the information available in these articles; ♣: Median [range]; ♠: Mean [range].

As shown in Table 2, 20 of the 58 studies included in this review did not find any evidence of an obesity paradox [17,27–29,36,39,42,43,46,47,49,50,53,56,59,62,63,65,68,69]. Of these 20 studies, 16 involved patients with no specific medical condition [17,28,29,36,39,42, 43,46,47,49,50,53,56,62,65,69]. One involved patients with chronic diseases [59], and two involved patients with type 2 diabetes mellitus [27,63]. Of the 58 studies, 34 used the threshold of BMI ≥ 25.0 kg/m^2 [11,12,14,16,19–22,24,26,30–32,34,38,40,41,44,45,51,52,54,55,57,58,60, 66–68]. A further 10 studies used a threshold different from 25 kg/m^2 and found evidence of the obesity paradox [13,18,23,25,33,35,37,48,61,64]. Regarding the time points, 9 studies looked at short-term mortality (less than 12-month mortality, ICU mortality, hospital mortality) [11,12,19,30,40,52,55,64,68]. All of these, except Yamamoto et al. [40] and Kananen et al. [68], found evidence of the obesity paradox. Of the 28 studies that examined longer-term mortality (time point ≥ 5 years) [13–15,20,22,27,28,32,34,36–39,42,44–46,49,53,56–63,66,67], 15 (54%) found evidence of the obesity paradox [13,14,20,22,32,34,37,38,44,45,57,58,60,61, 66,67]. In the studies that were conducted in people with a particular medical condition

(n = 24) [11,12,14,16,18,19,21,24–27,37,40,44,52,54,55,58–60,63,64,66,68], the obesity paradox appeared in 18 (75%) cases [11,12,14,16,18,19,21,24–26,37,40,44,52,54,55,58,60,64,66]. In the studies that were carried out among people with no specific medical condition (n = 34) [13,15,17,20,22,23,28–36,38,39,41–43,45–51,53,56,57,61,62,65,67], the obesity paradox appeared in 17 (50%) cases [22,23,30–35,38,41,45,48,51,57,61,67].

Table 2. Outcomes and association between body mass index group and mortality in aged adults.

Author(s), Year	Age (Mean ± SD)	Medical Condition	Outcome	Obesity Paradox	BMI Thresholds [#] (kg/m^2)
Kananen, 2022 [68]	x ± x	COVID-19	In-hospital mortality	No	18.5 < BMI < 25.0
Amin, 2021 [11]	x ± x	Hip fracture	30-day mortality	Yes	BMI ≥ 25.0 (No, if BMI > 40.0)
Danninger, 2021 [52]	x ± x	Sepsis	ICU mortality	Yes	BMI ≥ 30.0
El Moheb, 2021 [12]	75 ± x	Emergent Surgery	30-day mortality	Yes	BMI ≥ 25.0
Lin, 2021 [13]	74 ± 6	None specific	84-month mortality	Yes	BMI ≥ 24.0
Martinez-Tapia, 2021 [14]	81 ± 6	Cancer	12-month mortality (men) 12-month mortality (women) 60-month mortality (men) 60-month mortality (women)	Yes No Yes Yes	BMI ≥ 30.0 BMI ≥ 30.0 BMI ≥ 30.0
Lai, 2020 [15]	79 ± 8	None specific	72-month mortality	No	
Schneider, 2020 [16]	72 ± x	Glioblastoma	12-month mortality	Yes	BMI ≥ 30.0
Seino, 2020 [53]	72 ± 6	None specific	All-cause mortality (men) All-cause mortality (women)	No No	
Nishida, 2019 [17]	74 ± 5	None specific	36-month mortality	No	
Om, 2019 [18]	79 ± x	Aortic stenosis	12-month mortality	Yes	BMI ≥ 24.9
Tokarek, 2019 [54]	82 ± x	TAVI patients	12-month survival	Yes	BMI ≥ 30.0
Yoshihisa, 2019 [19]	x ± x	AHF	In-hospital mortality	Yes	BMI ≥ 25.0
Crotti, 2018 [20]	72 ± 5	None specific	68-month mortality	Yes	BMI ≥ 25.0 (No, if BMI > 30.0)
			68-month CVD mortality	No	
			68-month cancer mortality	No	
De Palma, 2018 [21]	83 ± 6	TAVI patients	12-month mortality 50-month mortality	Yes Yes	BMI ≥ 25.0 BMI ≥ 25.0
Keller, 2018 [55]	80 ± x	AMI	In-hospital mortality	Yes	BMI ≥ 30.0
Kim, 2018 [22]	72 ± 5	None specific	60-month mortality	Yes	BMI ≥ 25.0 (No, if BMI > 27.5)
Lee, 2018 [56]	72 ± 5	None specific	60-month mortality	No	
Lv, 2018 [23]	92 ± 8	None specific	36-month mortality	Yes	BMI ≥ 18.5
De Souto Barreto, 2017 [24]	86 ± 8	Dementia	18-month mortality (dementia) 18-month mortality (without dementia)	Yes Yes	BMI ≥ 25.0 BMI ≥ 25.0
Wu, 2017 [25]	x ± x	Atrial fibrillation	12-month mortality (65–74 years) 12-month mortality (≥75 years)	No Yes	BMI ≥ 24.0
Cheng, 2016 [57]	74 ± 5	None specific	132-month mortality	Yes	BMI ≥ 25.0 (No, if BMI ≥ 35.0)
		Diabetes		Yes	BMI ≥ 25.0 (No, if BMI ≥ 35.0)
		Hypertension		Yes	BMI ≥ 25.0 (No, if BMI ≥ 35.0)
		Dyslipidaemia		Yes	BMI ≥ 25.0 (No, if BMI ≥ 35.0)
Flodin, 2016 [26]	82 ± 7	Hip fracture	12-month survival	Yes	BMI > 26.0

Table 2. Cont.

Author(s), Year	Age (Mean ± SD)	Medical Condition	Outcome	Obesity Paradox	BMI Thresholds # (kg/m²)
Calabia, 2015 [58]	75 ± 6	Haemodialysis	120-month mortality	Yes	BMI = 30.0–34.9 (No, if BMI = 27.5–29.9 or BMI ≥ 35.0)
Kim, 2015 [59]	x ± x	Chronic diseases	108-month mortality	No	
Kubota, 2015 [60]	x ± x	T2DM	132-month ID mortality	Yes	BMI ≥ 25.0
Kuo, 2015 [27]	x ± x	T2DM	66-month mortality	No	
Shil hong, 2015 [61]	76 ± 9	None specific	72-month mortality	Yes	BMI ≥ 23.8
Buys, 2014 [28]	75 ± 7	None specific	102-month mortality	No	
Clark, 2014 [62]	77 ± 5	None specific	120-month mortality (Africans)	No	
			120-month mortality (African Americans)	No	
Ford, 2014 [29]	81 ± 4	None specific	40-month mortality	No	
Lang, 2014 [30]	85 ± 6	None specific	6-week mortality	Yes	BMI ≥ 30.0
			12-month mortality	Yes	BMI ≥ 25.0
			24-month mortality	Yes	BMI ≥ 25.0
Lee, 2014 [31]	73 ± 7	None specific	36-month mortality	Yes	BMI ≥ 25.0 (No, if BMI ≥ 30.0)
Murphy, 2014 [63]	77 ± x	T2DM	84-month mortality	No	
Wu, 2014 [32]	73 ± 7	None specific	60-month mortality	Yes	BMI ≥ 25.0 (No, if BMI ≥ 35.0)
			60-month CVD mortality		BMI ≥ 25.0 (No, if BMI ≥ 30.0)
Yamauchi, 2014 [64]	78 ± 7	COPD	In-hospital mortality	Yes	BMI ≥ 23.0
Chen, 2013 [33]	83 ± 5	None specific	18-month mortality	Yes	BMI ≥ 23.0
Dahl, 2013 [34]	80 ± 6	None specific	216-month mortality	Yes	BMI ≥ 25.0 (No, if BMI ≥ 30.0)
Nakazawa, 2013 [35]	84 ± 8	None specific	12-month mortality	Yes	BMI ≥ 23.6
Takata, 2013 [36]	80 ± 0	None specific	144-month mortality	No	
			144-month CVD mortality	No	
			144-month cancer mortality	No	
Tseng, 2013 [37]	x ± x	T2DM	144-month mortality	Yes	BMI ≥ 23.0
Veronese, 2013 [38]	81 ± 8	None specific	60-month	Yes	BMI ≥ 30.0
Woo, 2013 [39]	73 ± 5	None specific	84-month mortality	No	
Yamamoto, 2013 [40]	83 ± 7	TAVI patients	30-day mortality	No	
			12-month mortality	Yes	BMI ≥ 25.0
Zekry, 2013 [41]	85 ± 7	None specific	48-month mortality	Yes	BMI ≥ 30.0
de Hollander, 2012 [42]	73 ± 2	None specific	120-month mortality	No	
Kvamme, 2012 [43]	73 ± 5	None specific	12-month mortality (men)	No	
			12-month mortality (women)	No	
		Respiratory diseases	12-month mortality (men)	No	
			12-month mortality (women)	No	
		CVD	12-month mortality (men)	No	
			12-month mortality (women)	No	
		Cancer	12-month mortality (men)	No	
			12-month mortality (women)	No	
Mihel, 2012 [44]	x ± x	Hypertension	60-month mortality (men)	Yes	BMI ≥ 30.0
			60-month mortality (women)	No	

Table 2. Cont.

Author(s), Year	Age (Mean ± SD)	Medical Condition	Outcome	Obesity Paradox	BMI Thresholds # (kg/m²)
Tsai, 2012 [65]	x ± x	None specific	48-month mortality (65–74 y; men) 48-month mortality (≥75 y; men) 48-month mortality (65–74 y; women) 48-month mortality (≥75 y; women)	No No No No	
Cereda, 2011 [45]	84 ± 8	None specific	72-month mortality	Yes	BMI ≥ 25.0
Berraho, 2010 [46]	75 ± 7	None specific	156-month mortality	No	
Han, 2010 [47]	75 ± 8	None specific	42-month mortality	No	
Kitamura, 2010 [48]	84 ± 8	None specific	24-month mortality	Yes	BMI ≥ 17.1
Lea, 2009 [66]	77 ± x	AMI	125-month mortality	Yes	BMI ≥ 25.0 (No, if BMI > 40.0)
Luchsinger, 2008 [49]	78 ± 6	None specific	144-month mortality	No	
Locher, 2007 [50]	75 ± 7	None specific	36-month mortality	No	
Takata, 2007 [51]	80 ± 0	None specific	48-month mortality 48-month CVD mortality 48-month cancer mortality	Yes No No	BMI ≥ 25.0
Grabowski, 2001 [67]	77 ± 6	None specific	96-month mortality	Yes	BMI ≥ 28.5

BMI thresholds at which an obesity paradox was demonstrated. SD: Standard deviation; ICU: Intensive Care Unit; TAVI: Transcatheter Aortic Valve Implementation; COPD: Chronic Obstructive Pulmonary Disease; AHF: Acute Heart Failure; AMI: Acute Myocardial Infarction; T2DM: Type 2 Diabetes Mellitus; CVD: Cardiovascular disease; y, years. x: Missing information.

An appendix provides detailed information of the analyses and results of the relationship between BMI and mortality in aged adults. Of the analyses tested for the existence of an obesity paradox, 48 were adjusted for confounders, and 10 were unadjusted analyses (see Supplementary Materials).

The quality of the included studies, as assessed using the NOS, was considered high for all 58 studies (Table 3).

Table 3. Quality assessment of the different studies included in this systematic review, using the Newcastle–Ottawa scale (NOS).

Author, Year	Study Design	Selection	Comparability	Outcome	Total Score	Quality Rating
Kananen, 2022 [68]	Retrospective cohort	****	**	***	9	High
Amin, 2021 [11]	Prospective cohort	****	**	***	9	High
Danninger, 2021 [52]	Retrospective cohort	****	**	***	9	High
El Moheb, 2021 [12]	Prospective cohort	****	**	***	9	High
Lin, 2021 [13]	Prospective cohort	***	**	***	8	High
Martinez-Tapia, 2021 [14]	Prospective cohort	****	**	***	9	High
Lai, 2020 [15]	Prospective cohort	****	**	***	9	High
Schneider, 2020 [16]	Prospective cohort	****	**	***	9	High
Seino, 2020 [53]	Retrospective cohort	****	**	***	9	High
Nishida, 2019 [17]	Prospective cohort	****	**	***	9	High
Om, 2019 [18]	Prospective cohort	****	*	***	8	High
Tokarek, 2019 [54]	Retrospective cohort	****	*	***	8	High
Yoshihisa, 2019 [19]	Prospective cohort	****	*	***	8	High
Crotti, 2018 [20]	Prospective cohort	****	**	***	9	High
De Palma, 2018 [21]	Prospective cohort	****	*	***	8	High
Keller, 2018 [55]	Retrospective cohort	****	*	***	8	High
Kim, 2018 [22]	Prospective cohort	****	**	***	9	High

Table 3. *Cont.*

Author, Year	Study Design	Selection	Comparability	Outcome	Total Score	Quality Rating
Lee, 2018 [56]	Retrospective cohort	****	**	***	9	High
Lv, 2018 [23]	Prospective cohort	****	**	***	9	High
de Souto Barreto, 2017 [24]	Prospective cohort	****	**	***	9	High
Wu, 2017 [25]	Prospective cohort	****	**	***	9	High
Cheng, 2016 [57]	Retrospective cohort	****	**	***	9	High
Flodin, 2016 [26]	Prospective cohort	****	**	***	9	High
Calabia, 2015 [58]	Retrospective cohort	****	**	***	9	High
Kim, 2015 [59]	Retrospective cohort	****	**	***	9	High
Kubota, 2015 [60]	Retrospective study	****	**	***	9	High
Kuo, 2015 [27]	Prospective cohort	****	*	***	8	High
Shil Hong, 2015 [61]	Retrospective cohort	****	**	***	9	High
Buys, 2014 [28]	Prospective cohort	***	**	***	8	High
Clark, 2014 [62]	Retrospective cohort	****	**	***	9	High
Ford, 2014 [29]	Prospective cohort	***	**	***	8	High
Lang, 2014 [30]	Prospective cohort	****	**	***	9	High
Lee, 2014 [31]	Prospective cohort	****	**	***	9	High
Murphy, 2014 [63]	Retrospective cohort	****	**	***	9	High
Wu, 2014 [32]	Prospective cohort	****	**	***	9	High
Yamauchi, 2014 [64]	Retrospective cohort	****	**	***	9	High
Chen, 2013 [33]	Prospective cohort	***	**	***	8	High
Dahl, 2013 [34]	Prospective cohort	***	**	***	8	High
Nakazawa, 2013 [35]	Prospective cohort	****	**	***	9	High
Takata, 2013 [36]	Prospective cohort	***	**	***	8	High
Tseng, 2013 [37]	Prospective cohort	****	**	***	9	High
Veronese, 2013 [38]	Prospective cohort	***	**	***	8	High
Woo, 2013 [39]	Prospective cohort	****	**	***	9	High
Yamamoto, 2013 [40]	Prospective cohort	****	**	***	9	High
Zekry, 2013 [41]	Prospective cohort	****	**	***	9	High
de Hollander, 2012 [42]	Prospective cohort	***	**	***	8	High
Kvamme, 2012 [43]	Prospective cohort	****	**	***	9	High
Mihel, 2012 [44]	Prospective cohort	***	*	***	7	High
Tsai, 2012 [65]	Retrospective cohort	****	**	***	9	High
Cereda, 2011 [45]	Prospective cohort	***	**	***	8	High
Berraho, 2010 [46]	Prospective cohort	****	**	***	9	High
Han, 2010 [47]	Prospective cohort	****	**	***	9	High
Kitamura, 2010 [48]	Prospective cohort	****	**	***	9	High
Lea, 2009 [66]	Retrospective cohort	****	**	***	9	High
Luchsinger, 2008 [49]	Prospective cohort	****	**	***	9	High
Locher, 2007 [50]	Prospective cohort	****	**	***	9	High
Takata, 2007 [51]	Prospective cohort	****	**	***	9	High
Grabowski, 2001 [67]	Retrospective cohort	****	**	***	9	High

Each star is equal to one point. The sum of the stars gives the total score of the NOS. NOS score of ≥7 were considered as high quality studies, NOS score of 5–6 as moderate quality, and NOS Scores less than 5 as low quality.

4. Discussion

In this systematic review of studies exploring the relationship between BMI and mortality in patients aged 65 years or older, 28 out of the 58 studies included observed longer survival in patients with a BMI ≥ 25 kg/m^2 (the so-called obesity paradox) [11,12,14, 16,19–22,24,26,30–32,34,38,40,41,44,45,51,52,54,55,57,58,60,66,67]. Among these 28 studies,

16 involved patients with a specific or acute medical condition [11,12,14,16,19,21,24,26,40, 44,52,54,55,58,60,66]. Seven studies found improved survival in overweight and obese older people when focussing on short-term mortality [11,12,19,30,52,55,64,70]. One showed increased survival only in the oldest patients [25]. Two showed increased survival only in men [14,44]. Of the 23 studies that did not observe an obesity paradox [14,15,17,25,27–29, 36,39,40,42,43,46,47,49,50,53,56,59,62,63,65,68], 7 involved populations selected according to the presence of a particular medical condition [14,25,27,40,59,63,68].

Nearly two-thirds of the studies included in this work report better survival in overweight or obese older people. Several factors may influence the relationship between obesity and survival in the older population, including age, degree of obesity, presence or absence of comorbidities, and occurrence of an acute event.

Regarding age, the studies in this review that failed to show better survival in overweight or obese individuals included populations that were, on average, younger than those demonstrating an obesity paradox. Wu et al. [25], in their study of the impact of age on the association between BMI and all-cause mortality in patients with atrial fibrillation, found better survival in overweight or obese patients aged 75 years or older but not in patients aged between 65 and 74 years. Observations made in older populations must therefore take into account the intrinsic characteristics of the survivors. For the same BMI, patient profiles can be different, and this profile can influence survival. For instance, body composition may differ due to ethnicity, sex, or advancing age [71,72]. BMI does not provide information on body composition, and is less correlated with percentage of body mass or fat mass index, especially in younger people [72]. Abdominal obesity has direct metabolic consequences (adipose tissue inflammation, dysglycaemia, alteration of blood pressure regulation, etc.). Conversely, subcutaneous fat accumulation in the hips, for example, appears to have benign effects on cardiovascular risk. Other indicators, such as waist circumference or waist-to-hip ratio, are strongly associated with higher mortality risk [73,74]. Taking only BMI into account does not make it possible to differentiate between these situations [9]. In all studies included in this work, BMI was defined as an obesity index. If obesity is defined by "body adiposity", BMI level is probably not the best criterion [75]. The term "BMI paradox" may be more appropriate than "obesity paradox", as suggested by Antonopoulos et al. [9].

Obesity is a factor associated with higher mortality in younger populations [76–78], but it is also associated with an increased risk of developing and dying from a number of diseases [3], such as cancer [79,80], Some authors point to the obesity-related cellular and immune changes that make obese people more vulnerable, including an increased risk of infections [1]. Older obese people could be considered constitutionally more robust as they have survived the risk factor of obesity into adulthood. The degree of obesity could also be a factor. In this review, not all authors differentiated between different classes of obesity. However, the positive effect on survival in cases of overweight and obesity was not found for morbid obesity (BMI $\geq$ 35.0 kg/m^2) in 5 studies [11,32,57,58,66]. Furthermore, weight is not a reflection of body composition, in particular the muscle mass/fat mass ratio. Loss of muscle mass and strength (sarcopenia) is a factor associated with an increased risk of death. Tian et al. reported that obese people with sarcopenia have a higher risk of death than obese people without sarcopenia [81]. Obese people may be less frequently sarcopenic than non-obese people. In 1493 subjects aged 65 years or more (median age 74 $\pm$ 11 years), Sousa-Santos et al. [82] found a prevalence of 0.8% of obese sarcopenic individuals versus 11.6% of sarcopenic individuals of all BMI status.

The presence of a chronic pathology or an acute event may also influence survival. In this review, 20 studies [11,12,14,16,18,19,21,24–26,37,40,44,52,54,55,58,60,64,66] of the 38 which found a favourable effect of overweight or obesity on survival involved patients with a particular chronic condition or facing a specific medical event. This finding suggests that even moderately overweight older individuals with chronic disease or acute medical events have better survival. Obesity in older people with a chronic disease could be a sign of greater robustness or higher reserves (better appetite, less risk of undernutrition).

Overweight or obese older subjects would be less undernourished than the general older population. Cereda et al. [83], in their meta-analysis of the prevalence of undernutrition in an older population, found a prevalence of undernutrition ranging from 3.1 to 29.4%, depending on the setting. Sousa-Santos et al. [84] showed that 6% of obese elderly subjects (BMI $\geq$ 30 kg/m^2) were also undernourished or at risk of undernutrition. In the event of an acute event, obese elderly people may have a better chance of survival, particularly because of their greater functional reserves. This observation is also made in younger obese or overweight subjects. Akinnusi et al. [85] show in their meta-analysis of patients admitted to intensive care that obese subjects have a similar mortality to non-obese subjects. In 2013, the meta-analysis by Flegal et al. [76] confirmed in a population without any particular pathology that overweight people (BMI > 25 kg/m^2) (all types of obesity and all ages) had a higher overall mortality rate, whatever the cause. However, mildly overweight people (BMI $\geq$ 25 and <30 kg/m^2) had lower all-cause mortality than normal weight people (BMI < 25 kg/m^2). Thus, this advantage was found regardless of age.

Several mechanisms could explain "obesity paradox". Probably, there are "good adipose tissues" in elderly subjects. In the literature, overweight or obesity, defined by high level of BMI, is shown to have positive influence on prothrombotic factors, production of certain cytokines, or NT-proBNP levels. Adipokine produced by adipose tissue seems to be cardioprotective [86]. Obesity could have a protective effect against progression or consequences of some chronic diseases. High BMI could also reflect better nutritional status and adequate muscle reserves. Casas-Vara et al. [87] showed better nutritional status in overweight or obese elderly people with heart failure.

Our systematic review has limitations. Although the WHO has proposed thresholds for BMI, the authors used different thresholds in their respective studies. In addition, the outcomes were also different between the studies. This made it difficult to compare the studies, and precluded meta-analysis. The age variable was missing in 14.0% of cases (8/57).

However, this work covers a large number of studies, totalling more than 1,120,000 people aged 65 years or over, with varying medical conditions and in different settings. The follow-up time of the studies ranged from 30 days to 156 months (even though the majority of studies have a long-term follow-up). These differences in follow-up time may make comparison difficult. In addition, there is no information on BMI variation over time, especially for studies with long-term follow-up. Weight loss or gain between baseline measurement and death could have a significant impact. The fact that only studies conducted in subjects aged 65 years or older were selected gives a certain homogeneity to this systematic review in terms of population. Finally, all studies were evaluated for methodological quality using the NOS, and were found to be of high quality.

5. Conclusions

The findings of this systematic review are in favour of the existence of an obesity paradox, which could more specifically concern older subjects with a comorbidity and/or experiencing an acute event. Nevertheless, because BMI does not reflect body composition, the term "BMI paradox" would be more appropriate. The influence of the level of BMI remains unclear. These findings should help guide strategies for nutritional counselling in the older population.

Supplementary Materials: The following supporting information can be downloaded at: https://www.mdpi.com/article/10.3390/nu15071780/s1, Table S1: Outcome and results of association between body mass index groups and mortality in aged adults (detailed information).

Author Contributions: L.G. and M.D. conceived and designed the study, prepared the material, collected the data, and performed the analysis. They wrote the first draft of the manuscript, and approved the final manuscript. All authors have read and agreed to the published version of the manuscript.

Funding: The authors declare that no funds, grants, or other support were received during the preparation of this manuscript. The APC was funded by tht University Hospitals of Martinique.

Informed Consent Statement: Not applicable.

Data Availability Statement: Data could be made available on reasonable request at moustapha.drame@chu-martinique.fr.

Acknowledgments: Thanks to Fiona Ecarnot for editorial assistance.

Conflicts of Interest: This research did not receive any specific grant from funding agencies in the public, commercial, or not-for-profit sectors.

References

1. Frydrych, L.M.; Bian, G.; O'Lone, D.E.; Ward, P.A.; Delano, M.J. Obesity and type 2 diabetes mellitus drive immune dysfunction, infection development, and sepsis mortality. *J. Leukoc. Biol.* **2018**, *104*, 525–534. [CrossRef] [PubMed]
2. Liu, Z.; Sanossian, N.; Starkman, S.; Avila-Rinek, G.; Eckstein, M.; Sharma, L.K.; Liebeskind, D.; Conwit, R.; Hamilton, S. Adiposity and Outcome After Ischemic Stroke: Obesity Paradox for Mortality and Obesity Parabola for Favorable Functional Outcomes. *Stroke* **2021**, *52*, 144–151. [CrossRef] [PubMed]
3. Powell-Wiley, T.M.; Poirier, P.; Burke, L.E.; Després, J.-P.; Gordon-Larsen, P.; Lavie, C.J.; Lear, S.A.; Ndumele, C.E.; Neeland, I.J.; Sanders, P.; et al. Obesity and Cardiovascular Disease: A Scientific Statement From the American Heart Association. *Circulation* **2021**, *143*, e984–e1010. [CrossRef] [PubMed]
4. Hales, C.M.; Carroll, M.D.; Fryar, C.D.; Ogden, C.L. Prevalence of Obesity and Severe Obesity Among Adults: United States. 2017–2018. *NCHS Data Brief* **2020**, *360*, 1–8.
5. Ward, Z.J.; Bleich, S.N.; Cradock, A.L.; Barrett, J.L.; Giles, C.M.; Flax, C.; Gortmaker, S.L. Projected, U.S. State-Level Prevalence of Adult Obesity and Severe Obesity. *N. Engl. J. Med.* **2019**, *381*, 2440–2450. [CrossRef]
6. Kwon, Y.; Kim, H.J.; Park, S.; Park, Y.G.; Cho, K.H. Body mass index-related mortality in patients with type 2 diabetes and heterogeneity in obesity paradox studies: A dose-response meta-analysis. *PLoS ONE* **2017**, *12*, e0168247. [CrossRef]
7. Skinner, J.S.; Abel, W.M.; McCoy, K.; Wilkins, C.H. Exploring the "Obesity Paradox" as a Correlate of Cognitive and Physical Function in Community-dwelling Black and White Older Adults. *Ethn. Dis.* **2017**, *27*, 387–394. [CrossRef]
8. Yamazaki, K.; Suzuki, E.; Yorifuji, T.; Tsuda, T.; Ohta, T.; Ishikawa-Takata, K.; Doi, H. Is there an obesity paradox in the Japanese elderly population? A community-based cohort study of 13,280 men and women. *Geriatr. Gerontol. Int.* **2017**, *17*, 1257–1264. [CrossRef]
9. Antonopoulos, A.S.; Tousoulis, D. The molecular mechanisms of obesity paradox. *Cardiovasc. Res.* **2017**, *113*, 1074–1086. [CrossRef]
10. Wells, G.A.; Shea, B.; O'Connell, D.; Peterson, J.; Welch, V.; Losos, M.; Tugwell, P. The Newcastle-Ottawa Scale (NOS) for Assessing the Quality of Non-Randomised Studies in Meta-Analyses: The Ottawa Hospital. 2013. Available online: http://www.ohri.ca/programs/clinical_epidemiology/oxford.asp (accessed on 1 November 2022).
11. Amin, R.M.; Raad, M.; Rao, S.S.; Musharbash, F.; Best, M.J.; Amanatullah, D.F. Survival bias may explain the appearance of the obesity paradox in hip fracture patients. *Osteoporos. Int.* **2021**, *32*, 2555–2562. [CrossRef]
12. El Moheb, M.; Jia, Z.; Qin, H.; El Hechi, M.W.; Nordestgaard, A.T.; Lee, J.M.; Kaafarani, H.M. The Obesity Paradox in Elderly Patients Undergoing Emergency Surgery: A Nationwide Analysis. *J. Surg. Res.* **2021**, *265*, 195–203. [CrossRef] [PubMed]
13. Lin, Y.-K.; Wang, C.-C.; Yen, Y.-F.; Chen, L.-J.; Ku, P.-W.; Chen, C.-C.; Lai, Y.-J. Association of body mass index with all-cause mortality in the elderly population of Taiwan: A prospective cohort study. *Nutr. Metab. Cardiovasc. Dis. NMCD* **2021**, *31*, 110–118. [CrossRef] [PubMed]
14. Martinez-Tapia, C.; Diot, T.; Oubaya, N.; Paillaud, E.; Poisson, J.; Gisselbrecht, M.; Morisset, L.; Caillet, P.; Baudin, A.; Pamoukdjian, F.; et al. The obesity paradox for mid- and long-term mortality in older cancer patients: A prospective multicenter cohort study. *Am. J. Clin. Nutr.* **2020**, *113*, 129–141. [CrossRef] [PubMed]
15. Lai, K.-Y.; Wu, T.-H.; Liu, C.-S.; Lin, C.-H.; Lin, C.-C.; Lai, M.-M.; Lin, W.-Y. Body mass index and albumin levels are prognostic factors for long-term survival in elders with limited performance status. *Aging* **2020**, *12*, 1104–1113. [CrossRef]
16. Schneider, M.; Potthoff, A.-L.; Scharnböck, E.; Heimann, M.; Schäfer, N.; Weller, J.; Schaub, C.; Jacobs, A.H.; Güresir, E.; Herrlinger, U.; et al. Newly diagnosed glioblastoma in geriatric (65+) patients: Impact of patients frailty, comorbidity burden and obesity on overall survival. *J. Neurooncol.* **2020**, *149*, 421–427. [CrossRef]
17. Nishida, M.M.; Okura, M.; Ogita, M.; Aoyama, T.; Tsuboyama, T.; Arai, H. Two-Year Weight Loss but Not Body Mass Index Predicts Mortality and Disability in an Older Japanese Community-Dwelling Population. *J. Am. Med. Dir. Assoc.* **2019**, *20*, 1654.e11–1654.e18. [CrossRef]
18. Om, S.Y.; Ko, E.; Ahn, J.-M.; Kang, D.-Y.; Lee, K.; Kwon, O.; Lee, P.H.; Lee, S.-W.; Kim, H.J.; Kim, J.B.; et al. Relation of Body Mass Index to Risk of Death or Stroke in Patients Who Underwent Transcatheter Aortic Valve Implantation. *Am. J. Cardiol.* **2019**, *123*, 638–643. [CrossRef]
19. Yoshihisa, A.; Sato, T.; Kajimoto, K.; Sato, N.; Takeishi, Y. Acute Decompensated Heart Failure Syndromes i. Heterogeneous impact of body mass index on in-hospital mortality in acute heart failure syndromes: An analysis from the ATTEND Registry. *Eur. Heart J. Acute Cardiovasc. Care* **2019**, *8*, 589–598. [CrossRef]

20. Crotti, G.; Gianfagna, F.; Bonaccio, M.; Di Castelnuovo, A.; Costanzo, S.; Persichillo, M.; Iacoviello, L. Body Mass Index and Mortality in Elderly Subjects from the Moli-Sani Study: A Possible Mediation by Low-Grade Inflammation? *Immunol. Investig.* **2018**, *47*, 774–789. [CrossRef]
21. De Palma, R.; Ivarsson, J.; Feldt, K.; Saleh, N.; Ruck, A.; Linder, R.; Settergren, M. The obesity paradox: An analysis of pre-procedure weight trajectory on survival outcomes in patients undergoing transcatheter aortic valve implantation. *Obes. Res. Clin. Pract.* **2018**, *12*, 51–60. [CrossRef]
22. Kim, H.; Yoon, J.L.; Lee, A.; Jung, Y.; Kim, M.Y.; Cho, J.J.; Ju, Y.S. Prognostic effect of body mass index to mortality in Korean older persons. *Geriatr. Gerontol. Int.* **2018**, *18*, 538–546. [CrossRef] [PubMed]
23. Lv, Y.-B.; Liu, S.; Yin, Z.-X.; Gao, X.; Kraus, V.B.; Mao, C.; Yuan, J.-Q.; Zhang, J.; Luo, J.-S.; Chen, H.-S.; et al. Associations of Body Mass Index and Waist Circumference with 3-Year All-Cause Mortality Among the Oldest Old: Evidence from a Chinese Community-Based Prospective Cohort Study. *J. Am. Med. Dir. Assoc.* **2018**, *19*, 672–678.e4. [CrossRef]
24. de Souto Barreto, P.; Cadroy, Y.; Kelaiditi, E.; Vellas, B.; Rolland, Y. The prognostic value of body-mass index on mortality in older adults with dementia living in nursing homes. *Clin. Nutr.* **2017**, *36*, 423–428. [CrossRef] [PubMed]
25. Wu, S.; Yang, Y.-M.; Zhu, J.; Wan, H.-B.; Wang, J.; Zhang, H.; Shao, X.-H. Impact of Age on the Association Between Body Mass Index and All-Cause Mortality in Patients with Atrial Fibrillation. *J. Nutr. Heal. Aging* **2017**, *21*, 1125–1132. [CrossRef]
26. Flodin, L.; Laurin, A.; Lokk, J.; Cederholm, T.; Hedstrom, M. Increased 1-year survival and discharge to independent living in overweight hip fracture patients: A prospective study of 843 patients. *Acta Orthop.* **2016**, *87*, 146–151. [CrossRef]
27. Kuo, J.F.; Hsieh, Y.T.; Mao, I.C.; Lin, S.D.; Tu, S.T.; Hsieh, M.C. The Association Between Body Mass Index and All-Cause Mortality in Patients With Type 2 Diabetes Mellitus: A 5.5-Year Prospective Analysis. *Medicine* **2015**, *94*, e1398. [CrossRef] [PubMed]
28. Buys, D.R.; Roth, D.L.; Ritchie, C.S.; Sawyer, P.; Allman, R.M.; Funkhouser, E.M.; Locher, J.L. Nutritional risk and body mass index predict hospitalization, nursing home admissions, and mortality in community-dwelling older adults: Results from the UAB Study of Aging with 8.5 years of follow-up. *J. Gerontol. Biol. Sci. Med. Sci.* **2014**, *69*, 1146–1153. [CrossRef]
29. Ford, D.W.; Hartman, T.J.; Do, C.S.; Wood, C.; Mitchell, D.C.; Erickson, P.; Bailey, R.; Smiciklas-Wright, H.; Coffman, D.L.; Jensen, G.L. Body mass index, poor diet quality, and health-related quality of life are associated with mortality in rural older adults. *J. Nutr. Gerontol. Geriatr.* **2014**, *33*, 23–34. [CrossRef]
30. Lang, P.O.; Mahmoudi, R.; Novella, J.-L.; Tardieu, E.; Bertholon, L.-A.; Nazeyrollas, P.; Blanchard, F.; Jolly, D.; Dramé, M. Is obesity a marker of robustness in vulnerable hospitalized aged populations? Prospective, multicenter cohort study of 1306 acutely ill patients. *J. Nutr. Health Aging* **2014**, *18*, 66–74. [CrossRef]
31. Lee, Y.; Kim, J.; Han, E.S.; Ryu, M.; Cho, Y.; Chae, S. Frailty and body mass index as predictors of 3-year mortality in older adults living in the community. *Gerontology* **2014**, *60*, 475–482. [CrossRef]
32. Wu, C.Y.; Chou, Y.C.; Huang, N.; Chou, Y.J.; Hu, H.Y.; Li, C.P. Association of body mass index with all-cause and cardiovascular disease mortality in the elderly. *PLoS ONE* **2014**, *9*, e102589. [CrossRef]
33. Chen, L.; Peng, L.; Liu, L.; Lin, M.; Lan, C.; Chang, P. Body mass index, health status, and mortality of older Taiwanese men: Overweight good, underweight bad, obesity neutral. *J. Am. Geriatr. Soc.* **2013**, *61*, 2233–2234. [CrossRef] [PubMed]
34. Dahl, A.K.; Fauth, E.B.; Ernsth-Bravell, M.; Hassing, L.B.; Ram, N.; Gerstof, D. Body mass index, change in body mass index, and survival in old and very old persons. *J. Am. Geriatr. Soc.* **2013**, *61*, 512–518. [CrossRef] [PubMed]
35. Nakazawa, A.; Nakamura, K.; Kitamura, K.; Yoshizawa, Y. Association between body mass index and mortality among institutionalized elderly adults in Japan. *Environ. Health Prev. Med.* **2013**, *18*, 502–506. [CrossRef]
36. Takata, Y.; Ansai, T.; Soh, I.; Awano, S.; Nakamichi, I.; Akifusa, S.; Goto, K.; Yoshida, A.; Fujii, H.; Fujisawa, R.; et al. Body mass index and disease-specific mortality in an 80-year-old population at the 12-year follow-up. *Arch. Gerontol. Geriatr.* **2013**, *57*, 46–53. [CrossRef]
37. Tseng, C.H. Obesity paradox: Differential effects on cancer and noncancer mortality in patients with type 2 diabetes mellitus. *Atherosclerosis* **2013**, *226*, 186–192. [CrossRef] [PubMed]
38. Veronese, N.; De Rui, M.; Toffanello, E.D.; De Ronch, I.; Perissinotto, E.; Bolzetta, F.; D'Avanzo, B.; Cardin, F.; Coin, A.; Manzato, E.; et al. Body mass index as a predictor of all-cause mortality in nursing home residents during a 5-year follow-up. *J. Am. Med. Dir. Assoc.* **2013**, *14*, 53–57. [CrossRef] [PubMed]
39. Woo, J.; Yu, R.; Yau, F. Fitness, fatness and survival in elderly populations. *Age* **2013**, *35*, 973–984. [CrossRef] [PubMed]
40. Yamamoto, M.; Mouillet, G.; Oguri, A.; Gilard, M.; Laskar, M.; Eltchaninoff, H.; Fajadet, J.; Iung, B.; Donzeau-Gouge, P.; Leprince, P.; et al. Effect of body mass index on 30- and 365-day complication and survival rates of transcatheter aortic valve implantation (from the FRench Aortic National CoreValve and Edwards 2 [FRANCE 2] registry). *Am. J. Cardiol.* **2013**, *112*, 1932–1937. [CrossRef]
41. Zekry, D.; Herrmann, F.R.; Vischer, U.M. The association between the body mass index and 4-year all-cause mortality in older hospitalized patients. *J. Gerontol. Biol. Sci. Med. Sci.* **2013**, *68*, 705–711. [CrossRef]
42. de Hollander, E.L.; Van Zutphen, M.; Bogers, R.P.; Bemelmans, W.J.; De Groot, L.C. The impact of body mass index in old age on cause-specific mortality. *J. Nutr. Health Aging* **2012**, *16*, 100–106. [CrossRef]
43. Kvamme, J.M.; Holmen, J.; Wilsgaard, T.; Florholmen, J.; Midthjell, K.; Jacobsen, B.K. Body mass index and mortality in elderly men and women: The Tromso and HUNT studies. *J. Epidemiol. Community Health* **2012**, *66*, 611–617. [CrossRef] [PubMed]
44. Mihel, S.; Milanovic, S.M. Association of elevated body mass index and hypertension with mortality: The CroHort study. *Coll. Antropol.* **2012**, *36*, 183–188. [CrossRef] [PubMed]

45. Cereda, E.; Pedrolli, C.; Zagami, A.; Vanotti, A.; Piffer, S.; Opizzi, A.; Rondanelli, M.; Caccialanza, R. Body mass index and mortality in institutionalized elderly. *J. Am. Med. Dir Assoc.* **2011**, *12*, 174–178. [CrossRef] [PubMed]
46. Berraho, M.; Nejjari, C.; Raherison, C.; El Achhab, Y.; Tachfouti, N.; Serhier, Z.; Dartigues, J.F.; Barberger-Gateau, P. Body mass index, disability, and 13-year mortality in older French adults. *J. Aging Health* **2010**, *22*, 68–83. [CrossRef]
47. Han, S.S.; Kim, K.W.; Na, K.Y.; Chae, D.-W.; Kim, S.; Chin, H.J. Lean mass index: A better predictor of mortality than body mass index in elderly Asians. *J. Am. Geriatr. Soc.* **2010**, *58*, 312–317. [CrossRef]
48. Kitamura, K.; Nakamura, K.; Nishiwaki, T.; Ueno, K.; Hasegawa, M. Low body mass index and low serum albumin are predictive factors for short-term mortality in elderly Japanese requiring home care. *Tohoku J. Exp. Med.* **2010**, *221*, 29–34. [CrossRef]
49. Luchsinger, J.A.; Patel, B.; Tang, M.X.; Schupf, N.; Mayeux, R. Body mass index, dementia, and mortality in the elderly. *J. Nutr. Health Aging.* **2008**, *12*, 127–131. [CrossRef]
50. Locher, J.L.; Roth, D.L.; Ritchie, C.S.; Cox, K.; Sawyer, P.; Bodner, E.V.; Allman, R.M. Body mass index, weight loss, and mortality in community-dwelling older adults. *J. Gerontol. Biol. Sci. Med. Sci.* **2007**, *62*, 1389–1392. [CrossRef]
51. Takata, Y.; Ansai, T.; Soh, I.; Akifusa, S.; Sonoki, K.; Fujisawa, K.; Awano, S.; Kagiyama, S.; Hamasaki, T.; Nakamichi, I.; et al. Association between body mass index and mortality in an 80-year-old population. *J. Am. Geriatr. Soc.* **2007**, *55*, 913–917. [CrossRef]
52. Danninger, T.; Rezar, R.; Mamandipoor, B.; Dankl, D.; Koköfer, A.; Jung, C.; Wernly, B.; Osmani, V. Underweight but not overweight is associated with excess mortality in septic ICU patients. *Wien. Klin. Wochenschr.* **2021**, *134*, 139–147. [CrossRef] [PubMed]
53. Seino, S.; Kitamura, A.; Abe, T.; Taniguchi, Y.; Yokoyama, Y.; Amano, H.; Nishi, M.; Nofuji, Y.; Narita, M.; Ikeuchi, T.; et al. Dose-Response Relationships Between Body Composition Indices and All-Cause Mortality in Older Japanese Adults. *J. Am. Med. Dir. Assoc.* **2020**, *21*, 726–733.e4. [CrossRef]
54. Tokarek, T.A.; Dziewierz, A.; Sorysz, D.; Bagienski, M.; Rzeszutko, Ł.; Krawczyk-Ożóg, A.; Kleczyński, P. The obesity paradox in patients undergoing transcatheter aortic valve implantation: Is there any effect of body mass index on survival? *Kardiol. Pol.* **2019**, *77*, 190–197. [CrossRef] [PubMed]
55. Keller, K.; Munzel, T.; Ostad, M.A. Sex-specific differences in mortality and the obesity paradox of patients with myocardial infarction ages > 70 y. *Nutrition* **2018**, *46*, 124–130. [CrossRef]
56. Lee, S.H.; Kim, D.H.; Park, J.H.; Kim, S.; Choi, M.; Kim, H.; Park, Y.G. Association between body mass index and mortality in the Korean elderly: A nationwide cohort study. *PLoS ONE* **2018**, *13*, e0207508. [CrossRef]
57. Cheng, F.W.; Gao, X.; Mitchell, D.C.; Wood, C.; Still, C.D.; Rolston, D.; Jensen, G.L. Body mass index and all-cause mortality among older adults. *Obesity* **2016**, *24*, 2232–2239. [CrossRef] [PubMed]
58. Calabia, J.; Arcos, E.; Carrero, J.J.; Comas, J.; Valles, M. Does the obesity survival paradox of dialysis patients differ with age? *Blood Purif.* **2015**, *39*, 193–199. [CrossRef] [PubMed]
59. Kim, N.H.; Lee, J.; Kim, T.J.; Kim, N.H.; Choi, K.M.; Baik, S.H.; Choi, D.S.; Pop-Busui, R.; Park, Y.; Kim, S.G. Body Mass Index and Mortality in the General Population and in Subjects with Chronic Disease in Korea: A Nationwide Cohort Study (2002–2010). *PLoS ONE* **2015**, *10*, e0139924. [CrossRef]
60. Kubota, Y.; Iso, H.; Tamakoshi, A.; Group, J.S. Association of Body Mass Index and Mortality in Japanese Diabetic Men and Women Based on Self-Reports: The Japan Collaborative Cohort (JACC) Study. *J. Epidemiol.* **2015**, *25*, 553–558. [CrossRef]
61. Shil Hong, E.; Khang, A.R.; Roh, E.; Jeong Ku, E.U.; An Kim, Y.E.; Min Kim, K.; Lim, S. Counterintuitive relationship between visceral fat and all-cause mortality in an elderly Asian population. *Obesity* **2015**, *23*, 220–227. [CrossRef]
62. Clark, D.O.; Gao, S.; Lane, K.A.; Callahan, C.M.; Baiyewu, O.; Ogunniyi, A.; Hendrie, H.C. Obesity and 10-year mortality in very old African Americans and Yoruba-Nigerians: Exploring the obesity paradox. *J. Gerontol. Biol. Sci. Med. Sci.* **2014**, *69*, 1162–1169. [CrossRef] [PubMed]
63. Murphy, R.A.; Reinders, I.; Garcia, M.E.; Eiriksdottir, G.; Launer, L.J.; Benediktsson, R.; Gudnason, V.; Jonsson, P.V.; Harris, T.B. Adipose tissue, muscle, and function: Potential mediators of associations between body weight and mortality in older adults with type 2 diabetes. *Diabetes Care* **2014**, *37*, 3213–3219. [CrossRef]
64. Yamauchi, Y.; Hasegawa, W.; Yasunaga, H.; Sunohara, M.; Jo, T.; Matsui, H.; Fushimi, K.; Takami, K.; Nagase, T. Paradoxical association between body mass index and in-hospital mortality in elderly patients with chronic obstructive pulmonary disease in Japan. *Int. J. Chronic Obstr. Pulm. Dis.* **2014**, *9*, 1337–1346. [CrossRef] [PubMed]
65. Tsai, A.C.; Hsiao, M.L. The association of body mass index (BMI) with all-cause mortality in older Taiwanese: Results of a national cohort study. *Arch Gerontol. Geriatr.* **2012**, *55*, 217–220. [CrossRef] [PubMed]
66. Lea, J.P.; Crenshaw, D.O.; Onufrak, S.J.; Newsome, B.B.; McClellan, W.M. Obesity, end-stage renal disease, and survival in an elderly cohort with cardiovascular disease. *Obesity* **2009**, *17*, 2216–2222. [CrossRef]
67. Grabowski, D.C.; Ellis, J.E. High body mass index does not predict mortality in older people: Analysis of the Longitudinal Study of Aging. *J. Am. Geriatr. Soc.* **2001**, *49*, 968–979. [CrossRef]
68. Kananen, L.; Eriksdotter, M.; Boström, A.; Kivipelto, M.; Annetorp, M.; Metzner, C.; Jerlardtz, V.B.; Engström, M.; Johnson, P.; Lundberg, L.; et al. Body mass index and Mini Nutritional Assessment-Short Form as predictors of in-geriatric hospital mortality in older adults with COVID-19. *Clin. Nutr.* **2022**, *41*, 2973–2979. [CrossRef]
69. Lai, C.C.; Wang, C.Y.; Wang, Y.H.; Hsueh, S.C.; Ko, W.C.; Hsueh, P.R. Global epidemiology of coronavirus disease 2019: Disease incidence, daily cumulative index, mortality, and their association with country healthcare resources and economic status. *Int. J. Antimicrob. Agents* **2020**, *55*, 105946. [CrossRef]

70. Yaffe, K.; Fox, P.; Newcomer, R.; Sands, L.; Lindquist, K.; Dane, K.; Covinsky, K.E. Patient and caregiver characteristics and nursing home placement in patients with dementia. *JAMA* **2002**, *287*, 2090–2097. [CrossRef]
71. Heymsfield, S.B.; Peterson, C.M.; Thomas, D.M.; Heo, M.; Schuna, J.M., Jr. Why are there race/ethnic differences in adult body mass index-adiposity relationships? A quantitative critical review. *Obes. Rev.* **2016**, *17*, 262–275. [CrossRef]
72. Jeong, S.M.; Lee, D.H.; Rezende, L.F.M.; Giovannucci, E.L. Different correlation of body mass index with body fatness and obesity-related biomarker according to age, sex and race-ethnicity. *Sci Rep.* **2023**, *13*, 3472. [CrossRef] [PubMed]
73. Coutinho, T.; Goel, K.; de Sá, D.C.; Kragelund, C.; Kanaya, A.M.; Zeller, M.; Park, J.-S.; Kober, L.; Torp-Pedersen, C.; Cottin, Y.; et al. Central obesity and survival in subjects with coronary artery disease: A systematic review of the literature and collaborative analysis with individual subject data. *J. Am. Coll. Cardiol.* **2011**, *57*, 1877–1886. [CrossRef] [PubMed]
74. de Koning, L.; Merchant, A.T.; Pogue, J.; Anand, S.S. Waist circumference and waist-to-hip ratio as predictors of cardiovascular events: Meta-regression analysis of prospective studies. *Eur. Heart J.* **2007**, *28*, 850–856. [CrossRef] [PubMed]
75. Okorodudu, D.O.; Jumean, M.F.; Montori, V.M.; Romero-Corral, A.; Somers, V.K.; Erwin, P.J.; Lopez-Jimenez, F. Diagnostic performance of body mass index to identify obesity as defined by body adiposity: A systematic review and meta-analysis. *Int. J. Obes.* **2010**, *34*, 791–799. [CrossRef]
76. Flegal, K.M.; Kit, B.K.; Orpana, H.; Graubard, B.I. Association of all-cause mortality with overweight and obesity using standard body mass index categories: A systematic review and meta-analysis. *JAMA* **2013**, *309*, 71–82. [CrossRef]
77. Gao, F.; Wang, Z.J.; Shen, H.; Yang, S.W.; Nie, B.; Zhou, Y.J. Impact of obesity on mortality in patients with diabetes: Meta-analysis of 20 studies including 250,016 patients. *J. Diabetes Investig.* **2018**, *9*, 44–54. [CrossRef]
78. Zhao, X.; Gang, X.; He, G.; Li, Z.; Lv, Y.; Han, Q.; Wang, G. Obesity Increases the Severity and Mortality of Influenza and COVID-19: A Systematic Review and Meta-Analysis. *Front. Endocrinol.* **2020**, *11*, 595109. [CrossRef]
79. Golabek, T.; Bukowczan, J.; Szopinski, T.; Chlosta, P.; Lipczynski, W.; Dobruch, J.; Borowka, A. Obesity and renal cancer incidence and mortality–a systematic review of prospective cohort studies. *Ann. Agric. Environ. Med.* **2016**, *23*, 37–43. [CrossRef]
80. Liu, X.; Ju, W.; Huo, C.; Zhang, S.; Wang, X.; Huang, K. Overweight and Obesity as Independent Factors for Increased Risk of Hepatocellular Cancer-Related Mortality: A Meta-Analysis. *J. Am. Coll. Nutr.* **2021**, *40*, 287–293. [CrossRef]
81. Tian, S.; Xu, Y. Association of sarcopenic obesity with the risk of all-cause mortality: A meta-analysis of prospective cohort studies. *Geriatr. Gerontol. Int.* **2016**, *16*, 155–166. [CrossRef]
82. Sousa-Santos, A.R.; Afonso, C.; Borges, N.; Santos, A.; Padrão, P.; Moreira, P.; Amaral, T.F. Sarcopenia and Undernutrition Among Portuguese Older Adults: Results from Nutrition UP 65 Study. *Food Nutr. Bull.* **2018**, *39*, 487–492. [CrossRef] [PubMed]
83. Cereda, E.; Pedrolli, C.; Klersy, C.; Bonardi, C.; Quarleri, L.; Cappello, S.; Caccialanza, R. Nutritional status in older persons according to healthcare setting: A systematic review and meta-analysis of prevalence data using MNA((R)). *Clin. Nutr.* **2016**, *35*, 1282–1290. [CrossRef] [PubMed]
84. Sousa-Santos, A.R.; Afonso, C.; Borges, N.; Santos, A.; Padrão, P.; Moreira, P.; Amaral, T.F. Sarcopenia, physical frailty, undernutrition and obesity cooccurrence among Portuguese community-dwelling older adults: Results from Nutrition UP 65 cross-sectional study. *BMJ Open* **2020**, *10*, e033661. [CrossRef] [PubMed]
85. Akinnusi, M.E.; Pineda, L.A.; El Solh, A.A. Effect of obesity on intensive care morbidity and mortality: A meta-analysis. *Crit. Care Med.* **2008**, *36*, 151–158. [CrossRef]
86. Donini, L.M.; Pinto, A.; Giusti, A.M.; Lenzi, A.; Poggiogalle, E. Obesity or BMI Paradox? Beneath the Tip of the Iceberg. *Front. Nutr.* **2020**, *7*, 53. [CrossRef]
87. Casas-Vara, A.; Santolaria, F.; Fernandez-Bereciartua, A.; Gonzalez-Reimers, E.; Garcia-Ochoa, A.; Martinez-Riera, A. The obesity paradox in elderly patients with heart failure: Analysis of nutritional status. *Nutrition* **2012**, *28*, 616–622. [CrossRef]

Disclaimer/Publisher's Note: The statements, opinions and data contained in all publications are solely those of the individual author(s) and contributor(s) and not of MDPI and/or the editor(s). MDPI and/or the editor(s) disclaim responsibility for any injury to people or property resulting from any ideas, methods, instructions or products referred to in the content.

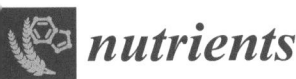

Article

Hypomagnesemia Is Associated with Excessive Daytime Sleepiness, but Not Insomnia, in Older Adults

Muhammed Tunc [1], Pinar Soysal [2,*], Ozge Pasin [3], Lee Smith [4], Masoud Rahmati [5], Veliye Yigitalp [2], Sevnaz Sahin [6] and Moustapha Dramé [7]

1. Division of Internal Medicine, Faculty of Medicine, Bezmialem Vakif University, Istanbul 34093, Türkiye; mtunc@bezmialem.edu.tr
2. Division of Geriatric Medicine, Faculty of Medicine, Bezmialem Vakif University, Istanbul 34093, Türkiye; yigitalpveliye@gmail.com
3. Division of Biostatistics, Faculty of Medicine, Bezmialem Vakif University, Istanbul 34093, Türkiye; ozgepasin90@yahoo.com.tr
4. Centre for Health, Performance, and Wellbeing, Anglia Ruskin University, Cambridge CB1 1PT, UK; lee.smith@aru.ac.uk
5. Division of Physical Education and Sport Sciences, Faculty of Literature and Human Sciences, Lorestan University, Khoramabad 68151-44316, Iran; rahmati.mas@lu.ac.ir
6. Division of Geriatrics, Department of Internal Medicine, Faculty of Medicine, Ege University, Izmir 35040, Türkiye; drsevnaz@gmail.com
7. Division of Clinical Research and Innovation, University Hospitals of Martinique, 97261 Fort-de-France, France; moustapha.drame@chu-martinique.fr
* Correspondence: dr.pinarsoysal@hotmail.com; Tel.: +90-212-4531700; Fax: +90-212-4531869

Abstract: The aim of this study was to investigate associations between serum magnesium levels with insomnia and excessive daytime sleepiness (EDS) in older adults. A total of 938 older outpatients were included in the study. Hypomagnesemia was defined as serum magnesium concentration below <1.6 mg/dL. Patients were divided into two groups: hypomagnesemia and normomagnesia (1.6–2.6 mg/dL). The Epworth Sleepiness Scale was implemented and scores of ≥ 11 points were categorized as EDS. The Insomnia Severity Index was implemented and scores of ≥ 8 indicated insomnia. The mean age was 81.1 ± 7.6 years. While the presence of EDS, hypertension, diabetes mellitus, and coronary artery disease were more common in the hypomagnesemia group than the normomagnesia group, Parkinson's disease was less common ($p < 0.05$). Hemoglobin and HDL cholesterol were lower, whereas HbA1c, triglyceride, and number of drugs used were higher in the hypomagnesemia group compared to the normomagnesia group ($p < 0.05$). In both univariate analysis and multivariate analysis adjusted for gender, age and all confounders, there were significant associations between hypomagnesemia and EDS [odds ratio (OR):1.7; 95% confidence interval (CI): 1.6–2.6, and OR: 1.9; 95%CI: 1.2–3.3, respectively ($p < 0.05$)]. There was no significant relationship between hypomagnesemia and insomnia ($p > 0.05$). The present study identified an association between hypomagnesemia and EDS in older adults. Therefore, it may be prudent to consider hypomagnesemia when evaluating older adults with EDS and vice versa.

Keywords: excessive daytime sleepiness; hypomagnesemia; insomnia; elderly

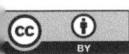

1. Introduction

Magnesium plays a role in the maintenance of vascular tone, thrombus formation, cardiac conduction, and neurotransmitter synthesis, as well as acting as a cofactor in many enzymatic reactions [1]. Hypomagnesemia, which is associated with chronic diseases, gastrointestinal system or renal loss, and low intake or alcohol use, is often neglected in clinical practice [1,2]. With aging, decreases in the total level of magnesium occur mainly owing to a decrease in oral magnesium intake as a result of consumption of less green vegetables, which are key sources of magnesium [3,4]. Decreased intestinal reabsorption of magnesium, increased urinary excretion, and drug interactions also contribute to magnesium deficiency in the geriatric population [2].

Magnesium is an essential element required for the regulation of various cellular and metabolic reactions, including ATP generation, DNA replication, and DNA repair. It is an important co-factor for the folate–methionine–neurotransmitter cycle; and thus, magnesium has a pivotal role in the neurotransmitter synthesis pathway [5]. The disruption of methylation processes leads to a build-up of homocysteine, thereby increasing the likelihood of inflammation, oxidative stress, and subsequent damage to mitochondria and DNA [6,7]. Additionally, telomeres are protective nucleoprotein structures at the ends of all chromosomes that provide genomic stability and prevent the loss of coding DNA, and impaired telomeric structure has a sensitivity to oxidative damage. The telomeric chromatin structure and integrity is impacted upon by magnesium biochemistry [8]. The effect of magnesium on cellular aging may be related to its interactions with telomere homeostasis, telomere maintenance, and activity of telomerase. A recent study showed that inadequate magnesium levels have an adverse impact on telomere attrition rate in older people with sleep disturbances [9]. Moreover, magnesium may also enhance melatonin secretion which promotes sleep onset [10]. Magnesium is important for the synthesis of N-acetyltransferase, which converts 5-hydroxytryptamine into N-acetyl-5-hydroxytryptamine, which can then be converted to melatonin [9]. Magnesium also contributes to the maintenance of a normal circadian rhythm and sleep quality and thus may reduce insomnia.

Findings from analyses of The National Health and Nutrition Examination's database have found that aging is a superposed risk factor for deficient magnesium consumption and that magnesium consumption has a progressive decrease with age [11]. Indeed, the literature has shown that intestinal magnesium absorption and bio-variability vary with age [12]. The change in intestinal absorption of magnesium in older people is usually exacerbated by the disruption of vitamin D homeostasis. Renal magnesium reabsorption is an active process that occurs in the loop of Henle and the proximal convoluted tubule. Decreased kidney functionality, which is also common in old age, is likely to be an additional cause of magnesium loss [12,13]. In epidemiological and clinical studies, magnesium deprivation has been associated with low serum magnesium levels. Moreover, low dietary magnesium intake has been found to be associated with low-grade systemic inflammation, increased levels of inflammatory markers, proinflammatory molecules, and increased production of free oxygen radicals [13]. Ageing is accompanied by a low-grade inflammatory condition called "inflammaging". A chronic magnesium deficiency and disruption of the redox state that expedites this inflammatory condition may have a significant impact on the development of age-related diseases and geriatric syndromes [2]. Moreover, magnesium acts as a crucial cofactor for both acquired and innate immune responses and is implicated in pathways that control the development and maintenance of immune cell activation and homeostasis [14]. There may be a relationship between magnesium deficiency and the condition of insulin resistance, T2DM, the emergence of the cardiometabolic syndrome, and prognosis of infectious clinical course [13]. Therefore, it can be hypothesized that maintaining an optimal magnesium balance throughout life may help prevent inflammation and related conditions associated with magnesium deficiency, thereby helping to prolong healthy life.

There are limited studies on the prevalence of hypomagnesemia in the elderly. However, a small number of studies have reported that the prevalence of hypomagnesemia is between 20–25% in the general population, and over 50% in hospitalized patients [15–17] Although hypomagnesemia is common, clinical symptoms or signs are often asymptomatic or are non-specific presentations, which can include fatigue, weakness, dizziness, depressive mood, anxiety, hyperemotionality, sleep disturbances, headache, myalgias, non-specific pain, and cramps. Severe hypomagnesemia can be more symptomatic, with presentations including muscle fasciculation, orthostatic hypotension, tremor, dysphagia, presence of Trousseau's sign and Chvostek's sign, and hypertension [18]. Chronic hypomagnesemia is often clinically undiagnosed, but it has many long-term negative outcomes [13]. It has been observed that hypomagnesemia is associated with an increased risk of delirium, geriatric depression, psychiatric disorders, Alzheimer's disease, other dementia, and mortality in the elderly [13,19].

One important implication of magnesium deficiency is subsequent sleep complications. Sleep disorders are a common health problem that negatively affect quality of life and functionality in older people [15]. Indeed, magnesium is considered to have important effects on sleep regulation and circadian rhythm as it is a natural antagonist of N-metil-D-aspartic acid (NMDA) receptors and an agonist of gamma-aminobutyric acid (GABA) receptors, as well as having important effects on the regulation of the central nervous system [20]. It is likely that magnesium acts as a relaxant and anti-depressant. Therefore, magnesium may increase melatonin and renin levels as well as reduce levels of cortisol [20]. Recent research has found that magnesium may play a crucial role in the regulation of cellular timekeeping, energy balance, and circadian rhythm, and consequently sleep regulation [20]. However, despite this, study findings on the relationship between magnesium levels and sleep quality or quantity are inconsistent. For example, in one study carried out on a sample of adults, dietary magnesium intake was found to be significantly higher in those with adequate sleep quality in comparison to those without [21]. In another study, it was observed that magnesium had no superiority on sleep quality over placebo [22]. Although magnesium supplements have been shown to have a positive effect on insomnia parameters such as sleep efficiency, sleep time and sleep onset latency, and early morning awakening in the elderly [23], to date, there is no study in which hypomagnesemia and insomnia and excessive daytime sleepiness (EDS), two common sleep disorders in the elderly, have been evaluated simultaneously.

Therefore, the aim of this study was to investigate whether there is a relationship between hypomagnesemia and insomnia or EDS in the elderly.

2. Materials and Methods

In the retrospective monocentric study, patients aged 60 years and older who applied to one University Hospital Geriatrics outpatient clinic in Türkiye between December 2018 and January 2023 were retrospectively screened. The patients were evaluated according to inclusion and exclusion criteria. The local Ethics in Research Committees of the institutes approved the study.

2.1. Inclusion Criteria

Accepting detailed geriatric evaluation: The patients who underwent insomnia severity index and Epworth Sleepiness Scale, and the patients whose file records were not incomplete and whose serum magnesium levels were checked on the same day, were included in our study. All patients who did not have an exclusion criterion were included in this study (Figure 1).

2.2. Exclusion Criteria

Those with moderate and severe dementia, those with severe visual or hearing impairment that prevented communication and understanding commands during the examination, those who refusde to participate in the examination, those who had a fatal illness, those who had a life-threatening illness in the last 6 months, or those who had been hospitalized for a major surgery were excluded from the present study. In addition, those who were determined to have an acute health problem (such as acute kidney failure, delirium, or stroke); those taking magnesium supplements or taking medications that may affect sleep, such as trazadone, mirtazapine, melatonin, antipsychotics, benzodiazepines, methylphenidate, and modafinil; and those with sleep disorders, such as sleep apnea syndrome, or central disorders of hypersomnolence, such as narcolepsy or restless leg syndrome, were also excluded. Those who were detected to have hypermagnesemia (≥ 2.6 mg/dL) according to serum magnesium values were also excluded [24].

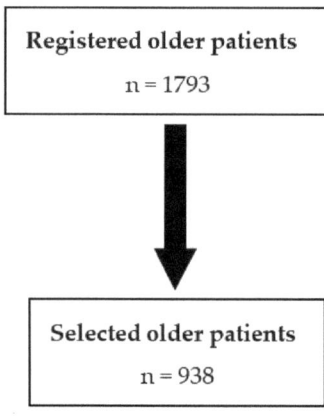

Figure 1. Study flow chart.

2.3. Compherensive Geriatric Assessment [14]

Patients were assessed by a geriatrician whereas study data were collected by a gerontologist. The following variables were reported: participant age in years, sex, education status, marital and living status, number of medications, and chronic comorbid diseases (hypertension, diabetes mellitus, chronic obstructive pulmonary disease, coronary artery disease, congestive heart disease, dementia, periferic artery disease, cerebrovascular event, Parkinson's disease, and osteoarthritis).

The Barthel Index (BADL) was used to evaluate the patients' basic activities of daily living, and the Lawton index was used to evaluate instrumental activities of daily living (IADL). BADL includes functional status and the level of independence in basic daily living activities for feeding, bathing, dressing, bowel or bladder control, using the toilet, transfers, mobility, and stair climbing. A total score of 100 indicates full independence, whereas a score of 0 shows dependency on another person. The IADL measures abilities, including food preparation, shopping, handling finances, the use of a telephone, taking own medication, laundry, transportation and housekeeping. A total score of 23 indicates complete independence, whereas a score of 0 shows complete dependency on another person for IADL [25].

Information on nocturia was collected and nocturia was defined by the International Continence Society [26]. "Overall, in the last 30 days, how many times have you usually urinated from going to bed to waking up in the morning?" Urination at least once a night was considered as nocturia. The mean number of nocturia episodes of the patients was recorded [26]. Urinary incontinence was considered to be present in the individuals who had involuntary urinary incontinence in the last 3 months, except in cases without urinary tract infection and similar temporary conditions. Depression was diagnosed using the Geriatric Depression Scale-15. A score of ≥ 5 on the Geriatric Depression Scale-15 was classified as depression [27].

2.4. Evaluation of Insomnia

The Insomnia Severity Index includes seven self-reported items. These items assess symptoms of insomnia as well as the daytime impact, and were designed in accordance with criteria from the Diagnostic and Statistical Manual of Mental Disorders, Fifth Edition. The Insomnia Severity Index scores range from 0 (no insomnia) to 28 (severe insomnia). The Insomnia Severity Index scores for the present study were categorised as follows: mild (14–19), moderate (20–26), and severe (22–28) [28].

2.5. Evaluation of Excessive Daytime Sleepiness

The Epworth Sleepiness Scale was employed to examine EDS. The Epworth Sleepiness Scale is composed of eight items and the participant self-reports responses on a 4-point Likert scale. The patient is asked to report the possibility of "napping" while watching television, lying down to rest, and traveling in a vehicle. Scores for each item range from 0 (no chance of napping) to 3 (high probability of napping). The total score for Epworth Sleepiness Scale is based on a scale of 0 to 24, with a score ≥ 11 indicating [29].

2.6. Laboratory Findings

The following laboratory assessments were carried out: biochemical, metabolic, and nutritional status of patients; complete blood count; kidney and liver function; thyroid-stimulating hormone; HbA1c; albumin; calcium; phosphorus; ferritin; vitamin B12; folate; and vitamin D (25-hydroxy D3). All the biochemical tests were analyzed by using the Diagnostic Modular Systems (Roche E170 and P-800) autoanalyzer.

2.7. Serum Magnesium Level

Hypomagnesemia with serum magnesium level below 1.6 mg/dL and those with 1.6–2.6 mg/dL were considered normomagnesemic [18]. If serum magnesisum level was >2.6, it was accepted as hypermagnesemia, and older patients with hypermagnesemia were excluded.

2.8. Statistical Analysis

Descriptive statistics of categorical variables were reported as frequencies and percentages, while descriptive statistics of quantitative variables were given as mean, median, standard deviation, minimum and maximum values. Pearson chi-square was used to compare group ratios of categorical variables. The conformity of quantitative variables to normal distribution was examined with the Kolmogorov–Smirnov test. The assumption of homogeneity of variances was tested with the Levene test. In the mean comparison of two independent groups, t-test (Student t) was used in independent groups. The Mann–Whitney U test was used for the median comparison of two independent groups. In order to examine the multivariate effects of variables on hypomagnesemia, the variables that were significant in univariate analyzes and considered to be clinically significant were added to the binary logistic regression model as independent variables, and odds ratio values were obtained. These variables were hypertension, diabetes mellitus, coronary artery disease, Parkinson's disease, hemoglobin, HDL cholesterol, HbA1c, triglyceride, and number of drugs used; 95% confidence intervals are given for odds ratio values. The Backward LR (likelihood ratio) method was used as a variable selection method in the model. Model explanatory power was examined with the Nagelkerke R square value, and the fit of the model was examined with the Hosmer and Lemeshow test. The statistical significance level was taken as 0.05 in the calculations and IBM SPSS Statistics for Windows, Version 26 (IBM Corp, Armonk, NY, USA) was used.

3. Results

A total of 938 older patients were included in the study. The mean age of the sample was 81.1 ± 7.6 years and 70.3% were female. The prevalence of hypomagnesemia, insomnia, and EDS was 14.3%, 54.1%, and 21.1%, respectively.

The comparison of the characteristics of the patients with hypomagnesemia and normomagnesemia is shown in Table 1. While the presence of EDS, hypertension, diabetes mellitus, and coronary artery disease was more common, Parkinson's disease was less common in the hypomagnesemia group than the normomagnesia group ($p < 0.05$). There was no difference in insomnia between the two groups ($p > 0.05$). Hemoglobin and HDL cholesterol were lower, whereas HbA1c, triglyceride, and number of drugs used were higher in the hypomagnesemia group compared to the normomagnesia group ($p < 0.05$) (Table 1).

Table 1. Characteristics of patients according to magnesium status.

	Hypomagnesemia	Normomagnesemia	p Value
Age, years	82.03 ± 7.42	80.96 ± 7.62	0.132 *
Female, (%)	73.9	69.8	0.359 **
Education, year	5 (0–28)	5 (0–24)	0.224 ***
Comorbidities (%)			
Hypertension	82.8	68.5	0.001 **
Diabetes Mellitus	68.7	32.7	0.001 **
Coronary Artery Disease	26.9	17.7	0.013 **
COPD	7.5	7.2	1.000 **
Cerebrovascular Events	11.9	10.4	0.650 **
Congestive Heart Disease	13.4	9.7	0.217 **
Peripheric Artery Disease	2.2	2.7	0.790 **
Parkinson's Disease	3.7	9.3	0.043 **
Dementia	22.4	28.1	0.175 **
Osteoarthritis	21.6	16.9	0.220 **
Laboratory Findings			
Hemoglobin, g/dL	12.04 ± 1.52	12.56 ± 1.69	<0.001 *
HbA1c, %	6.5 (4.79–11.64)	5.95 (4.30–14)	0.001 ***
Ferritin, ng/mL	55.91 (4.31–1146.43)	57.55 (2.18–1897.39)	0.349 ***
Folate, ng/mL	6.45 (1.70–24)	6.6 (1.8–24)	0.909 ***
Vitamin B12, ng/mL	382 (95–2000)	371 (83–2000)	0.127 ***
Vitamin D, ng/mL	25.65 (5.30–97.40)	22.30 (3.90–118.9)	0.273 ***
GFR, mL/min/1.73 m^2	60.64 ± 17.14	61.70 ± 18.96	0.524 *
Albumin, g/dL	4.2 (2.70–45)	4.3 (2.5–41.9)	0.486 ***
Triglycerides, mg/dL	137.5 (6–470)	120 (18–988)	0.034 ***
HDL cholesterol, mg/dL	12.04 ± 1.52	51.7 (17.9–102.7)	0.001 ***
LDL cholesterol mg/dL	6.5 (4.79–11.64)	128.1 (36.40–338)	0.134 ***
Calcium, mg/dL	55.91 (4.31–1146.43)	9.4 (7.6–12.6)	0.097 ***
Phosphorus, mg/dL	6.45 (1.70–24)	3.4 (1.5–8.7)	0.596 ***
TSH, mIU/L	382 (95–2000)	1.3 (0.01–26.15)	0.647 ***
Comprehensive geriatric assessment			
Urinary Incontinence, %	58.2	56.0	0.640 **
Nocturia episodes, number	2 (0–10)	2 (0–10)	0.101 ***
Number of drugs used	7 (0–15)	6 (0,25)	0.001 ***
Geriatric Depression Scale–15	4 (0–15)	4 (0–15)	0.382 ***
BADL	85 (0–100)	88 (0–100)	0.171 ***
IADL	13 (0–23)	14 (0–23)	0.101 ***
ISI	10 (0–28)	8 (0–28)	0.976 ***
Insomnia, %	56.7	53.6	0.514 **
Severe Insomnia, %	36.6	36.3	1.000 **
ESS	7 (0–24)	4 (0–24)	0.004 ***
EDS	%29.9	%19.7	0.009 **

BADL (Barthel Activities of Daily Living); COPD (Chronic obstructive pulmonary disease); EDS (Excessive Daytime Sleepiness); ESS (Epworth Sleepiness Scale); GFR (Glomerular filtration rate); HDL (High-Density Lipoprotein); IADL (Instrumental Activities of Daily Living); ISI (Insomnia Severity Index); LDL (Low-Density lipoprotein); TSH (Thyroid-stimulating hormone).* Student's *t*-test was used. Descriptive statistics were given as mean and standard deviation.** Pearson's chi square test was used.*** Mann–Whitney U test was used. Descriptive statistics were given as median (minimum–maximum).

In both univariate analysis and multivariate analysis adjusted for gender, age, and all confounders, there were significant associations between hypomagnesemia and EDS [odds ratio (OR):1.7, 95% confidence interval (CI):1.6–2.6, and OR:1.9, 95% CI:1.2–3.3, respectively ($p < 0.05$)] (Table 2). While there was a relationship between diabates mellitus and hypomagnesemia in both univariate and multivariate analysis, age was significant only in multivariate analysis ($p < 0.05$). There were no significant relationships between hypomagnesemia and insomnia ($p > 0.05$).

Table 2. Predictors of hypomagnesemia.

Parameters	Univariate Analysis		Multivariate Analysis	
	OR, %95 CI	p Value	OR, %95 CI	p Value
Age	1.02 (0.99–1.04)	0.132	1.051 (1.014–1.089)	0.007
Female	1.23 (0.81–1.85)	0.336		
HT	2.21 (1.38–3.56)	<0.001	1.91 (0.97–3.75)	0.062
DM	4.49 (3.03–6.66)	<0.001	4.87 (2.82–8.42)	<0.001
CAD	1.71 (1.12–2.61)	0.013		
PD	2.65 (1.05–6.59)	0.038	0.380 (0.128–1.135)	0.088
TG	1.00 (1.00–1.01)	0.042		
HDL	0.97 (0.95–0.98)	<0.001	0.982 (0.96–1.001)	0.066
HbA1c	1.44 (1.24–1.67)	<0.001		
Number of Drugs	1.12 (1.07–1.18)	<0.001		
Hemoglobin	0.83 (0.74–0.93)	<0.001		
Insomnia	1.13 (0.78–1.64)	0.504		
EDS	1.74 (1.16–2.62)	0.008	1.96 (1.15–3.33)	0.013

Binary logistic regression analysis was used. The variables that were statistically significant in univariate analysis were included in the multivariate analysis. The backward LR variable selection method was used, and the final results were given in multivariate analysis. CAD: Coronary Artery Disease; CI: Confidence Interval; DM: Diabetes Mellitus, EDS: Excessive Daytime Sleepiness; HDL: High-Density Lipoprotein; HT: Hypertension; PD: Parkinson's Disease; TG: Triglyceride. Nagelkerke R square value was obtained as 0.215. Hosmer and Lemeshow test p value was obtained as 0.250.

4. Discussion

In this study, the frequency of hypomagnesemia in the elderly patients admitted to the outpatient hospital was 14.3%, in whom the frequency of hypertension, diabetes mellitus, and coronary artery disease was higher compared to those with normomagnesemia, but the frequency of Parkinson's disease was lower. Triglyceride and HbA1c levels were higher, while hemoglobin and HDL levels were lower. In addition, drug use was higher in patients with hypomagnesemia. There was no relationship between insomnia and hypomagnesemia. EDS was present in one out of five older adults, the frequency of which was 1.9 times higher in those with hypomagnesemia than in those with normomagnesemia.

In our study, the prevalence of hypomagnesemia was 14.3%, which was lower than in other studies conducted in older people [15–17]. The possible reason for this may be that our study included older adults who were outpatients and were relatively healthy compared to those in other studies, and the cut-off values for hypomagnesemia somewhat differed between studies. For example, the prevalence was reported to be 24.3% in a study in which a value below 1.8 mg/dl was considered as hypomagnesemia and in hospitalized elderly people [15]. In another study using the same criteria for hypomagnesemia as the present study, but in medical settings including units such as geriatrics, oncology, and intensive care, the prevalence was 59.0% [17]. In the present study, frail patients such as moderate and advanced dementia patients were excluded, since ISI and ESS scales were required to be applied to the participants; this may account for the lower frequency of hypomagnesemia. In a similar study conducted in Türkiye where the same cut-off was used, but the mean age was 78 (81.1% in this study), hypomagnesemia was found to be 8.8% [30]. Magnesium intake, which may vary depending on geographical and ethnic differences, may also account for the differences in the prevalence of hypomagnesemia [31].

Magnesium is the second most important intracellular element after potassium in the cell. Magnesium activates more than 300 enzymes and is a co-factor of many enzymes, especially in carbohydrate metabolism [13]. For example, hypomagnesemia may cause insulin resistance by disrupting the function of the tyrosine kinase enzyme located in insulin receptors and increasing intracellular calcium, and, accordingly, disrupting blood sugar regulation and triggering oxidative stress [32,33]. Insulin resistance itself also leads to dyslipidemia; HDL decreases, while triglyceride increases [34]. In support of the previous literature, the present study identified a negative association between magnesium concentrations and HbA1c, which may be accounted for by decreased tubular reabsorption caused by hyperglycemia and/or hyperfiltration [33]. These above-mentioned mechanisms may explain why diabetes mellitus was higher, levels of HbA1c and triglycerides were higher, and HDL was lower in the hypomagnesemic elderly in our study. In addition, HT and CAD were also higher in those with hypomagnesemia. The reason for this may be that the positive effects of magnesium on endothelial function, regulation of vascular tone, regulation of catecholamine release, and renin angiotension aldosterone system are decreased in hypomagnesemics [32]. Another reason may be that the use of multiple drugs (for example, loop diuretics, thiazides, proton pump inhibitors, digoxin, some antidiabetics) may cause hypomagnesemia in patients with cardiovascular disease and diabetes mellitus [32,33,35]. According to our results, the number of drugs used in patients with hypomagnesemia was high. However, in our study, only the number of drugs was examined and individual drug groups could not be evaluated.

In this study, the main aim of which was to investigate the relationship between hypomagnesemia with insomnia and EDS, it was important to eliminate the influence of the factors mentioned above and other confounders, because factors such as diabetes mellitus, impaired blood sugar regulation, metabolic syndrome, CAD, multiple drug use, and anemia, which are excessive in hypomagnesemics, also affect sleep disorders [36,37]. Indeed, the present study demonstrated that hypomagnesemia was not associated with insomnia, but increased EDS by 1.9 times. However, results of studies investigating the effects of magnesium on sleep health (few of them carried out in the elderly) are conflicting [14]. For example, a cross-sectional study indicated that magnesium consumption was significantly higher in individuals with better sleep quality than in those with poor sleep quality [21]. In another cross-sectional study of 3304 female Japanese dietetics students aged 18–20 years, the midpoint of sleep was negatively associated with dietary magnesium intake [38]. However, the serum magnesium level of the participants in these two studies was not reported. This positive effect on sleep has not been demonstrated in randomized controlled trials. One study including 12 older adults (60 to 80 years) examined the relationship between oral magnesium supplementation and sleep. Magnesium was administered to the patients in 10 mmol doses and 20 mmol doses each for 3 days, and this was followed by 30 mmol doses for 2 weeks (i.e., 14 days). It was observed that wakefulness was reduced; however, this finding did not reach a level of significance [39]. Moreover, a recent crossover randomized double-blind placebo-controlled trial that included a total of 42 participants (average age 61.6 years) observed no effect on sleep disorders caused by nocturnal leg cramps when oral magnesium citrate was administered twice a day for one month [40]. In these studies, serum magnesium levels were evaluated neither at baseline nor after magnesium replacement. Therefore, it may have made no sense to replace magnesium in a normomagnesemic person initially. However, in a randomized controlled study conducted by Abbasi et al., they found that among the two groups in which there was no difference between serum magnesium levels at baseline, those who received magnesium replacement improved insomnia parameters in parallel with the increased serum magnesium level compared to placebo [23]. Nevertheless, it may be a limitation that EDS, which is one of the factors that frequently causes insomnia in the elderly, was not evaluated simultaneously in this study. In the present study, we showed that hypomagnesemia was associated with EDS rather than insomnia.

In a study similar to the present, Lai et al. showed that there was a negative correlation between serum magnesium levels and EDS in peritoneal dialysis patients; and in multivariate regression analysis, urinary magnesium was an independent predictor of EDS [41]. Previous evidence suggests that magnesium regulates sleep; because it acts as an NMDA and a GABA agonist, sleep architecture is closely associated with the glutamatergic and GABAergic system [20,39]. Indeed, the use of glutamatergic and GABAergic system modulators in the treatment of EDS has been of recent interest [42]. Moreover, healthy eating habits are impaired in the elderly with EDS, and thus those with EDS are at a higher risk of malnutrition [29]. Therefore, the elderly with EDS may have decreased magnesium intake and a higher frequency of hypomagnesemia. Additionally, EDS may lead to a reduction in leptin, an adiponectin that has been shown to decrease appetite. It is thus possible that there is a reduction in food intake owing to loss of appetite and skipped meals as a consequence of time asleep during the day; this may subsequently result in a higher risk of nutritional deficiencies [43]. Consequently, a bi-directional relationship between hypomagnesemia and EDS may occur. However, future studies are now required to test these hypotheses.

EDS, which is referred to as the condition of being sleepy during the day when an individual needs to be active and awake, is the second most common sleep disorder among sleep disorders, the importance of which has increased in recent years [44]. The decrease in the amplitude of the circadian rhythm with increasing age causes the frequency of night awakenings to increase [44]. Nonetheless, alterations in sleep physiology, such as decreased duration of slow-wave sleep (stages 3 and 4), increased compensatory stage 1 and 2 slow-wave sleep, and shortened rapid eye movement sleep, may give rise to EDS in older people [44]. For this reason, advancing age is a factor that increases the prevalence of EDS. Despite the fact that the prevalence of EDS between the ages of 30–60 is 11.0% in women and 6.7% in men, this rate increases in approximately 1 out of 3 people in both sexes over the age of 80 [45]. In our study, one out of every five elderly people was shown to have EDS and the rate was similar to the results of previous studies. The studies demonstrated that EDS was associated with adverse health conditions such as cognitive impairment, falls, sarcopenia, inability to perform activities of daily living, malnutrition, dysphagia, Vitamin D deficiency, depression, and cardiovascular events [29,46]. Even though EDS is associated with common and significant health problems, it is a condition that may be missed if it is not questioned in the evaluation of elderly patients in daily clinical practice. EDS is also common in neurodegenerative diseases, particularly dementia. Indeed, EDS is considered to be both an early indicator for future dementia and a risk factor. In our study, the determination of the relationship between hypomagnesemia and EDS suggests that magnesium replacement may also be beneficial in preventing negative health outcomes of EDS.

Findings from the present study must be interpreted in light of its limitations. First, the present study was cross-sectional in nature. Therefore, it is not known whether EDS leads to hypomagnesemia or vice versa. It is possible that the relationship is bidirectional. Second, self-reported scales were employed to assess EDS and insomnia, potentially introducing recall and social desirability bias into the findings; it would be prudent for future studies to employ objective measures of sleep, such as actigraphy. The strengths of our study are as follows: the number of adequate samples; evaluating both the presence of EDS and insomnia, and simultaneous evaluation of detailed comorbidities and comprehensive geriatric assessment parameters (e.g., nocturia, urinary incontinence, and functional status) which may affect sleep. To the best of the authors' knowledge, this is the first study to evaluate hypomagnesaemia and EDS and insomnia simultaneously in older adults.

5. Conclusions

Hypomagnesemia is associated with hypertension, diabetes mellitus, coronary artery disease, low hemoglobin, and HDL cholesterol; and high HbA1c, triglyceride, and number of drugs used. Regardless of these factors, there was a significant relationship between hypomagnesemia and EDS in the elderly, but not insomnia. Therefore, hypomagnesemia or vice versa should be considered when evaluating an elderly patient with EDS. However, further longitudinal studies and intervention trials are needed to elucidate the complex pathophysiology of EDS and hypomagnesemia in older adults.

Author Contributions: M.T. and P.S. designed the research; P.S. and V.Y. performed the experiment; O.P. analyzed the data; M.T., P.S., L.S. and M.R. wrote the paper; and S.S. and M.D. revised the manuscript. All authors have read and agreed to the published version of the manuscript.

Funding: This research received no external funding.

Institutional Review Board Statement: The local Ethics in Research Committees of the institutes approved the study. (Approval number:E-54022451-050.05.04-95076). The ethical approval date was 31 January 2023.

Informed Consent Statement: Not applicable.

Data Availability Statement: The data that support the findings of this research are available from the corresponding author upon reasonable request.

Conflicts of Interest: The authors declare no conflict of interest.

References

1. Morris, M.E. Brain and CSF magnesium concentrations during magnesium deficit in animals and humans: Neurological symptoms. *Magnes. Res.* **1992**, *5*, 303–313.
2. Barbagallo, M.; Belvedere, M.; Dominguez, L.J. Magnesium homeostasis and aging. *Magnes. Res.* **2009**, *22*, 235–246. [CrossRef]
3. Ford, E.S. Race, education and dietary cations: Findings form the Third National Health and Nutrition Examination Survey. *Ethn. Dis.* **1998**, *8*, 10–20. [PubMed]
4. Padro, L.; Benacer, R.; Foix, S.; Maestre, E.; Murillo, S.; Sanviçens, E.; Somoza, D.; Ngo, J.; Cervera, P. Assessment of dietary adequacy for an elderly population based on a Mediterranean model. *J. Nutr. Health Aging* **2002**, *6*, 31–33. [PubMed]
5. Killilea, D.W.; Ames, B.N. Magnesium deficiency accelerates cellular senescence in cultured human fibroblasts. *Proc. Natl. Acad. Sci. USA* **2008**, *15*, 5768–5773. [CrossRef] [PubMed]
6. Christensen, K.E.; Mirza, I.A.; Berghuis, A.M.; Mackenzie, R.E. Magnesium and phosphate ions enable NAD binding to methylenetetrahydrofolate dehydrogenase-methenyltetrahydrofolate cyclohydrolase. *J. Biol. Chem.* **2005**, *7*, 34316–34323. [CrossRef]
7. Botturi, A.; Ciappolino, V.; Delvecchio, G.; Boscutti, A.; Viscardi, B.; Brambilla, P. The Role and the Effect of Magnesium in Mental Disorders: A Systematic Review. *Nutrients* **2020**, *12*, 1661. [CrossRef]
8. Rowe, W.J. Correcting magnesium deficiencies may prolong life. *Clin. Interv. Aging* **2012**, *7*, 51–54. [CrossRef]
9. Dhillon, V.S.; Deo, P.; Thomas, P.; Fenech, M. Low Magnesium in Conjunction with High Homocysteine and Less Sleep Accelerates Telomere Attrition in Healthy Elderly Australian. *Int. J. Mol. Sci.* **2023**, *24*, 982. [CrossRef]
10. Peuhkuri, K.; Sihvola, N.; Korpela, R. Diet promotes sleep duration and quality. *Nutr. Res.* **2012**, *32*, 309–319. [CrossRef]
11. Ford, E.S.; Mokdad, A.H. Dietary magnesium intake in a national sample of US adults. *J. Nutr.* **2003**, *133*, 2879–2882. [CrossRef] [PubMed]
12. Coudray, C.; Feillet-Coudray, C.; Rambeau, M.; Tressol, J.C.; Gueux, E.; Mazur, A.; Rayssiguier, Y. The effect of aging on intestinal absorption and status of calcium, magnesium, zinc, and copper in rats: A stable isotope study. *J. Trace Elem. Med. Biol.* **2006**, *20*, 73–81. [CrossRef] [PubMed]
13. Barbagallo, M.; Veronese, N.; Dominguez, L.J. Magnesium in Aging, Health and Diseases. *Nutrients* **2021**, *13*, 463. [CrossRef] [PubMed]
14. Mazur, A.; Maier, J.A.; Rock, E.; Gueux, E.; Nowacki, W.; Rayssiguier, Y. Magnesium and the inflammatory response: Potential physiopathological implications. *Arch. Biochem. Biophys.* **2007**, *458*, 48–56. [CrossRef]
15. Boccardi, V.; Ercolani, S.; Serra, R.; Bubba, V.; Piccolo, A.; Scamosci, M.; Villa, A.; Ruggiero, C.; Mecocci, P. Hypomagnesemia and incident delirium in hospitalized older persons. *Aging Clin. Exp. Res.* **2023**, *35*, 847–853. [CrossRef]
16. Windsant-van den Tweel, A.V.; Annemieke, M.; Derijks, H.J.; Gadiot, N.P.P.M.; Keijsers, C.J.P.W. Proton Pump Inhibitors and Hypomagnesemia in Older Inpatients: An Observational Study. *Sr. Care Pharm.* **2022**, *37*, 623–630. [CrossRef]
17. Catalano, A.; Bellone, F.; Chilà, D.; Loddo, S.; Morabito, N.; Basile, G.; Benvenga, S.; Corica, F. Rates of hypomagnesemia and hypermagnesemia in medical settings. *Magnes. Res.* **2021**, *34*, 1–8. [CrossRef]

18. Flink, E.B. Magnesium deficiency. Etiology and clinical spectrum. *Acta Med. Scand. Suppl.* **1981**, *647*, 125–137. [CrossRef]
19. Wolf, F.; Hilewitz, A. Hypomagnesaemia in patients hospitalised in internal medicine is associated with increased mortality. *Int. J. Clin. Pract.* **2014**, *68*, 111–116. [CrossRef]
20. Arab, A.; Rafie, N.; Amani, R.; Shirani, F. The Role of Magnesium in Sleep Health: A Systematic Review of Available Literature. *Biol. Trace Elem. Res.* **2023**, *201*, 121–128. [CrossRef]
21. Cakir, B.; Kılınç, F.N.; Uyar, G.Ö.; Özenir, Ç.; Ekici, E.M.; Karaismailoğlu, E. The relationship between sleep duration, sleep quality and dietary intake in adults. *Sleep Biol. Rhythm.* **2020**, *18*, 49–57. [CrossRef]
22. Roguin Maor, N.; Alperin, M.; Shturman, E.; Khairaldeen, H.; Friedman, M.; Karkabi, K.; Milman, U. Effect of Magnesium Oxide Supplementation on Nocturnal Leg Cramps: A Randomized Clinical Trial. *JAMA Intern. Med.* **2017**, *177*, 617–623. [CrossRef] [PubMed]
23. Abbasi, B.; Kimiagar, M.; Sadeghniiat, K.; Shirazi, M.M.; Hedayati, M.; Rashidkhani, B. The effect of magnesium supplementation on primary insomnia in elderly: A double-blind placebo-controlled clinical trial. *J. Res. Med. Sci.* **2012**, *17*, 1161–1169. [PubMed]
24. Millart, H.; Durlach, V.; Durlach, J. Red blood cell magnesium concentrations: Analytical problems and significance. *Magnes. Res.* **1995**, *8*, 65–76.
25. Soysal, P.; Koc Okudur, S.; Uslu, F.; Smith, L. Functional loss and worsening geriatric assessment parameters are more common in dementia with Lewy bodies than Alzheimer's disease. *Psychogeriatrics* **2023**, *23*, 77–85. [CrossRef] [PubMed]
26. Dutoglu, E.; Soysal, P.; Smith, L.; Arik, F.; Kalan, U.; Kazancioglu, R.T.; Isik, A.T. Nocturia and its clinical implications in older women. *Arch. Gerontol. Geriatr.* **2019**, *85*, 103917. [CrossRef]
27. Ates Bulut, E.; Soysal, P.; Isik, A.T. Frequency and coincidence of geriatric syndromes according to age groups: Single-center experience in Turkey between 2013 and 2017. *Clin. Interv. Aging* **2018**, *13*, 1899–1905. [CrossRef]
28. Soysal, P.; Smith, L.; Dokuzlar, O.; Isik, A.T. Relationship between nutritional status and insomnia severity in older adults. *J. Am. Med. Dir. Assoc.* **2019**, *20*, 1593–1598. [CrossRef]
29. Koc Okudur, S.; Soysal, P. Excessive daytime sleepiness is associated with malnutrition, dysphagia, and vitamin D deficiency in older adults. *J. Am. Med. Dir. Assoc.* **2021**, *22*, 2134–2139. [CrossRef]
30. Heybeli, C.; Tan, S.G.; Kazancioglu, R.; Smith, L.; Soysal, P. Prevalence of Electrolyte Impairments among Outpatient Elderly Subjects. *Bezmialem Sci.* **2022**, *10*, 305–311. [CrossRef]
31. Jackson, S.E.; Smith, L.; Grabovac, I.; Haider, S.; Demurtas, J.; López-Sánchez, G.F.; Soysal, P.; Redsell, S.; Isik, A.T.; Yang, L. Ethnic Differences in Magnesium Intake in U.S. Older Adults: Findings from NHANES 2005–2016. *Nutrients* **2018**, *10*, 1901. [CrossRef] [PubMed]
32. Dominguez, L.; Veronese, N.; Barbagallo, M. Magnesium and Hypertension in Old Age. *Nutrients* **2020**, *13*, 139. [CrossRef] [PubMed]
33. Waanders, F.; Dullaart, R.P.F.; Vos, M.J.; Hendriks, S.H.; van Goor, H.; Bilo, H.J.G.; van Dijk, P.R. Hypomagnesaemia and its determinants in a contemporary primary care cohort of persons with type 2 diabetes. *Endocrine* **2020**, *67*, 80–86. [CrossRef]
34. Guerrero-Romero, F.; Rodríguez-Morán, M. Hypomagnesemia is linked to low serum HDL-cholesterol irrespective of serum glucose values. *J. Diabetes Complicat.* **2000**, *14*, 272–276. [CrossRef] [PubMed]
35. Chrysant, S.G.; Chrysant, G.S. Adverse cardiovascular and blood pressure effects of drug-induced hypomagnesemia. *Expert Opin. Drug Saf.* **2020**, *19*, 59–67. [CrossRef]
36. Tian, M.; Ma, H.; Shen, J.; Hu, T.; Cui, H.; Huangfu, N. Causal association between sleep traits and the risk of coronary artery disease in patients with diabetes. *Front. Cardiovasc. Med.* **2023**, *10*, 1132281. [CrossRef]
37. Kara, O.; Elibol, T.; Koc Okudur, S.; Smith, L.; Soysal, P. Associations between anemia and insomnia or excessive daytime sleepiness in older adults. *Acta Clin. Belg.* **2022**, *29*, 223–228. [CrossRef]
38. Sato-Mito, N.; Sasaki, S.; Murakami, K.; Okubo, H.; Takahashi, Y.; Shibata, S.; Yamada, K.; Sato, K. Freshmen in Dietetic Courses Study II group. The midpoint of sleep is associated with dietary intake and dietary behavior among young Japanese women. *Sleep Med.* **2011**, *12*, 289–294. [CrossRef]
39. Held, K.; Antonijevic, I.A.; Künzel, H.; Uhr, M.; Wetter, T.C.; Golly, I.C.; Steiger, A.; Murck, H. Oral Mg^{2+} supplementation reverses age-related neuroendocrine and sleep EEG changes in humans. *Pharmacopsychiatry* **2002**, *35*, 135–143. [CrossRef]
40. Frusso, R.; Zárate, M.; Augustovski, F.; Rubinstein, A. Magnesium for the treatment of nocturnal leg cramps: A crossover randomized trial. *J. Fam. Pract.* **1999**, *48*, 868–871.
41. Lai, X.; Chen, W.; Bian, X.; Wang, T.; Li, J.; Wang, H.; Guo, Z. Predictors of poor sleep quality and excessive daytime sleepiness in peritoneal dialysis patients. *Ren. Fail.* **2015**, *37*, 61–65. [CrossRef]
42. Pérez-Carbonell, L. Treatment of Excessive Daytime Sleepiness in Patients with Narcolepsy. *Curr. Treat. Options Neurol.* **2019**, *21*, 57. [CrossRef] [PubMed]
43. Mota, M.C.; Waterhouse, J.; De-Souza, D.A.; Rossato, L.T.; Silva, C.M.; Araújo, M.B.; Tufik, S.; de Mello, M.T.; Crispim, C.A. Sleep pattern is associated with adipokine levels and nutritional markers in resident physicians. *Chronobiol. Int.* **2014**, *31*, 1130–1138. [CrossRef] [PubMed]
44. Littner, M.R.; Kushida, C.; Wise, M.; Davila, D.G.; Morgenthaler, T.; Lee-Chiong, T.; Hirshkowitz, M.; Daniel, L.L.; Bailey, D.; Berry, R.B.; et al. Standards of Practice Committee of the American Academy of Sleep Medicine. Practice parameters for clinical use of the multiple sleep latency test and the maintenance of wakefulness test. *Sleep* **2005**, *28*, 113–121. [CrossRef]

45. Hayley, A.C.; Williams, L.J.; Kennedy, G.A.; Berk, M.; Brennan, S.L.; Pasco, J.A. Prevalence of excessive daytime sleepiness in a sample of the Australian adult population. *Sleep Med.* **2014**, *15*, 348–354. [CrossRef]
46. Soysal, P.; Smith, L.; Tan, S.G.; Capar, E.; Veronese, N.; Yang, L. Excessive daytime sleepiness is associated with an increased frequency of falls and sarcopenia. *Exp. Gerontol.* **2021**, *15*, 111364. [CrossRef] [PubMed]

Disclaimer/Publisher's Note: The statements, opinions and data contained in all publications are solely those of the individual author(s) and contributor(s) and not of MDPI and/or the editor(s). MDPI and/or the editor(s) disclaim responsibility for any injury to people or property resulting from any ideas, methods, instructions or products referred to in the content.

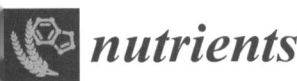

Article

Correlates of Undernutrition in Older People in Guadeloupe (French West Indies): Results from the KASADS Study

Nadine Simo-Tabue [1,*], Denis Boucaud-Maitre [2], Laurys Letchimy [1], Jeff Guilhem-Decleon [3], Jeannie Helene-Pelage [3], Guillaume T. Duval [4,5] and Maturin Tabue-Teguo [1,5,6,*]

1. Pôle Gériatrie-Gérontologie, CHU de Martinique, 97261 Fort-de-France, France; laurys.letchimy@chu-martinique.fr
2. Centre Hospitalier le Vinatier, 69500 Bron, France; denis.boucaud@gmail.com
3. Department of Geriatric Medicine, Angers University, CHU de Guadeloupe, 97110 Pointe-à-Pitre, France; jeff.gd@live.fr (J.G.-D.); jeannie.pelage@wanadoo.fr (J.H.-P.)
4. Department of Geriatric, FWI University, CHU d'Angers, 49100 Angers, France; guillaume.duval@chu-angers.fr
5. Equipe EpiCliV, Université des Antilles, 34095 Montpellier, France
6. Equipe ACTIVE, INSERM 1219, Université de Bordeaux, 33600 Pessac, France
* Correspondence: nadine_tabue@yahoo.fr (N.S.-T.); tabue.maturin@gmail.com (M.T.-T.)

Abstract: **Objectives**: This study aimed to determine the risk factors for undernutrition in community-dwelling older adults in Guadeloupe (Caribbean islands). **Methods**: We used data from the KArukera Study of Aging-Drugs Storage (KASADS), an observational cross-sectional study of community-dwelling older people living in Guadeloupe. The Mini Nutritional Assessment (MNA) was used to assess the risk of undernutrition. An MNA-short form (SF) score ≤11 defined the risk of undernutrition. Depression was assessed using the Center for Epidemiologic Studies Depression (CES-D) scale, cognitive function was assessed using the Mini Mental State Examination (MMSE), frailty was assessed using the Study of Osteoporotic Fractures index (SOF), and dependency was assessed using Lawton's instrumental activities of daily living (IADL) scale. Bivariate and multivariate analyses were used to determine the correlates of undernutrition. **Results**: The study sample comprised 115 patients aged 65 years or older; 67.8% were women, and the mean age was 76 ± 7.8 years. The prevalence of undernutrition was 21.7% (95% CI = 15.2–30.1%). In our bivariate analysis, the risk of undernutrition was associated with MMSE score, IADL score, frailty, and CES-D score. We found no significant relation between nutrition risk and other variables, such as marital status, pain, or polypharmacy. In the multivariate analysis, the factors associated with the risk of undernutrition were MMSE score (Odd-Ratio (OR): 0.74 (0.58–0.97)) and CES-D score (OR: 1.13 (1.02–1.27)). **Conclusions**: Cognitive decline and the risk of depression were independently associated with the risk of undernutrition in community-dwelling older people in Guadeloupe. Although we cannot imply causality in this relation, the detection of these three key geriatric syndromes in community-dwelling elders is essential to prevent adverse health outcomes. Further studies are warranted to confirm these findings.

Keywords: risk factors; undernutrition; aged; older adults; Guadeloupe

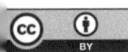

1. Introduction

Undernutrition is a frequent and serious geriatric syndrome that is a major contributor to vulnerability in older adults. Undernutrition is defined as a state resulting from deficiencies, excesses, or imbalances in a person's food intake and expenditure of energy and/or nutrients. It leads to a reduction in lean and cellular mass [1]. Undernutrition is multifactorial, and reported risk factors include social isolation, financial precariousness, psychological factors, and socio-demographic status, among others [2]. It is known to be associated with various clinical conditions such as low body mass index (BMI), infection, cancer, diabetes, renal function, acute kidney injury, pulmonary disease, gastrointestinal disorders, depression, cognitive or functional disorders, and comorbidities and polypharmacy [3]. Undernutrition is also associated with an increased risk of adverse health outcomes, including infection, impaired health-related quality of life (HRQoL), falls, longer length of stay when hospitalized, bedsores, and mortality [4,5]. The prevalence of undernutrition rises with increasing age [6], and in France, it ranges from 6.4% in rural areas to 18.5% in urban zones [4]. It is estimated that 32% of elderly people living at home suffer from malnutrition [6]. In France, new diagnostic criteria to measure undernutrition in the elderly were to be taken in consideration by the High Authority of Health and the French Nutrition Federation in 2019. In summary, to diagnose undernutrition, it is necessary to combine at least one phenotypic criterion (weight loss $\geq$ 5% in 1 month or $\geq$10% in 6 months or $\geq$10% compared with the usual weight before the onset of the disease; BMI < 22 kg/m^2; confirmed sarcopenia) and an etiological criterion (reduction in food intake $\geq$50% for more than 1 week or any reduction in intake for more than 2 weeks compared with usual food intake and/or protein-energy requirements; reduced absorption (malabsorption/maldigestion), as well as a pathological situation (with or without inflammatory syndrome). Despite the fact that MNA, as well as its short form, MNA-SF (a validated tool to estimate nutritional status), allows us to identify the risk of undernutrition, it is not considered as a criterion to diagnose undernutrition. The MNA-SF comprises six questions relating to nutritional, functional, and cognitive status. It is quick and easy to administer, and shows a strong correlation and good agreement with the full-length MNA in older adults. The MNA-SF accurately identifies people at risk of and suffering from undernutrition in the community [7]. As with the majority of geriatric syndromes, people with undernutrition do not always receive the attention of primary care healthcare providers [8]. However, since 2019, the World Health Organization program for integrated care for older people (ICOPE), which aims to promote primary prevention initiatives, has highlighted nutritional status as an intrinsic capacity that is necessary for successful ageing [9,10]. By 2030, the population of Guadeloupe (a French territory in the Caribbean) is expected to decline. This is due to an ageing population. The proportion of people over 65 years old could account for 28% of the total population (INSEE projections). At the same time, there will be a considerable increase (the double) in the number of dependent elderly people. Studies reveal that this part of the population will have to face age-related medical problems and an increase in the prevalence of chronic pathologies (hypertension, diabetes, cancer) or neuropsychiatric diseases. Other consequences will be a growing number of avoidable hospitalizations. On the other hand, the island of Guadeloupe faces numerous challenges. Some diseases are prevalent and above the national (France) level with regards to ethnic and genetic characteristics. There are also specific social and economic characteristics. In addition to this, the geographical location of the island in terms of access to care is also challenging. In the current context, the economic, medical, social, and human stakes are considerable, and the question that needs to be addressed is to what extent does living in Guadeloupe have an impact on the care of the elderly population [11,12]. It is of particular importance to identify the factors associated with undernutrition in this context, especially since certain modifiable risk factors are susceptible to influence by the geographic, psycho-socio-cultural, and ethno-anthropological environment. To the best of our knowledge, to date, no study has investigated the risk factors for undernutrition in older adults living in the Caribbean islands. The aim of this study was to identify the correlates of undernutrition in older people in Guadeloupe.

2. Methods
2.1. Study Design

This observational, cross-sectional study in Guadeloupe, a French overseas department situated in the Caribbean sea, used data from the Karukera Study Aging-Drug Storage (KASADS) [11]. In the KASADS cohort, the selected patients were contacted over the phone by two medical school students. The two interviewers were trained in standardized geriatric assessment tools (falls, dementia, depression, undernutrition, confusion, psychosocial vulnerabilities, etc.) by the geriatrics team at the CHU de Guadeloupe. A total of 15 GPs from the region took part in recruiting participants (i.e., a maximum of 10 patients per GP). GPs systematically offered patients who met the inclusion criteria a chance to participate in the study until our quota of 8 patients was reached. The two investigators acquired verbal consent from all participants. The investigators visited the participants' homes to collect the various parameters. Subjects who had not been correctly selected by the GPs were excluded upon home visitation.

All consenting participants received a study information leaflet explaining the study procedures, and all participants provided written informed consent.

The study was approved by the Ethics Committee of the University Hospital of Guadeloupe (A6_19_10_01_KASADS).

2.2. Data Recorded

The validated French-language version of the MNA-SF was used to assess the nutritional status of all patients [7]. Each participant was evaluated based on the following: food intake, weight loss, mobility, psychological stress or acute disease, neuropsychological problems (only dementia), and BMI. The final score was used to classify individuals as undernourished (0 to 7 points), at risk of undernutrition (8 to 11 points), or as having a normal nutritional status (13 to 14 points). For the purposes of this study, we considered all those with an MNA-SF score ≤ 11 to be at risk of undernutrition.

In the KASADS cohort, functional status was assess using Lawton's instrumental activities of daily living (IADLs) [13] and Katz's ADL scale [14]. Lawton's IADL scale measures four dimensions: using the telephone, using transport, managing medications, and managing finances. Scores range from 0 to 4; a score of 0 indicates total autonomy, while a score of 4 indicates total dependency. Katz's ADL scale measures 6 dimensions: bathing, toileting, transferring, eating, dressing, and continence. It appears that when there is an alteration of one or more ADLs, the elderly loses functional independence. The ADL provides a rating of each of the 6 items on a binary scale (0/1), with 1 indicating independence and 0 indicating dependency. The total score varies between 0 and 6. Cognitive function was assessed using the Mini Mental-State Examination [15]. This 30-item instrument evaluates cognitive function in terms of orientation, repetition, verbal recall, attention and calculation, language, and visual construction. Scores range from 0 to 30, and scores of 24/30 or lower indicate impaired cognitive function. Pain and HRQoL were evaluated using a visual analog scale (VAS). We also recorded socio-demographic characteristics (age, sex, level of education, marital status), usual alcohol intake (non-drinker, former drinker and current drinker) and tobacco consumption (non-smoker, former smoker current smoker), comorbidities (presence or absence of diabetes, hypertension, dyslipidemia), and BMI (calculated as the weight divided the square of the height in meters). We recorded all current medications, and polypharmacy was defined as the concomitant use of ≥ 5 different drugs per day [16].

Frailty syndrome was assessed using the Study of Osteoporotic Fractures index (SOF) [17], which comprises 3 items: involuntary weight loss of 5 kg or more, inability to rise from a chair 5 times without using the arms, and reduced energy level (answer "no" to the question "Do you feel full of energy?"). Meeting two or more criteria indicates frailty; 1/3 indicates pre-or-intermediate frailty; 0/3 indicates non-frail patients. Depression was evaluated using the Center for Epidemiologic Studies-Depression (CES-D) scale [18], which is a self-reported questionnaire comprising 20 items asking how often over the past week the person experienced symptoms associated with depression. Scores range from 0 to 60, with higher scores indicating greater depressive symptoms.

2.3. Statistical Analysis

Quantitative variables are expressed as mean ± standard deviation, and qualitative variables are expressed as either numbers or percentages. In our study population, no patient had an MNA-SF score <8, corresponding to undernutrition. Therefore, the variable MNA-SF was dichotomized, with individuals having a score > 11 considered not at risk and those with a score ≤ 11 considered at risk of undernutrition. Physical frailty (assessed by the SOF index scale) was studied by categorizing the SOF score into two groups: those with a score of 1 or 2 were considered frail, and those with a score of 0 were considered robust. Variables were compared between those at risk and those not at risk of undernutrition using the chi-square or Student's t-test as appropriate. Variables at a 20% threshold in the univariate analysis were considered in a multivariable analysis using logistic regression. At last, the relation between MNA-SF and other variables was investigated in a multivariable analysis using a logistic regression model to identify the factors independently associated with risk of undernutrition. We excluded BMI score, considering that BMI is already part of the MNA assessment scale. No imputation was used to account for missing data. A p-value of <0.05 was considered statistically significant. All analyses were performed with RStudio software (v.3.0.2. 21).

3. Results

The study sample comprised 115 community-dwelling individuals aged 65 and older. The mean age of the participants was 76.0 ± 7.8 years; the mean BMI was 26.8 ± 5.3, and 67.8% were women. In total, 43.5% had diabetes, 87.0% had hypertension, 45.2% had dyslipidemia, and 21.7% (25/115 participants) were at risk of undernutrition. The mean HRQoL score was 66.2 ± 20.3, and for pain, the score was 51.6 ± 21.7. The mean IADL score was 3.4 ± 1.0, and the mean ADL score was 5.79 ± 0.83 (Table 1).

Table 1. Comparison of population characteristics according to risk of undernutrition.

	Total Sample n = 115	MNA-SF ≤ 11 (n = 25)	MNA-SF > 11 (n = 90)	p
Age, years—mean (±SD)	76.0 (±7.8)	78.9 ± 8.5	75.2 ± 7.5	0.040
Men	37 (32.2%)	8 (32.0%)	29 (32.2%)	0.983
BMI, Kg/m² —mean (±SD)	26.8 (±5.3)	22.3 ± 3.9	28.0 ± 5.1	<0.001
No diploma	39 (33.9%)	10 (40.0%)	29 (32.2%)	0.467
Lives alone	67 (58.3%)	16 (64.0%)	51 (56.7%)	0.511
Diabetes	50 (43.5%)	7 (28.0%)	43 (47.8%)	0.078
Hypertension	100 (87.0%)	23 (92.0%)	77 (85.6%)	0.397
Dyslipidemia	52 (45.2%)	10 (40.0%)	42 (46.7%)	0.553
Tobacco consumption	8 (7.0%)	1 (4.0%)	7 (7.8%)	0.511
Alcohol consumption	16 (13.9%)	1 (4.0%)	15 (16.7%)	0.105
Polypharmacy	72 (62.6%)	14 (56.0%)	58 (64.4%)	0.440
HRQoL/100—mean (±SD)	66.2 (±20.3)	61.8 ± 20.2	67.5 ± 20.3	0.217
Pain/100—mean (±SD)	51.6 (±21.7)	57.2 ± 27.6	50.0 ± 19.6	0.142
IADL/4—mean (±SD)	3.4 (±1.0)	2.8 ± 1.4	3.6 ± 0.8	<0.001
Frailty (SOF index)	35 (30.4%)	12 (48.0%)	23 (25.6%)	0.031
MMSE—mean (±SD)	23.7 (±3.6)	22.2 ± 3.8	24.1 ± 3.4	0.015
CES-D—mean (±SD)	9.2 (±7.0)	13.8 ± 7.9	7.9 ± 6.1	<0.001

SD: Standard deviation; BMI: Body Mass Index; HRQoL: Health-Related Quality of Life; IADL: Instrumental Activities of Daily Living; SOF, Study of Osteoporotic Fractures Index; MMSE: Mini Mental State Examination; MNA-SF: Mini Nutritional Assessment Short Form; CES-D: Center for Epidemiologic Studies Depression Scale.

Table 1 presents the population characteristics according to nutritional status. On average, individuals at risk of undernutrition were older and more dependent. They were also more frequently pre-frail or frail compared to those with normal nutritional status (48.0% vs. 25.6%, respectively; p = 0.031). In bivariate analysis, those at risk of undernutrition more frequently were considered to be in cognitive decline (MMSE score 22.2 ± 3.8 vs. 24.1 ± 3.4; p = 0.015), have a higher CES-D score (13.8 ± 7.9 vs. 7.9 ± 6.1; p < 0.001), a lower BMI (22.3± 3.9 vs. 28.0 ± 5.1), and a lower IADL score (2.8 ± 1.4 vs. 3.6 ± 0.8). No significant relation was observed between the risk of undernutrition and the other variables, such as marital status, alcohol and tobacco consumption, pain, or polypharmacy. Table 2 shows the factors found to be significantly associated with the risk of undernutrition by multivariate analysis. The risk of undernutrition was associated with a low MMSE ($p = 0.015$) and CES-D score ($p = 0.020$). No significant association between age, IADL score, pain, physical frailty, alcohol consumption, and risk of undernutrition was found. We also did not observe any significant interaction effect between cognitive impairment and depressive symptoms on the risk of undernutrition ($p = 0.741$).

Table 2. Factors associated with the risk of undernutrition by multivariate logistic regression.

Variable	Estimate	p	OR (95%CI)
Age	0.04	0.467	-
MMSE score	−0.29	0.015	0.74 (0.58–0.97)
Pain score	0.03	0.061	1.03 (1.00–1.06)
IADL score	0.43	0.313	-
Frailty (=yes)	0.03	0.808	-
CES-D score (depression)	0.13	0.020	1.13 (1.02–1.27)
Alcohol consumption (=yes)	−0.96	0.431	-

OR: odds ratio; IADL: Instrumental Activities of Daily Living; MMSE: Mini Mental State Examination; CES-D: Center for Epidemiologic Studies Depression Scale.

4. Discussion

In this study, cognitive decline assessed using the MMSE score and depressive symptoms (using the CES-D score) were both associated with an increased risk of undernutrition among community-dwellers aged 65 years and over in Guadeloupe. Our results are consistent with the data found in the literature on this subject. Different studies have already shown a correlation between cognitive impairment and risk of undernutrition. A study by an Italian pharmacovigilance group (Agencia Italiana del ARmaco) showed an association between cognitive disorders and certain markers of malnutrition, such as albuminemia and low BMI. In a prospective study with 32 years of follow-up, Stewart et al. reported that weight loss in participants preceded the onset of mild cognitive decline in the diagnostic trajectory of dementia [19–21]. This involuntary weight loss could be associated with both a loss of muscle mass and a loss of muscle strength, characteristics of sarcopenia, which seems to be more frequent in the elderly [22]. Several hypotheses have been proposed to explain undernutrition in people with cognitive disorders, particularly in people with Alzheimer's disease [20]. Old people who suffer from cognitive decline have difficulty eating, shopping, or preparing meals. Atrophy of the mesial temporal cortex can lead to a loss of appetite [23]. Finally, other neurobiological factors have also been mentioned, such as a decrease in demanding hormones, such as neuropeptide Y or norepinephrine [24,25]. In our study, we also observed an association between depressive symptoms and undernutrition. This has also previously been described in studies performed in various contexts [26–29]. Weight loss, which is a contributing factor to MNA score, is listed as a possible symptom of depression in the Diagnostic and Statistical Manual of Mental Disorders 5th edition (DSM-5), apart from when it is attributable to a general condition. The possible explanations for this relate to the symptomatology of depression, which includes loss of appetite, general asthenia, and a loss of interest or pleasure in daily activities. However, a bi-directional relationship was also suggested by Lee et al. [26], whereby diseases that led to undernutrition could also be the cause of depressive symptoms. Depression is also thought to induce neuroendocrine modifications that disturb the regulation of food intake [29,30]. We observed a borderline significant link between pain and undernutrition ($p = 0.06$). Findings reported in the literature are conflicting with regard to this relationship, with some studies reporting that pain is a risk factor for undernutrition; however, few studies have specifically investigated this point. One Austrian study reported a link between severe pain and malnutrition risk in hospitalized patients [31]. Other studies have suggested a link between the intensity of pain and perceived alterations in appetite while accounting for Geriatric Depression Scale score, the number of painkillers one takes, and opioid use [32]. It has also been pointed out that side effects of painkillers, especially opiates, include reduced appetite, nausea, vomiting, or constipation [33]. Several elements could explain the lack of a statistically significant association in our study, notably the profile of the study population and the tools used to evaluate pain (a VAS) and depression (the CES-D instrument). Our data preclude any identification of the etiology or type of pain, which are key pieces of information guiding pain management. For example, cancer-related pain can be accompanied by hypercatabolism, which alone could account for undernutrition, whereas neuropathic pain or pain related to arthritis cannot. In our study, marital status was not found to be associated with nutritional status, although a meta-analysis published in 2020 including 16 cross-sectional studies showed an increased risk of malnutrition in those who were single, widowed, or divorced [2]. This could be due to a loss of pleasure in eating or poor dietary habits. A further explanation proposed was the lack of cooking experience in this generation of older men when they found themselves alone and having to cook for themselves. Given the lack of a statistical reason, there may be a cultural explanation for our findings. Indeed, the majority of studies to date that have reported a link between malnutrition and marital status were performed in western countries with populations who differed compared with ours, notably in terms of a culture of family solidarity and intergenerational interactions [12]. No link between nutritional status and polypharmacy was observed in our study. Again, the literature is discordant on this point. A meta-analysis of six longitudinal studies by Streicher et al. found no association with polypharmacy [34], while Zadak et al. underlined the difficulty of identifying a clear relationship between these two syndromes due to the abundance of confounding factors [35]. The lack of a significant relation in our study could be due to the different measurements used compared to other studies investigating polypharmacy and nutritional status. Indeed, contrary to other studies, we considered polypharmacy as the concomitant use of 5 or more drugs per day, whereas other studies considered hyper-polypharmacy, with a threshold at 10 drugs per day. In our study, alcohol consumption was also not found to be associated with nutritional status, which, although seemingly counter-intuitive, is congruent with previous reports. It is known that alcohol use can lead to deficiencies in micronutrients [36], but a risk of protein-energy malnutrition in older individuals has not been clearly described. In their review of the literature, van der Pols-Vijlbrief et al. included 28 observational studies of the risk factors for malnutrition, and no effect of alcohol was reported [37]. The proposed explanations include malabsorption, prolonged periods of fasting during hospitalization for complications of cirrhosis, and iatrogenic causes [36]. However, in our population, the majority of alcohol users reported only moderate consumption (one glass per day, with only three participants reporting an intake of more than three glasses of alcohol daily). Therefore, it is possible that only a very minute proportion would reach the stage of advanced liver disease. We could also hypothesize that, given the high average age of the patients in our study, any severe and chronic alcoholics would already have died since their life expectancy is shorter, leading to a potential survival bias [38].

Our results provide a good opportunity to underline the utility of performing systematic evaluations of depression risk and cognitive function during home visits and primary care consultations, either by GPs or nurses. Both depression and cognition can have a deleterious influence on nutritional status; therefore, early management is essential, especially considering that both are often underdiagnosed in older adults. In view of our findings and literature data, the MNA-SF scale appears to be an effective, user-friendly tool that would be easy to implement in routine practice. Furthermore, early intervention for depression or cognitive decline in older individuals before they begin to affect nutrition is an objective that is closely aligned with the practice and goals of GPs in primary care.

Our study has some limitations. The study design precluded the identification of any causal relationship between the risk of undernutrition on the one hand and depression or cognitive decline on the other hand. The few patients at risk of undernutrition limits the statistical power of the analyses. Nevertheless, despite a relatively small sample size (n = 115), the participants were representative of the general population of older individuals in the region in terms of comorbidities. Also, the MNA-SF is an instrument designed to capture the multidimensional nature of undernutrition. Our results are concordant with strategies designed to promote healthy nutritional status in older people, a key challenge and goal for GPs.

5. Conclusions

In this study of 115 community-dwelling individuals aged 65 years and older in Guadeloupe, we found that cognitive decline and depression were independently associated with the risk of undernutrition. Although our study design precludes concluding a causal relation, the detection of these three geriatric syndromes in older community-dwelling individuals is crucial for the prevention of adverse health outcomes. Further studies are required to confirm and expand on these findings.

Author Contributions: N.S.-T. and M.T.-T. designed the study. J.G.-D. and N.S.-T. collected the data. D.B.-M. and M.T.-T. developed the data analysis strategy. D.B.-M. analyzed the data. D.B.-M., M.T.-T., N.S.-T., G.T.D., L.L. and J.H.-P. interpreted the results and drafted the manuscript. All authors have read and agreed to the published version of the manuscript.

Funding: This research received no external funding.

Institutional Review Board Statement: All participants provided informed consent at baseline. The study was approved by the Ethics Committee of the University Hospital of Guadeloupe (Ref: A6_19_10_01_KASADS).

Informed Consent Statement: All authors discussed the findings and approved the final version of the manuscript.

Data Availability Statement: The datasets used and/or analyzed during the current study are available from the corresponding author upon reasonable request.

Acknowledgments: We would like to thank the Conseil Départemental de la Guadeloupe, ARS Guadeloupe and Saint Martin and Saint Barthelemy for their support.

Conflicts of Interest: The authors declare no conflict of interest.

References

1. Delarue, J.; Guillerme, S. Definition, epidemiology and prognosis of undernutrition in adults. *Rev. Prat.* **2022**, *72*, 850–857. [PubMed]
2. Besora-Moreno, M.; Llauradó, E.; Tarro, L.; Solà, R. Social and Economic Factors and Malnutrition or the Risk of Malnutrition in the Elderly: A Systematic Review and Meta-Analysis of Observational Studies. *Nutrients* **2020**, *12*, 737. [CrossRef] [PubMed]
3. Drevet, S.; Gavazzi, G. Undernutrition of the elderly. *Rev. Med. Interne* **2019**, *40*, 664–669. [CrossRef] [PubMed]
4. Torres, M.J.; Dorigny, B.; Kuhn, M.; Berr, C.; Barberger-Gateau, P.; Letenneur, L. Nutritional Status in Community-Dwelling Elderly in France in Urban and Rural Areas. *PLoS ONE* **2014**, *9*, e105137. [CrossRef] [PubMed]
5. Derbie, L.; Oumer, A.; Ayele, K.; Berhane, A. Determinants of Nutritional Status among Old Age Population in Eastern Ethiopia: A General Linear Model Approach. *J. Nutr. Sci.* **2022**, *11*, e70. [CrossRef]
6. Ferede, Y.M.; Derso, T.; Sisay, M. Prevalence of Malnutrition and Associated Factors among Older Adults from Urban and Rural Residences of Metu District, Southwest Ethiopia. *BMC Nutr.* **2022**, *8*, 52. [CrossRef]
7. Lilamand, M.; Kelaiditi, E.; Cesari, M.; Raynaud-Simon, A.; Ghisolfi, A.; Guyonnet, S.; Vellas, B.; van Kan, G.A.; Toulouse Frailty Platform Team. Validation of the Mini Nutritional Assessment-Short Form in a Population of Frail Elders without Disability. Analysis of the Toulouse Frailty Platform Population in 2013. *J. Nutr. Health Aging* **2015**, *19*, 570–574. [CrossRef]
8. Tabue-Teguo, M.; Grasset, L.; Avila-Funes, J.A.; Genuer, R.; Proust-Lima, C.; Péres, K.; Féart, C.; Amieva, H.; Harmand, M.G.-C.; Helmer, C.; et al. Prevalence and Co-Occurrence of Geriatric Syndromes in People Aged 75 Years and Older in France: Results From the Bordeaux Three-City Study. *J. Gerontol. A Biol. Sci. Med. Sci.* **2017**, *73*, 109–116. [CrossRef]
9. Cesari, M.; Sumi, Y.; Han, Z.A.; Perracini, M.; Jang, H.; Briggs, A.; Thiyagarajan, J.A.; Sadana, R.; Banerjee, A. Implementing Care for Healthy Ageing. *BMJ Glob. Health* **2022**, *7*, e007778. [CrossRef]
10. Sum, G.; Lau, L.K.; Jabbar, K.A.; Lun, P.; George, P.P.; Munro, Y.L.; Ding, Y.Y. The World Health Organization (WHO) Integrated Care for Older People (ICOPE) Framework: A Narrative Review on Its Adoption Worldwide and Lessons Learnt. *Int. J. Environ. Res. Public Health* **2022**, *20*, 154. [CrossRef]

11. Simo, N.; Boucaud-Maitre, D.; Gebhard, P.; Villeneuve, R.; Rinaldo, L.; Dartigues, J.-F.; Drame, M.; Tabue-Teguo, M. Correlates of Health-Related Quality of Life in Community-Dwelling Older Adults in Guadeloupe (French West Indies): Results from the KASADS Study. *Int. J. Environ. Res. Public Health* **2023**, *20*, 3004. [CrossRef]
12. Tabue-Teguo, M.; Simo, N.; Lorenzo, N.; Rinaldo, L.; Cesari, M. Frailty Syndrome among Elderly in Caribbean Region. *J. Am. Med. Dir. Assoc.* **2017**, *18*, 547–548. [CrossRef]
13. Lawton, M.P.; Brody, E.M. Assessment of Older People: Self-Maintaining and Instrumental Activities of Daily Living. *Gerontologist* **1969**, *9*, 179–186. [CrossRef]
14. Katz, S.; Ford, A.B.; Moskowitz, R.W.; Jackson, B.A.; Jaffe, M.W. Studies of illness in the aged. The index of ADL: A standardized measure of biological and psychosocial function. *JAMA* **1963**, *185*, 914–919. [CrossRef] [PubMed]
15. Folstein, M.F.; Folstein, S.E.; McHugh, P.R. "Mini-Mental State". A Practical Method for Grading the Cognitive State of Patients for the Clinician. *J. Psychiatr. Res.* **1975**, *12*, 189–198. [CrossRef]
16. Gnjidic, D.; Hilmer, S.N.; Blyth, F.M.; Naganathan, V.; Waite, L.; Seibel, M.J.; McLachlan, A.J.; Cumming, R.G.; Handelsman, D.J.; Le Couteur, D.G. Polypharmacy Cutoff and Outcomes: Five or More Medicines Were Used to Identify Community-Dwelling Older Men at Risk of Different Adverse Outcomes. *J. Clin. Epidemiol.* **2012**, *65*, 989–995. [CrossRef] [PubMed]
17. Ensrud, K.E.; Ewing, S.K.; Taylor, B.C.; Fink, H.A.; Cawthon, P.M.; Stone, K.L.; Hillier, T.A.; Cauley, J.A.; Hochberg, M.C.; Rodondi, N.; et al. Comparison of 2 Frailty Indexes for Prediction of Falls, Disability, Fractures, and Death in Older Women. *Arch. Intern. Med.* **2008**, *168*, 382–389. [CrossRef] [PubMed]
18. Radloff, L.S. The CES-D Scale: A Self-Report Depression Scale for Research in the General Population. *Appl. Psychol. Meas.* **1977**, *1*, 385–401. [CrossRef]
19. Stewart, R.; Masaki, K.; Xue, Q.-L.; Peila, R.; Petrovitch, H.; White, L.R.; Launer, L.J. A 32-Year Prospective Study of Change in Body Weight and Incident Dementia: The Honolulu-Asia Aging Study. *Arch. Neurol.* **2005**, *62*, 55–60. [CrossRef]
20. Gillette Guyonnet, S.; Abellan Van Kan, G.; Andrieu, S.; Barberger Gateau, P.; Berr, C.; Bonnefoy, M.; Dartigues, J.F.; de Groot, L.; Ferry, M.; Galan, P.; et al. IANA Task Force on Nutrition and Cognitive Decline with Aging. *J. Nutr. Health Aging* **2007**, *11*, 132–152.
21. Gillette-Guyonnet, S.; Lauque, S.; Ousset, P.-J. Nutrition and Alzheimer's disease. *Psychol. Neuropsychiatr. Vieil.* **2005**, *3* (Suppl. 1), S35–S41. [PubMed]
22. Tan, V.M.H.; Pang, B.W.J.; Lau, L.K.; Jabbar, K.A.; Seah, W.T.; Chen, K.K.; Ng, T.P.; Wee, S.-L. Malnutrition and Sarcopenia in Community-Dwelling Adults in Singapore: Yishun Health Study. *J. Nutr. Health Aging* **2021**, *25*, 374–381. [CrossRef] [PubMed]
23. Grundman, M.; Corey-Bloom, J.; Jernigan, T.; Archibald, S.; Thal, L.J. Low Body Weight in Alzheimer's Disease Is Associated with Mesial Temporal Cortex Atrophy. *Neurology* **1996**, *46*, 1585–1591. [CrossRef] [PubMed]
24. Smitka, K.; Papezova, H.; Vondra, K.; Hill, M.; Hainer, V.; Nedvidkova, J. The Role of "Mixed" Orexigenic and Anorexigenic Signals and Autoantibodies Reacting with Appetite-Regulating Neuropeptides and Peptides of the Adipose Tissue-Gut-Brain Axis: Relevance to Food Intake and Nutritional Status in Patients with Anorexia Nervosa and Bulimia Nervosa. *Int. J. Endocrinol.* **2013**, *2013*, 483145. [CrossRef] [PubMed]
25. Wham, C.A.; McLean, C.; Teh, R.; Moyes, S.; Peri, K.; Kerse, N. The BRIGHT Trial: What Are the Factors Associated with Nutrition Risk? *J. Nutr. Health Aging* **2014**, *18*, 692–697. [CrossRef]
26. Lee, J.-H.; Park, S.K.; Ryoo, J.-H.; Oh, C.-M.; Choi, J.-M.; McIntyre, R.S.; Mansur, R.B.; Kim, H.; Hales, S.; Jung, J.Y. U-Shaped Relationship between Depression and Body Mass Index in the Korean Adults. *Eur. Psychiatry J. Assoc. Eur. Psychiatr.* **2017**, *45*, 72–80. [CrossRef]
27. Pérez Cruz, E.; Lizárraga Sánchez, D.C.; Martínez Esteves, M.D.R. Association between malnutrition and depression in elderly. *Nutr. Hosp.* **2014**, *29*, 901–906. [CrossRef]
28. van Bokhorst-de van der Schueren, M.A.E.; Lonterman-Monasch, S.; de Vries, O.J.; Danner, S.A.; Kramer, M.H.H.; Muller, M. Prevalence and Determinants for Malnutrition in Geriatric Outpatients. *Clin. Nutr. Edinb. Scotl.* **2013**, *32*, 1007–1011. [CrossRef]
29. Ghimire, S.; Baral, B.K.; Pokhrel, B.R.; Pokhrel, A.; Acharya, A.; Amatya, D.; Amatya, P.; Mishra, S.R. Depression, Malnutrition, and Health-Related Quality of Life among Nepali Older Patients. *BMC Geriatr.* **2018**, *18*, 191. [CrossRef]
30. Grippo, A.J.; Cushing, B.S.; Carter, C.S. Depression-like Behavior and Stressor-Induced Neuroendocrine Activation in Female Prairie Voles Exposed to Chronic Social Isolation. *Psychosom. Med.* **2007**, *69*, 149–157. [CrossRef]
31. Bauer, S.; Hödl, M.; Eglseer, D. Association between Malnutrition Risk and Pain in Older Hospital Patients. *Scand. J. Caring Sci.* **2021**, *35*, 945–951. [CrossRef]
32. Hunt, L.J.; Covinsky, K.E.; Yaffe, K.; Stephens, C.E.; Miao, Y.; Boscardin, W.J.; Smith, A.K. Pain in Community-Dwelling Older Adults with Dementia: Results from the National Health and Aging Trends Study. *J. Am. Geriatr. Soc.* **2015**, *63*, 1503–1511. [CrossRef] [PubMed]
33. Bosley, B.N.; Weiner, D.K.; Rudy, T.E.; Granieri, E. Is Chronic Nonmalignant Pain Associated with Decreased Appetite in Older Adults? Preliminary Evidence. *J. Am. Geriatr. Soc.* **2004**, *52*, 247–251. [CrossRef] [PubMed]
34. Streicher, M.; van Zwienen-Pot, J.; Bardon, L.; Nagel, G.; Teh, R.; Meisinger, C.; Colombo, M.; Torbahn, G.; Kiesswetter, E.; Flechtner-Mors, M.; et al. Determinants of Incident Malnutrition in Community-Dwelling Older Adults: A MaNuEL Multicohort Meta-Analysis. *J. Am. Geriatr. Soc.* **2018**, *66*, 2335–2343. [CrossRef]
35. Zadak, Z.; Hyspler, R.; Ticha, A.; Vlcek, J. Polypharmacy and Malnutrition. *Curr. Opin. Clin. Nutr. Metab. Care* **2013**, *16*, 50–55. [CrossRef] [PubMed]

36. McClain, C.J.; Barve, S.S.; Barve, A.; Marsano, L. Alcoholic Liver Disease and Malnutrition. *Alcohol. Clin. Exp. Res.* **2011**, *35*, 815–820. [CrossRef] [PubMed]
37. van der Pols-Vijlbrief, R.; Wijnhoven, H.A.H.; Schaap, L.A.; Terwee, C.B.; Visser, M. Determinants of Protein-Energy Malnutrition in Community-Dwelling Older Adults: A Systematic Review of Observational Studies. *Ageing Res. Rev.* **2014**, *18*, 112–131. [CrossRef]
38. Ranabhat, C.L.; Park, M.-B.; Kim, C.-B. Influence of Alcohol and Red Meat Consumption on Life Expectancy: Results of 164 Countries from 1992 to 2013. *Nutrients* **2020**, *12*, 459. [CrossRef]

Disclaimer/Publisher's Note: The statements, opinions and data contained in all publications are solely those of the individual author(s) and contributor(s) and not of MDPI and/or the editor(s). MDPI and/or the editor(s) disclaim responsibility for any injury to people or property resulting from any ideas, methods, instructions or products referred to in the content.

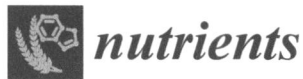 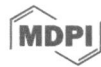

Article

The Effects of 12 Weeks Colostrum Milk Supplementation on the Expression Levels of Pro-Inflammatory Mediators and Metabolic Changes among Older Adults: Findings from the Biomarkers and Untargeted Metabolomic Analysis

Theng Choon Ooi [1], Azizan Ahmad [2], Nor Fadilah Rajab [1] and Razinah Sharif [1,*]

[1] Centre for Healthy Ageing and Wellness, Faculty of Health Science, Universiti Kebangsaan Malaysia, Kuala Lumpur 50300, Malaysia; ooithengchoon@ukm.edu.my (T.C.O.); nfadilah@ukm.edu.my (N.F.R.)
[2] School of Chemical Science and Food Technology, Universiti Kebangsaan Malaysia, Bangi 43600, Malaysia; azizan@ukm.edu.my
* Correspondence: razinah@ukm.edu.my; Tel.: +60-392897459

Abstract: Senescence is a normal biological process that is accompanied with a series of deteriorations in physiological function. This study aimed to investigate the effects of bovine colostrum milk supplementation on metabolic changes and the expression of various biomarkers on inflammation, antioxidant and oxidative damage, nutrient metabolism, and genomic stability among older adults. Older adults (50–69 years old) who participated in the 12-week randomized, double-blinded, placebo-controlled trial were instructed to consume the IgCo bovine colostrum-enriched skim milk or regular skim milk (placebo) twice daily. Following 12 weeks of intervention, participants in the intervention group had lower expression levels in pro-inflammatory mediators (CRP, IL-6, and TNF-α), with significant ($p < 0.05$) interaction effects of the group and time observed. However, no significant interaction effect was observed in the vitamin D, telomerase, 8-OHdG, MDA, and SOD activities. UPLC-MS-based untargeted metabolomics analysis revealed that 22 metabolites were upregulated and 11 were downregulated in the intervention group compared to the placebo group. Glycerophospholipid metabolism, along with cysteine and methionine metabolism were identified as the potential metabolic pathways that are associated with bovine colostrum milk consumption. In conclusion, consuming bovine colostrum milk may induce metabolic changes and reduce the expression of various pro-inflammatory mediators, thus improving the immune function in older adults.

Keywords: biomarkers; colostrum; inflammation; metabolomics; older adults

Citation: Ooi, T.C.; Ahmad, A.; Rajab, N.F.; Sharif, R. The Effects of 12 Weeks Colostrum Milk Supplementation on the Expression Levels of Pro-Inflammatory Mediators and Metabolic Changes among Older Adults: Findings from the Biomarkers and Untargeted Metabolomic Analysis. *Nutrients* 2023, 15, 3184. https://doi.org/10.3390/nu15143184

Academic Editor: Daniel König

Received: 4 May 2023
Revised: 31 May 2023
Accepted: 5 June 2023
Published: 18 July 2023

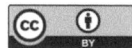

Copyright: © 2023 by the authors. Licensee MDPI, Basel, Switzerland. This article is an open access article distributed under the terms and conditions of the Creative Commons Attribution (CC BY) license (https://creativecommons.org/licenses/by/4.0/).

1. Introduction

The aging trend is a global phenomenon, with every region of the world experiencing increases in the proportion of older individuals. According to the United Nations, the global population aged 65 and older has been projected to reach 1.5 billion by 2050, indicating an increase from 9.3% to 16% of the worldwide population aged 65 years and above [1]. This trend is a consequence of declining fertility rates and increasing life expectancies, which have led to a significant shift in the age structure of many societies. The global aging trend represents a major demographic shift with wide-ranging implications for both societies and economies worldwide. One major challenge is its strain on healthcare systems, as older individuals are more likely to require medical attention and long-term care [2]. Additionally, aging populations may pressure social security systems and pension plans, as fewer working-age individuals support retired individuals [3]. As the proportion of older individuals continues to increase, policymakers and individuals alike need to anticipate and address the challenges and opportunities presented by this trend.

Aging and inflammation are strongly associated with each other. As we age, our body undergoes several changes, including a gradual decline in immune function, which results in chronic low-grade inflammation [4]. Inflammation is a natural response of the body's immune system to injury, infection, or tissue damage. However, this response can become prolonged and excessive in older adults, leading to age-related diseases such as cardiovascular disease, cancer, and neurodegenerative diseases [5]. Inflammation is characterized by the increased production of pro-inflammatory cytokines, reactive oxygen species (ROS), and other immune system molecules [6]. Lifestyle factors such as a poor diet, sedentary behavior, and stress can further exacerbate this chronic inflammation [7]. Thus, targeting inflammation may offer promising interventions to strengthen immune function, prevent age-related diseases, and thus improve the health span.

Colostrum milk, also known as "first milk", is a highly nutritious and specialized type of milk produced by mammals during the first few days after giving birth [8]. Colostrum milk is packed with essential nutrients, including proteins, carbohydrates, and vitamins, as well as high levels of antibodies and immune factors that help in protecting newborns from infections and illnesses [8,9]. In addition to its immune-boosting properties, colostrum milk has been found to support gut health and improve athletic performance [8–10]. Bovine colostrum contains a variety of growth factors that can help support tissue repair and regeneration, making it an attractive supplement for athletes and individuals recovering from injury [8–10]. Moreover, bovine colostrum has been shown to exert antioxidant properties due to the presence of antioxidative enzymes (such as glutathione peroxidase, superoxide dismutase, and catalase), low molecular antioxidants and proteins (such as lactoperoxidase, lactoferrin, and ceruloplasmin), vitamins (including vitamins A, C, and E) and minerals (such as selenium and zinc) [11,12]. Supplementation with bovine colostrum has been demonstrated to exert its antioxidative effects in an intestinal ischemia/reperfusion rat model and in the skeletal muscle of mice after performing exercise [13,14]. Since aging is consistently associated with various age-related degenerative diseases due to redox imbalance and a declination in immune function [4,5,15], we postulated that consuming bovine colostrum milk may help to boost the immune system, alleviate the oxidative condition, and support the overall health of older adults, hence promoting successful aging in their late life. Therefore, this double-blind, randomized control trial aimed to investigate the effects of bovine colostrum-enriched skim milk on the expression of various biomarkers on inflammation, antioxidant and oxidative damage, nutrient metabolism, and genomic stability. In addition, metabolomics analysis was also conducted to examine the metabolic changes following the consumption of bovine colostrum-enriched skim milk, thus increasing our understanding of the mechanisms underlying the beneficial effects of consuming bovine colostrum among older adults.

2. Materials and Methods

2.1. Ethics Approval and Informed Consent

This study protocol was approved by the Medical Research and Ethics Committee of Universiti Kebangsaan Malaysia (JEP-2021-174) and was conducted in accordance with the Declaration of Helsinki and Good Clinical Practice Guidelines. Written informed consent was obtained from all the participants before data collection.

2.2. Study Design and Participants

The study was a 12-week randomized, double-blinded, placebo-controlled trial. The sample size calculation was performed using GPower software version 3.0.10. This study used the mixed model analysis of variance (ANOVA) and repeated measures to analyze the time, group, and interaction effects of the intervention. Therefore, the F-test (ANOVA: repeated measure, within-between interactions) was chosen. The study power was set at 80%, the alpha value at 0.05, and the medium effect size = 0.4, respectively. Based on these parameters, a minimum sample of 52 subjects was required. After considering the 20% dropout rate, a total of 66 participants was required, with 33 subjects in each arm. Older adults aged between 50–69 years were included in this study.

Meanwhile, the exclusion criteria for this study were participants who had a current or past history of cancer or were on a chemotherapeutic regimen, allergic/intolerant to dairy products, chronic kidney diseases/kidney failure, uncontrolled hypertension or diabetes, and heart or cardiovascular disease. After screening for eligibility, a total of 66 participants were recruited. The participants were then randomly divided into two groups using computer-generated software based on their gender: the IgCo bovine colostrum supplement group ($n = 33$) and the placebo group ($n = 33$). There were 14 dropouts, with seven each in both the intervention and placebo groups, either due to a loss in interest in following the study or contracting COVID-19 infection during the intervention period, thus being unable to continue with the investigation. Hence, only 52 participants ($n = 52$) were included in the present analysis, with 26 participants in the intervention and placebo groups, respectively. The consort flow chart of the study is shown in Figure 1. Then, ten age- and gender-matched participants were randomly selected from each group and were subjected to metabolomics analysis.

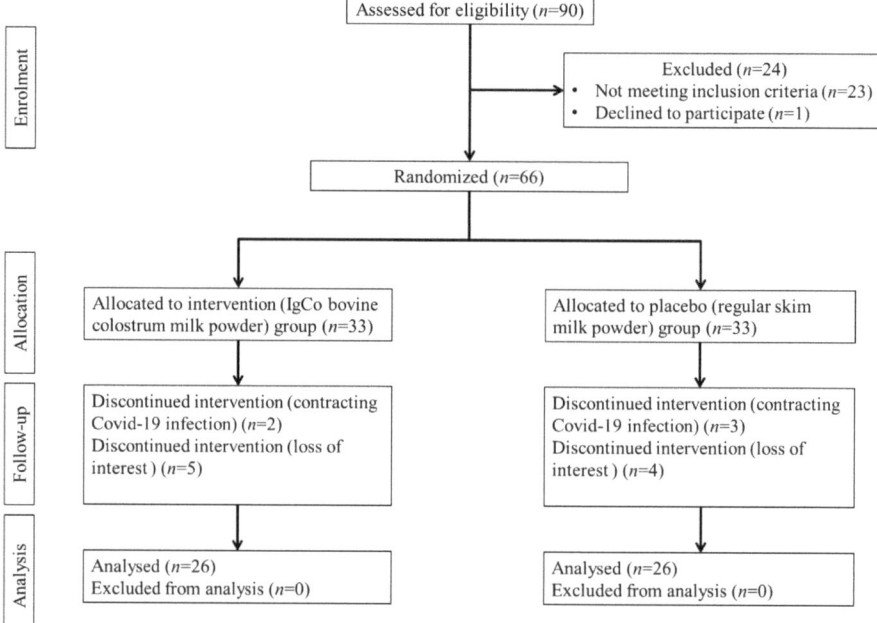

Figure 1. The consort study flow chart. After screening for eligibility, a total of 66 participants who agreed to participate in the study were randomized into the IgCo bovine colostrum supplement group ($n = 33$) and the placebo group ($n = 33$), respectively. There were 14 dropouts, with seven each in both the intervention and placebo groups during follow-up. Hence, only 52 participants ($n = 52$) were included in the analysis, with 26 participants in the intervention and placebo groups, respectively.

2.3. *Investigational Product*

The investigational product of this trial was IgCo bovine colostrum-enriched skim milk powder, which contains 150 mg of IgG in every sachet (15 g) in the form of pasteurized milk powder. Meanwhile, the placebo for this study was regular skim milk powder (15 g per sachet). The IgCo bovine colostrum and placebo skim milk powder were produced and sponsored by the company SNI SDN BHD. The IgCo bovine colostrum and placebo skim milk were identical in both appearance and taste. Each participant was instructed to consecutively consume the IgCo bovine colostrum or placebo skim milk in two sachets daily for 12 weeks. The nutrition composition of the IgCo bovine colostrum and placebo skim milk is available in the Supplementary Materials.

2.4. Data Collection

The investigators, enumerators, and study participants were blinded from knowing the intervention group allocation throughout the study and during data collection. The participants were interviewed face-to-face by well-trained enumerators to collect the required information, such as sociodemographic factors and self-reported medical history using a standardized questionnaire. Meanwhile, the participants' height, weight, and circumference of the waist and hip were measured using a SECA 206 portable body meter (Seca, Hamburg, Germany), Tanita digital lithium weighing scale (Tanita, Tokyo, Japan) and Lufkin tape, respectively [16,17]. The body mass index (BMI) of the participants was then calculated by using the formula "body weight (kg)/height (m)^2. Meanwhile, the systolic and diastolic blood pressure was taken twice using an automatic digital blood pressure monitor (OMRON, Kyoto, Japan) to obtain the average reading.

2.5. Blood Samples Collection and Clinical Laboratory Testing

A trained phlebotomist collected fasted venous blood samples from each participant during the baseline and 12th week of intervention. Participants were instructed to fast for at least 8 h prior to blood collection. Following centrifugation, plasma samples were separated from the blood and stored in a $-80\ °C$ freezer until further analysis [18,19].

2.6. Biomarkers Detection

A total of 8 biomarkers of interest under different categories of biological process were investigated in this study, including antioxidant and oxidative damage [including superoxide dismutase (SOD) activity, malondialdehyde (MDA), and 8-hydroxy-2'-deoxyguanosine (8-OHdG)], inflammation [C-reactive protein (CRP), interleukin 6 (IL-6), and tumor necrosis factor α (TNF-α)], nutrient metabolism [vitamin D], and genomic stability [telomerase]. Commercially available metabolism assay kits that were used for the detection of SOD activity and MDA levels, as well as the ELISA kits that were used for the detection of 8-OHdG, CRP, IL-6, TNF-α, vitamin D, and telomerase, were all purchased from Elabscience Biotechnology Co., Ltd. (Wuhan, China). The metabolism assays and the ELISA tests were conducted based on the protocol stated in the user manual.

2.7. Untargeted Metabolomics Analysis

2.7.1. Samples Preparation

A total of 100 μL of each plasma sample was mixed with 700 μL of extractant containing internal standard (methanol: acetonitrile: water in the ratio of 4:2:1 $v/v/v$). After shaking for 1 min, the mixtures were placed in a $-20\ °C$ refrigerator for 2 h. After centrifugation at 25,000× g and 4 °C for 15 min, the supernatants were separated, and 600 μL of each supernatant was transferred into a new microcentrifuge tube. The transferred samples were then dried using a drying machine. The samples were reconstituted by adding 180 μL of methanol: pure water (1:1 v/v) and mixed for 10 min via vortexing. The samples were centrifuged at 25,000× g and 4 °C for 15 min, and the supernatants were then transferred to a new microcentrifuge tube. Lastly, 20 μL of each sample was mixed with the QC samples before proceeding to UPLC-MS analysis.

2.7.2. UPLC-MS Analysis

This experiment used Waters 2777c UPLC (Waters, Mildford, MA, USA) in series with the Q Exactive HF high-resolution mass spectrometer (Thermo Fisher Scientific, Waltham, MA, USA) to separate and detect the metabolites. Briefly, chromatographic separation was performed on a Waters ACQUITY UPLC BEH C18 column (1.7 μm, 2.1 mm × 100 mm; Waters, Mildford, MA, USA), and the column temperature was maintained at 45 °C. The mobile phase composition for the positive mode consisted of 0.1% formic acid (A) and acetonitrile (B); whereas, for the negative mode, it comprised 10 mM ammonium formate (A) and acetonitrile (B). The gradient conditions were as follows: 0–1 min, 2% B; 1–9 min, 2–98% B; 9–12 min, 98% B; 12–12.1 min, 98% B to 2% B; and 12.1–15 min, 2% B, respectively.

The flow rate was 0.35 mL/min, and the injection volume was 5 µL. Then, primary and secondary mass spectrometry data acquisition was performed using Q Exactive HF (Thermo Fisher Scientific, USA). The full scan range was 70–1050 m/z with a resolution of 120,000, and the automatic gain control (AGC) target for MS acquisitions was set to 3×10^6 with a maximum ion injection time of 100 ms. The top 3 precursors were selected for subsequent MS/MS fragmentation with a maximum ion injection time of 50 ms and resolution of 30,000, and the AGC was set to 1×10^5, respectively. The stepped normalized collision energy was set to 20, 40, and 60 eV, respectively. The ESI parameters setting was as follows: the sheath gas flow rate was 40, the aux gas flow rate was 10, the positive-ion mode spray voltage(|KV|) was 3.80, the negative-ion mode spray voltage(|KV|) was 3.20, the capillary temperature was 320 °C, and the aux gas heater temperature was 350 °C, respectively.

2.7.3. Metabolite Ion Peak Extraction and Metabolite Identification

After importing the off-line data of mass spectrometry into Compound Discoverer 3.3 (Thermo Fisher Scientific, San Jose, CA, USA) software and analyzing the mass spectrometry data in combination with the BGI metabolome database, mzCloud database, and ChemSpider online database, a data matrix containing information such as metabolite peak area and identification results was obtained.

2.7.4. Bioinformatics Analysis

The result files from the Compound Discoverer were transferred to R software package metaX (BGI Shenzhen, Guangdong, China) for data pre-processing and further analysis. During pre-processing, the data were normalized to obtain the relative peak areas by probabilistic quotient normalization (PQN). Then, the batch effects were corrected using quality control-based robust LOESS signal correction. Metabolites with a coefficient of variation larger than 30% on their relative peak area in QC samples were then removed from further analysis. Subsequently, multivariate statistical and univariate analyzes were used to screen different metabolites between the groups, with slight modifications from the previously described methods [20]. The pre-processed data was log-transformed and auto-scaled in the Pareto scale. Then, principal component analysis (PCA) was performed to reflect the actual distribution of samples and to observe the separation trend between the sample groups. Partial least squares-discriminant analysis (PLS-DA), a supervised statistical method used to enhance the differentiation between the classification groups, was subsequently conducted. The PLS-DA model was established between the comparative analysis groups (two groups of samples), and a 5-fold cross-validation was used to validate when building the model. Then, the orthogonal partial least squares discriminant analysis (OPLS-DA) was performed on two groups of biological samples. The purpose was to establish the relationship model between the metabolite expression and sample categories, thereby allowing for the modelling and prediction of these sample categories. At the same time, the ability of each metabolite to classify and distinguish each group of samples was measured by calculating the variable important for the projection (VIP). For the screening of metabolic biomarkers, it is generally considered that a VIP greater than 1 indicates that the variable significantly affects the differentiation of the sample categories.

For univariate analysis of the data, the differences in metabolite concentration were evaluated in terms of fold change, and statistical comparison was conducted using the independent t-test. The displayed metabolites with a p-value < 0.05 indicated significant differences in the fold-change values. Only the statistically significant metabolites were considered as differential metabolites. Metabolites with a VIP value ≥ 1, fold change ≥ 1.2 or ≤ 0.8, or p-value < 0.05 were considered as differential metabolites.

After the differential metabolites were screened, the expression patterns of the differential metabolites were analyzed by clustering analysis, correlation clustering, and network analysis. Additionally, biological functions were explored through pathway annotation and pathway enrichment analysis. Using the Euclidean distance method, Hierarchical cluster analysis (HCA) was applied to examine the expression levels of the differential metabolites in the two different groups. The identified metabolites' taxonomic and functional annotations were performed by comparing the KEGG and HMDB databases. Afterward, enrichment and pathway analyzes were conducted using the MetaboAnalyst 5.0 software.

2.8. Statistical Analysis

Statistical Package for Social Science (SPSS) version 26 software was used to conduct all statistical analyzes at a significance level of $p < 0.05$. Descriptive analysis was performed using the independent t-test and chi-square test for continuous and categorical data, respectively. Then, the paired sample t-test was employed to examine the effects of the intervention on the expression levels of various biomarkers within the same treatment group by comparing the measurements before and after the treatment. Lastly, a two-way repeated measure ANOVA analysis was used to study the effects of IgCo bovine colostrum milk supplementation on biomarker outcomes, specifically the impact of time, group, and interactions between them. After the Bonferroni correction, the model was adjusted for various potential confounding factors including age and sex.

3. Results

3.1. The Baseline Attributes of Participants

Table 1 shows the baseline attributes of the participants. The mean age of all the participants was 61.71 ± 7.14, with the majority of the participants being female (55.8%), married (96.2%), non-smokers (96.2%), having BMI of 27.19 ± 4.61 kg/m^2, waist circumference of 90.32 ± 10.20 cm, hip circumference of 102.60 ± 8.80 cm, systolic blood pressure of 133.78 ± 16.13 mmHg, and diastolic blood pressure of 82.61 ± 9.79 mmHg, respectively. None of the aforementioned parameters showed significant differences across the intervention and placebo groups ($p > 0.05$). Regarding medical history, 21.2% of participants had diabetes, 28.8% had hypertension, and 32.7% had hypercholesterolemia, respectively. The distribution of comorbidities was found to be non-significant across the groups.

Table 1. The baseline attributes of participants, total and by intervention group.

Parameters	n (%) or Mean ± SD			p-Value
	Total 52 (100.0)	Bovine Colostrum Milk 26 (50.0)	Placebo 26 (50.0)	
Age	61.71 ± 7.14	60.46 ± 7.07	62.96 ± 7.13	0.210
Sex				0.780
Male	23 (44.2)	11 (42.3)	12 (46.2)	
Female	29 (55.8)	15 (57.7)	14 (53.8)	
Marital status				0.149
Single/Divorced	2 (3.8)	0 (0.0)	2 (7.7)	
Married	50 (96.2)	26 (100.0)	24 (92.3)	
Smoking status	2 (3.8)	1 (3.8)	1 (3.8)	1.000
BMI (kg/m^2)	27.19 ± 4.61	26.55 ± 5.16	27.84 ± 3.99	0.318
Waist circumference (cm)	90.32 ± 10.20	88.03 ± 11.15	92.81 ± 8.60	0.098
Hip circumference (cm)	102.60 ± 8.80	100.49 ± 8.62	104.89 ± 8.58	0.077
Systolic pressure (mmHg)	133.78 ± 16.13	130.65 ± 13.94	136.90 ± 17.79	0.165
Diastolic pressure (mmHg)	82.61 ± 9.79	81.37 ± 10.14	83.85 ± 9.45	0.366
Medical history				
Diabetes	11 (21.2)	4 (15.4)	7 (26.9)	0.308
Hypercholesterolemia	17 (32.7)	9 (34.6)	8 (30.8)	0.768
Hypertension	15 (28.8)	7 (26.9)	8 (30.8)	0.760

Note: Data were presented as mean ± SD or n (%). Descriptive analysis was performed using the independent t-test and chi-square test for continuous and categorical data, respectively. No significant differences were detected between the intervention and placebo groups ($p > 0.05$) in all the baseline attributes.

3.2. The Effects of 12 Weeks Intervention on the Expression of Biomarkers

Table 2 shows the effects of 12 weeks IgCo bovine colostrum milk supplementation on the levels of various biomarkers among the participants. Our current findings show that following 12 weeks of intervention, there were significant interaction effects observed between the group and time ($p < 0.05$) in the expression of various inflammatory biomarkers, namely the CRP, IL-6, and TNF-α. Specifically, there was a significant reduction ($p < 0.05$) observed in the expression levels of CRP (5.03 ± 3.26 to 3.34 ± 2.00 ng/mL), IL-6 (3.32 ± 1.19 to 2.67 ± 1.13 pg/mL), and TNF-α (91.88 ± 56.80 to 51.31 ± 44.07 pg/mL) among participants who consumed the IgCo bovine colostrum milk. It is noted that participants in the placebo group also showed a significant reduction in TNF-α expression levels (80.26 ± 46.85 to 64.51 ± 37.03 pg/mL, respectively) after the intervention. However, no significant interaction effects of the group and time were observed in the levels of vitamin D, telomerase, and antioxidant and oxidative damage biomarkers (8-OHdG, MDA, and SOD activities).

Table 2. The effects of 12 weeks of IgCo bovine colostrum milk supplementation on biomarkers among participants.

		Bovine Colostrum Milk ($n = 26$)	Placebo ($n = 26$)	Group Effect			Time Effect			Group × Time Effect		
				p	Partial Eta Squared	Power	p	Partial Eta Squared	Power	p	Partial Eta Squared	Power
Vitamin D (μmol/L)												
Baseline		105.74 ± 53.61	142.22 ± 60.79	0.012 *	0.125	0.729	0.265	0.026	0.197	0.119	0.050	0.343
Post		60.64 ± 24.05 ###	70.28 ± 50.52 ###									
MDA (μmol/L)												
Baseline		0.74 ± 0.40	1.14 ± 0.91	0.047 *	0.080	0.515	0.586	0.006	0.084	0.490	0.010	0.105
Post		1.11 ± 0.48 ##	1.31 ± 0.75									
SOD activity (U/mL)												
Baseline		122.23 ± 12.42	122.88 ± 25.13	0.306	0.022	0.173	0.002	0.175	0.879	0.942	0.000	0.051
Post		113.12 ± 11.36 ##	117.04 ± 20.47									
8-OHdG (ng/mL)												
Baseline		37.16 ± 36.43	30.03 ± 15.18	0.842	0.001	0.054	0.163	0.040	0.285	0.196	0.035	0.251
Post		42.76 ± 38.95	45.83 ± 44.50									
CRP (ng/mL)												
Baseline		5.03 ± 3.26	4.70 ± 1.91	0.640	0.005	0.075	0.657	0.004	0.072	0.015 *	0.117	0.694
Post		3.34 ± 2.00 ##	4.55 ± 2.16									
IL-6 (pg/mL)												
Baseline		3.32 ± 1.19	3.45 ± 1.43	0.082	0.062	0.413	0.156	0.041	0.292	0.018 *	0.111	0.671
Post		2.67 ± 1.13 #	3.64 ± 1.49									
TNF-α (pg/mL)												
Baseline		91.88 ± 56.80	80.26 ± 46.85	0.898	0.000	0.052	0.717	0.003	0.065	0.008 **	0.138	0.774
Post		51.31 ± 44.07 ###	64.51 ± 37.03 #									
Telomerase (ng/mL)												
Baseline		456.29 ± 179.56	465.68 ± 193.06	0.915	0.000	0.051	0.070	0.067	0.443	0.819	0.001	0.056
Post		495.59 ± 185.98	500.60 ± 229.12									

Note: The two-way repeated measured ANOVA model was adjusted with confounding factors such as age and gender. Abbreviation: 8-OHdG, 8-hydroxy-2-deoxyguanosine; CRP, C-reactive protein; IL-6, interleukin 6; MDA, malondialdehyde; SOD, superoxide dismutase; and TNF-α, tumor necrosis factor α. * $p < 0.05$; ** $p < 0.01$, significant different in two-way repeated measured ANOVA. # $p < 0.05$; ## $p < 0.01$; ### $p < 0.001$, significant differences before and after the intervention within the same treatment group.

3.3. Metabolic Profiles of Bovine Colostrum Supplemented Group and Placebo Group

To determine the metabolic changes following the consumption of IgCo colostrum milk, untargeted metabolomics analysis was conducted using the UPLC-MS approach. The serum profiles of the IgCo supplemented (G2) and placebo (S2) groups were analyzed using the multivariate data analyzes approach to provide a global view of the metabolic alterations. PCA was used to perform unsupervised multivariate analysis of the serum groups. The results showed an apparent separation between the IgCo-supplemented and placebo groups on the scores plot of PCA (Figure 2A). All the samples in each group were located in a 95% confidence interval. Based on findings from the OPLS-DA analysis, the first predictive component T score[1] (x-axis) explained 36.4% of the variation between the groups, while the orthogonal T score[1] (y-axis) accounted for 19.0% of the variation within the groups. The OPLS-DA model encompasses a good internal cumulative cross-validation of the goodness of fit and a good predictive ability (R2Y = 0.818, Q2 = 0.782). The discrete clusters by PC1 are shown in Figure 2B. From the OPLS-DA score plot, it can be observed that the IgCo supplemented (G2) and placebo (S2) groups were clearly distinguishable from each other by the first predictive component T score[1] (x-axis).

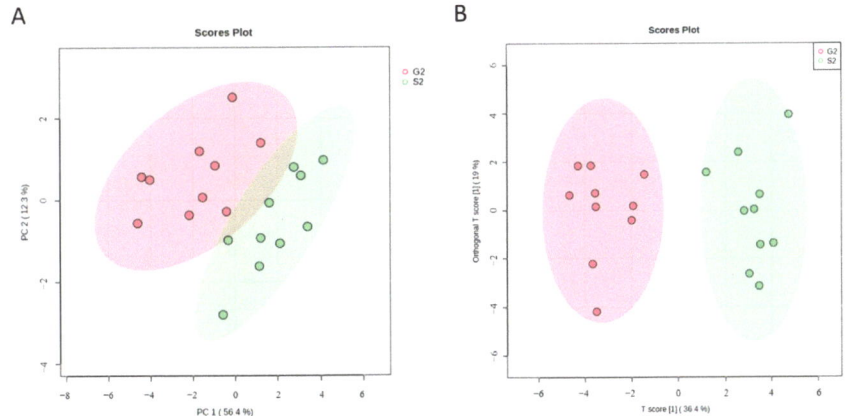

Figure 2. (**A**) PCA and (**B**) OPLS-DA score plot of the placebo group (red color) and the treatment group (green color) in plasma samples after 12 weeks of intervention. For clarity, the ellipses show the 95% confidence region.

3.4. Detection and Identification of Metabolic Markers

A total of 33 differential metabolites between the intervention and placebo groups were identified, with 22 metabolites upregulated (2,4,12-Octadecatrienoic acid isobutylamide, 4,4′-diapolycopenedial, docosanamide, ethyl acetate, gamma-glutamylglutamic acid, gamma-linolenic acid, glycerophosphocholine, indolepyruvate, isovaleric acid, leukotriene C5, leukotriene E3, linoleamide, LysoPC(16:1(9Z)), LysoPC(18:3(9Z,12Z,15Z)), LysoPE(18:0/0:0), N,N-dimethylsphingosine, N-arachidonoyl dopamine, n-butyl acetate, N-oleoylethanolamine, octadecanamide, oleamide and propionic acid) and 11 metabolites were downregulated (3-hydroxybutyric acid, 3-oxododecanoic acid, But-2-enoic acid, etiocholanolone, PC(o-18:1(9Z)/16:0), PE(O-18:1(1Z)/20:4(5Z,8Z,11Z,14Z)), PE(P-16:0/20:3(8Z,11Z,14Z)), PE(P-18:0/18:2(9Z,12Z)), PE(P-18:0/22:6(4Z,7Z,10Z,13Z,16Z,19Z)), PE(P-18:1(9Z)/22:6(4Z,7Z,10Z,13Z,16Z,19Z)), and ubiquinone-4) in the intervention group compared to the placebo group. The fold change, state, *p*-value, and VIP value of each differential metabolite are depicted in Table 3. The variation of these identified differential metabolites among the two groups was extended through the HCA analysis, as shown in Figure S1.

Table 3. Relative quantification of the major serum metabolites between the intervention and placebo groups post-intervention.

Metabolite	Fold Change	State	p-Value	VIP
Propionic acid	18.634	Up	0.001	5.251
Isovaleric acid	9.308	Up	0.003	4.594
n-butyl acetate	31.712	Up	0.004	4.464
Ethyl acetate	43.492	Up	0.016	4.306
Gamma-glutamylglutamic acid	10.617	Up	0.010	3.876
Linoleamide	2.749	Up	0.000	3.250
4,4'-diapolycopenedial	2.678	Up	0.000	3.012
Oleamide	2.247	Up	0.000	2.882
2,4,12-octadecatrienoic acid isobutylamide	2.563	Up	0.000	2.702
Leukotriene E3	2.268	Up	0.000	2.511
Gamma-linolenic acid	1.937	Up	0.001	2.240
N-oleoylethanolamine	2.049	Up	0.017	2.121
Etiocholanolone	0.467	Down	0.037	1.934
Glycerophosphocholine	1.832	Up	0.002	1.913
Octadecanamide	1.733	Up	0.000	1.911
N,N-dimethylsphingosine	1.747	Up	0.007	1.807
N-arachidonoyl dopamine	1.755	Up	0.004	1.775
Leukotriene C5	1.668	Up	0.013	1.759
3-oxododecanoic acid	0.689	Down	0.036	1.700
PE(P-18:0/18:2(9Z,12Z))	0.480	Down	0.018	1.605
PE(O-18:1(1Z)/20:4(5Z,8Z,11Z,14Z))	0.629	Down	0.014	1.552
But-2-enoic acid	0.563	Down	0.046	1.479
3-hydroxybutyric acid	0.694	Down	0.035	1.462
PE(P-18:0/22:6(4Z,7Z,10Z,13Z,16Z,19Z))	0.652	Down	0.003	1.407
LysoPC(18:3(9Z,12Z,15Z))	1.319	Up	0.004	1.405
LysoPE(18:0/0:0)	1.350	Up	0.006	1.368
Ubiquinone-4	0.725	Down	0.023	1.266
PC(o-18:1(9Z)/16:0)	0.673	Down	0.005	1.212
LysoPC(16:1(9Z))	1.383	Up	0.040	1.161
PE(P-16:0/20:3(8Z,11Z,14Z))	0.663	Down	0.028	1.141
PE(P-18:1(9Z)/22:6(4Z,7Z,10Z,13Z,16Z,19Z))	0.713	Down	0.039	1.111
Indolepyruvate	1.500	Up	0.038	1.071
Docosanamide	1.396	Up	0.002	1.055

Note: The differences in metabolite concentration were evaluated in terms of fold change, and statistical comparison was conducted using the t-test. The displayed metabolites with a p-value < 0.05 indicate significant differences in fold-change values between the groups. Only metabolites with VIP value $\geq$ 1, fold change $\geq$ 1.2 or $\leq$ 0.8, or p-value < 0.05 were considered differential metabolites. Up: a relatively higher concentration compared to the placebo group. Down: a relatively lower concentration compared to the placebo group.

Furthermore, to determine the within-group differences in the metabolic markers, the differential metabolites within the IgCo bovine colostrum milk-supplemented and placebo groups pre- and post-intervention were also determined, as shown in Tables S2 and S3, respectively. Overall, 48 (21 upregulated and 27 downregulated) and 37 (16 upregulated and 21 downregulated) differential metabolites were identified in the IgCo bovine colostrum milk-supplemented and placebo groups pre- and post-intervention, respectively.

3.5. Characterization and Functional Analysis of Metabolic Pathways

Metabolic pathways were defined with an online MetPa system (MetaboAnalyst 5.0). Nine suggested metabolic pathways were found to be associated with the consumption of IgCo bovine colostrum milk compared to the regular skim milk in the placebo group. The potential metabolic pathway was identified based on impact value > 0.1 and a p-value less than 0.05. Out of the nine suggested metabolic pathways, only the glycerophospholipid metabolism pathway fulfilled the criteria mentioned above and was determined as the potential metabolic pathway in this model. Table 4 shows the output of pathway analysis from the MetPa system, and the findings are summarized in Figure 3. Meanwhile, the potential metabolic pathway before and after consuming the IgCo bovine colostrum milk and regular skim milk were depicted in Tables S4 and S5, respectively. The possible metabolic pathways associated with bovine colostrum milk consumption were glycerophospholipid metabolism and cysteine and methionine metabolism. Meanwhile, sphingolipid and glycerolipid metabolism were found to be the potential metabolic pathways related to regular skim milk consumption.

Table 4. Pathway analysis results (IgCo bovine colostrum milk vs. placebo post-intervention) with the MetPA system (MetaboAnalyst 5.0).

Pathway Name	Hits	Raw p	$-\log(p)$	Holm Adjust	FDR	Impact
Glycerophospholipid metabolism	3	0.0004	3.4391	0.0029	0.0016	0.1700
Steroid hormone biosynthesis	1	0.0024	2.6193	0.0120	0.0038	0.0052
Glycosylphosphatidylinositol (GPI)-anchor biosynthesis	1	2.52×10^{-5}	4.5993	0.0002	0.0002	0.0040
Synthesis and degradation of ketone bodies	1	0.0007	3.1494	0.0050	0.0016	0.0000
Butanoate metabolism	1	0.0007	3.1494	0.0050	0.0016	0.0000
Propanoate metabolism	1	0.0025	2.6011	0.0120	0.0038	0.0000
Biosynthesis of unsaturated fatty acids	1	0.0806	1.0936	0.2418	0.1037	0.0000
Ether lipid metabolism	1	0.2411	0.6177	0.4823	0.2713	0.0000
Tryptophan metabolism	1	0.5021	0.2992	0.5021	0.5021	0.0000

Note: The potential metabolic pathway was identified based on an impact value > 0.1 and a p-value less than 0.05.

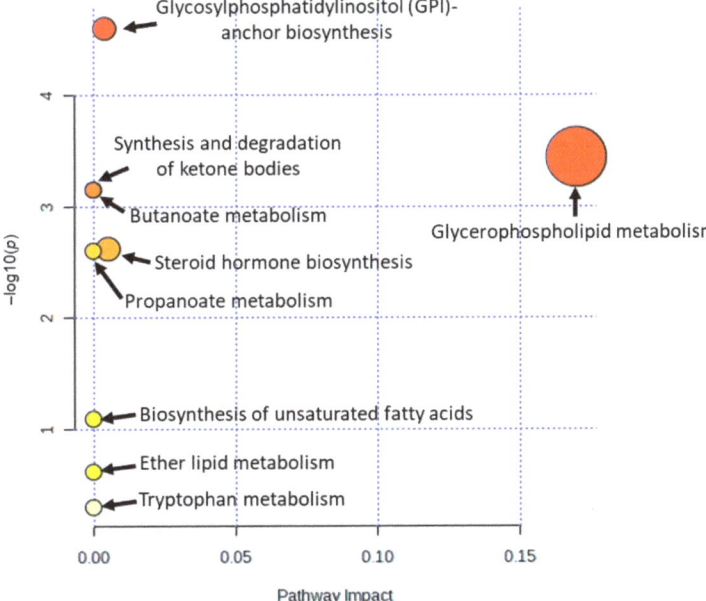

Figure 3. The summary of pathway analysis with the MetPA system (MetaboAnalyst 5.0). The metabolic pathways were represented as circles according to their $-\log(p)$ value at the y-axis and their pathway impact at the x-axis. The darkness and size of each circle corresponds to the $-\log(p)$ value and impact score of the metabolic pathway, respectively.

4. Discussion

This study aimed to investigate the effects of bovine colostrum-enriched skim milk on the expression of various biomarkers on inflammation, antioxidant and oxidative damage, nutrient metabolism, and genomic stability. Our current findings show a significant reduction in the expression of various pro-inflammatory mediators, such as the CRP, IL-6, and TNF-α following the consumption of IgCo bovine colostrum milk, suggesting that it can help in the regulation of immune function and improve the inflammatory conditions in the body. However, consumption of bovine colostrum milk did not have any significant interaction effects of the group and time in relation to the levels of vitamin D, telomerase, 8-OHdG, MDA, and SOD activity. Moreover, the untargeted metabolomics analysis using the UPLC-MS approach revealed that consuming bovine colostrum milk may be associated with alterations in glycerophospholipid metabolism and cysteine and methionine metabolism.

Bovine colostrum is a rich source of bioactive molecules, including immunoglobulins, growth factors, cytokines, and peptides that have anti-inflammatory properties [8–10]. The anti-inflammatory effects of bovine colostrum have been attributed to several mechanisms, including the modulation of immune responses, inhibition of pro-inflammatory cytokines and enzymes, and promotion of tissue repair [8,9,21]. One of the key bioactive molecules in bovine colostrum is lactoferrin, which has been shown to have anti-inflammatory effects [21,22]. Lactoferrin can bind to bacterial and viral cell walls, preventing them from attaching to host cells and reducing the production of pro-inflammatory cytokines [22]. In addition, lactoferrin can modulate the immune system by increasing the number and activity of natural killer cells, which play a crucial role in eliminating the infected cells [23]. Bovine colostrum also contains a variety of growth factors, including insulin-like growth factor 1 (IGF-1), transforming growth factor beta (TGF-β), and epidermal growth factor (EGF) [8]. These growth factors can promote tissue repair and regeneration, which is essential in resolving inflammation.

Furthermore, bovine colostrum contains peptides that have been shown to have anti-inflammatory properties. One of these peptides is lactoperoxidase, which has been shown to inhibit the pro-inflammatory hydrogen peroxide-induced IL-8 secretion in Caco-2 cells [24]. Deleting the lactoperoxidase gene has been demonstrated to cause inflammation in various organs of mice [25]. Meanwhile, another peptide known as lactoferrin has been shown to have an immunomodulatory function and exert anti-inflammatory properties by engaging with diverse cell receptors and activating various cell signaling pathways, frequently facilitated by iron-dependent mechanisms [26]. Moreover, human chondrocytes treated with lactoferrin from exogenous sources have been proven to inhibit the activation of the NF-κB signal transduction pathway, cyclooxygenase-2 expression, and prostaglandin E2 production following IL-1β-stimulation [27]. Previously, orally administered colostrum polyvalent immunoglobulins have been demonstrated to decrease the secretion of IL-1β, IL-6, interferon (IFN)-γ, TNF-α, and IL-12 inflammatory cytokines in patient-derived peripheral blood mononuclear cells (PBMCs) [28]. Additionally, the supplementation of bovine colostrum concentrate among male endurance athletes have been found to inhibit the secretion of TNF, IL-6, and IL-4 from PBMCs in the early phase after adding lipopolysaccharide (LPS) [29]. Hence, suppressing the expression of pro-inflammatory cytokines after consuming bovine colostrum milk may improve immune function.

Glycerophospholipids are a type of phospholipid that form the structural basis of cell membranes [30]. Previous studies have suggested that glycerophospholipid metabolism is implicated in overall systemic immune function and low-grade inflammation, with phospholipids potentially acting as mediators of inflammation [31,32]. Glycerophospholipids play a crucial role in regulating inflammation by serving as precursors for a wide range of signaling molecules, including prostaglandins, leukotrienes, and platelet-activating factors (PAF) [33,34]. These lipid mediators are synthesized by a series of enzymatic reactions that are tightly regulated in response to cellular signals. Research has shown that alterations in the composition of glycerophospholipids can profoundly affect the inflammatory response. For example, studies have indicated that supplementation with glycerophospholipid phosphatidylcholine (PC) can decrease the production of inflammatory cytokines in response to LPS, which is a potent activator of the immune system [35].

In addition, glycerophospholipids have been found to play a role in inflammation by modulating the activity of immune cells and regulating the production of inflammatory mediators. Glycerophospholipids may contribute to inflammation by interacting with toll-like receptors (TLR), thus inhibiting the activation of TLR2 and TLR4 induced by pathogen-associated molecular patterns [36]. In addition, studies have proven that phospholipids, such as PC and phosphatidylethanolamine (PE), can be subjected to hydrolysis by the enzyme phospholipase A2 (PLA2) to release arachidonic acid from cell membranes [37]. Arachidonic acid is a precursor to various inflammatory mediators, including prostaglandins and leukotrienes [38]. Furthermore, the dysregulation in the glycerophospholipid metabolism pathway has been shown to affect the inflammatory response and has been implicated in the development of various diseases associated with chronic inflammation, such as Behçet's disease, allergic airway disease, and rheumatoid arthritis [39–41]. Interestingly, a previous study found that most PCs or Pes were negatively correlated with the inflammatory index, particularly those containing more polyunsaturated acyl chains [42]. Conversely, those with lower levels of polyunsaturated acyl chains were more likely to correlate positively with inflammation. As most of the identified PCs and PEs in this present study were those with lower levels of polyunsaturated acyl chains, the reduction in the expression of the pro-inflammatory biomarkers may be due to the alterations in such PC and PE metabolites following the consumption of the IgCo bovine colostrum milk.

In addition to the glycerophospholipid metabolism pathway, our current findings also demonstrate that cysteine and methionine metabolism is one of the potential metabolic pathways associated with bovine colostrum milk consumption pre- and post-intervention. Following the intervention, a decrease in the expression of methionine, one of the metabolites involved in the cysteine and methionine metabolism, was observed. Methionine is an essential amino acid that plays a vital role in protein synthesis and many other metabolic processes including immunity [43,44]. It has also been linked to inflammation, with several studies suggesting that high levels of methionine intake may contribute to chronic inflammation. One way methionine may contribute to inflammation is through the generation of homocysteine, a toxic amino acid that can damage cells and tissues [45]. Elevated homocysteine levels have been found to be associated with increased inflammation, oxidative stress, and a higher risk of cardiovascular disease [45–47]. Furthermore, methionine metabolism can also lead to the production of S-adenosylmethionine (SAMe), a methyl donor involved in various cellular processes, including the regulation of gene expression. Studies have shown that alterations in the SAMe levels can affect the activation of the mitogen-activated protein kinase (MAPK) signaling pathway, thus reducing the production of TNF-α, IL-6, and interferon-β, respectively [48]. Moreover, a previous study demonstrated that consuming a methionine restriction diet can mitigate the inflammation associated with aging and obesity in the liver, visceral, and subcutaneous white adipose tissue [49]. Thus, the reduction in the expression levels of these pro-inflammatory mediators may be due to the decrease in the methionine levels following the consumption of IgCo bovine colostrum milk.

5. Conclusions

In conclusion, consuming IgCo bovine colostrum-enriched skim milk may help reduce the expression levels of various pro-inflammatory mediators, such as the CRP, IL-6, and TNF-α. Findings from the untargeted metabolomics analysis revealed that consuming bovine colostrum may induce alterations in the glycerophospholipid metabolism and cysteine and methionine metabolism pathways, thus improving the immune function in older adults. Our current findings suggest that bovine colostrum milk has the potential to be used as one of the nutraceutical foods in promoting healthy and successful aging.

Supplementary Materials: The following supporting information can be downloaded at: https://www.mdpi.com/article/10.3390/nu15143184/s1, Figure S1: Heat map of the identified plasma metabolites of individuals in IgCo supplemented group and placebo group after 12 weeks of intervention; Table S1: Nutritional information of IgCo bovine colostrum milk and placebo (regular skim milk); Table S2: Relative quantification of the major serum metabolites within the IgCo supplemented group pre- and post-intervention; Table S3: Relative quantification of the major serum metabolites within the placebo group pre- and post-intervention; Table S4: Results of pathway analysis (IgCo colostrum milk pre- vs post-intervention) with MetPA system (MetaboAnalyst 5.0); Table S5: Results of pathway analysis (Placebo pre- vs. post-intervention) with MetPA system (MetaboAnalyst 5.0).

Author Contributions: Conceptualization, R.S., N.F.R. and A.A.; methodology, T.C.O.; software, T.C.O.; validation, T.C.O., R.S., N.F.R. and A.A.; formal analysis, T.C.O.; investigation, T.C.O. and R.S.; resources, T.C.O. and R.S.; data curation, T.C.O.; writing—original draft preparation, T.C.O.; writing—review and editing, R.S., N.F.R. and A.A.; visualization, T.C.O.; supervision, R.S., N.F.R. and A.A.; project administration, T.C.O.; funding acquisition, R.S. All authors have read and agreed to the published version of the manuscript.

Funding: This work was funded by the SNI SDN BHD (NN-2020-093) and Universiti Kebangsaan Malaysia (DPK-2021-016).

Institutional Review Board Statement: The study was conducted in accordance with the Declaration of Helsinki and approved by the Medical Research and Ethics Committee of Universiti Kebangsaan Malaysia with code JEP-2021-174 on 24 May 2021. The trial was registered at ISRCTN registry (ISRCTN15330940).

Informed Consent Statement: Informed consent was obtained from all subjects involved in the study.

Data Availability Statement: The data presented in this study are available from the corresponding author on reasonable request.

Acknowledgments: We thank all the enumerators for their support and assistance in the study. We want to thank all the participants for participating in this study.

Conflicts of Interest: The authors declare no conflict of interest.

References

1. United Nations Department of Economic and Social Affairs, Population Division. *World Population Ageing 2020 Highlights: Living Arrangements of Older Persons (ST/ESA/SER.A/451)*; United Nations Publication: New York, NY, USA, 2020; ISBN 978-92-1-148347-5.
2. Fulmer, T.; Reuben, D.B.; Auerbach, J.; Fick, D.M.; Galambos, C.; Johnson, K.S. Actualizing Better Health and Health Care For Older Adults. *Health Aff.* **2021**, *40*, 219–225. [CrossRef]
3. Valls Martínez, M.; Santos-Jaén, J.M.; Amin, F.U.; Martín-Cervantes, P.A. Pensions, Ageing and Social Security Research: Literature Review and Global Trends. *Mathematics* **2021**, *9*, 3258. [CrossRef]
4. Chung, H.Y.; Kim, D.H.; Lee, E.K.; Chung, K.W.; Chung, S.; Lee, B.; Seo, A.Y.; Chung, J.H.; Jung, Y.S.; Im, E.; et al. Redefining Chronic Inflammation in Aging and Age-Related Diseases: Proposal of the Senoinflammation Concept. *Aging Dis.* **2019**, *10*, 367–382. [CrossRef] [PubMed]
5. Ferrucci, L.; Fabbri, E. Inflammageing: Chronic Inflammation in Ageing, Cardiovascular Disease, and Frailty. *Nat. Rev. Cardiol.* **2018**, *15*, 505–522. [CrossRef]
6. Chen, L.; Deng, H.; Cui, H.; Fang, J.; Zuo, Z.; Deng, J.; Li, Y.; Wang, X.; Zhao, L. Inflammatory Responses and Inflammation-Associated Diseases in Organs. *Oncotarget* **2018**, *9*, 7204–7218. [CrossRef]
7. Huston, P. A Sedentary and Unhealthy Lifestyle Fuels Chronic Disease Progression by Changing Interstitial Cell Behaviour: A Network Analysis. *Front. Physiol.* **2022**, *13*, 904107. [CrossRef] [PubMed]
8. Playford, R.J.; Weiser, M.J. Bovine Colostrum: Its Constituents and Uses. *Nutrients* **2021**, *13*, 265. [CrossRef]
9. Arslan, A.; Kaplan, M.; Duman, H.; Bayraktar, A.; Ertürk, M.; Henrick, B.M.; Frese, S.A.; Karav, S. Bovine Colostrum and Its Potential for Human Health and Nutrition. *Front. Nutr.* **2021**, *8*, 651721. [CrossRef]
10. Główka, N.; Woźniewicz, M. Potential Use of Colostrum Bovinum Supplementation in Athletes—A Review. *Acta Sci. Pol. Technol. Aliment.* **2019**, *18*, 115–123. [CrossRef]
11. Przybylska, J.; Albera, E.; Kankofer, M. Antioxidants in Bovine Colostrum. *Reprod. Domest. Anim.* **2007**, *42*, 402–409. [CrossRef]
12. Albera, E.; Kankofer, M. Antioxidants in Colostrum and Milk of Sows and Cows. *Reprod. Domest. Anim.* **2009**, *44*, 606–611. [CrossRef]
13. Kwon, O.Y.; Lee, J.S.; Choi, H.S.; Hong, H.P.; Jang, K.H.; Paek, J.H.; Ah Kan, S.; Ko, Y.G. Antioxidant and Anticytokine Effects of Bovine Colostrum in Intestinal Ischemia/Reperfusion Injured Rat Model. *Food Sci. Biotechnol.* **2010**, *19*, 1295–1301. [CrossRef]
14. Appukutty, M.; Radhakrishnan, A.K.; Ramasamy, K.; Ramasamy, R.; Abdul Majeed, A.B.; Noor, M.I.; Safii, N.S.; Koon, P.B.; Chinna, K.; Haleagrahara, N. Colostrum Supplementation Protects against Exercise—Induced Oxidative Stress in Skeletal Muscle in Mice. *BMC Res. Notes* **2012**, *5*, 649. [CrossRef]
15. Liguori, I.; Russo, G.; Curcio, F.; Bulli, G.; Aran, L.; Della-Morte, D.; Gargiulo, G.; Testa, G.; Cacciatore, F.; Bonaduce, D.; et al. Oxidative Stress, Aging, and Diseases. *Clin. Interv. Aging* **2018**, *13*, 757–772. [CrossRef]
16. Ooi, T.C.; Singh, D.K.A.; Shahar, S.; Rajab, N.F.; Vanoh, D.; Sharif, R.; Tan, M.P. Incidence and Multidimensional Predictors of Occasional and Recurrent Falls among Malaysian Community-dwelling Older Persons. *BMC Geriatr.* **2021**, *21*, 154. [CrossRef]

17. Ooi, T.C.; Ishak, W.S.; Sharif, R.; Shahar, S.; Rajab, N.F.; Singh, D.K.A.; Mukari, S.Z.M.S. Multidimensional Risk Factors of Age-Related Hearing Loss among Malaysian Community-Dwelling Older Adults. *Clin. Interv. Aging* **2021**, *16*, 2033–2046. [CrossRef]
18. Ooi, T.C.; Singh, D.K.A.; Shahar, S.; Sharif, R.; Rivan, N.F.M.; Meramat, A.; Rajab, N.F. Higher Lead and Lower Calcium Levels Are Associated with Increased Risk of Mortality in Malaysian Older Population: Findings from the LRGS-TUA Longitudinal Study. *Int. J. Environ. Res. Public Health* **2022**, *19*, 6955. [CrossRef]
19. Ooi, T.C.; Singh, D.K.A.; Shahar, S.; Rajab, N.F.; Sharif, R. Higher Levels of Lead and Aluminium Are Associated with Increased Risk of Falls among Community-Dwelling Older Adults: An 18-Month Follow-up Study. *Geriatr. Gerontol. Int.* **2021**, *21*, 1026–1032. [CrossRef]
20. Ooi, T.C.; Meramat, A.; Rajab, N.F.; Shahar, S.; Ismail, I.S.; Azam, A.A.; Sharif, R. Intermittent Fasting Enhanced the Cognitive Function in Older Adults with Mild Cognitive Impairment by Inducing Biochemical and Metabolic Changes: A 3-Year Progressive Study. *Nutrients* **2020**, *12*, 2644. [CrossRef]
21. Gomes, R.D.S.; Anaya, K.; Galdino, A.B.S.; Oliveira, J.P.F.; Gama, M.A.S.; Medeiros, C.A.C.X.; Gavioli, E.C.; Porto, A.L.F.; Rangel, A.H.N. Bovine Colostrum: A Source of Bioactive Compounds for Prevention and Treatment of Gastrointestinal Disorders. *NFS J.* **2021**, *25*, 1–11. [CrossRef]
22. Superti, F. Lactoferrin from Bovine Milk: A Protective Companion for Life. *Nutrients* **2020**, *12*, 2562. [CrossRef]
23. Kell, D.B.; Heyden, E.L.; Pretorius, E. The Biology of Lactoferrin, an Iron-Binding Protein That Can Help Defend Against Viruses and Bacteria. *Front. Immunol.* **2020**, *11*, 1221. [CrossRef] [PubMed]
24. Matsushita, A.; Son, D.O.; Satsu, H.; Takano, Y.; Kawakami, H.; Totsuka, M.; Shimizu, M. Inhibitory Effect of Lactoperoxidase on the Secretion of Pro-inflammatory Cytokine Interleukin-8 in Human Intestinal Epithelial Caco-2 Cells. *Int. Dairy J.* **2008**, *18*, 932–938. [CrossRef]
25. Yamakaze, J.; Lu, Z. Deletion of the Lactoperoxidase Gene Causes Multisystem Inflammation and Tumors in Mice. *Sci. Rep.* **2021**, *11*, 12429. [CrossRef]
26. Kruzel, M.L.; Zimecki, M.; Actor, J.K. Lactoferrin in a Context of Inflammation-Induced Pathology. *Front. Immunol.* **2017**, *8*, 1438. [CrossRef]
27. Rasheed, N.; Alghasham, A.; Rasheed, Z. Lactoferrin from Camelus Dromedarius Inhibits Nuclear Transcription Factor-kappa B Activation, Cyclooxygenase-2 Expression and Prostaglandin E2 Production in Stimulated Human Chondrocytes. *Pharmacogn. Res.* **2016**, *8*, 135–141. [CrossRef]
28. Gasser, M.; Lissner, R.; Nawalaniec, K.; Hsiao, L.-L.; Waaga-Gasser, A.M. KMP01D Demonstrates Beneficial Anti-Inflammatory Effects on Immune Cells: An Ex Vivo Preclinical Study of Patients with Colorectal Cancer. *Front. Immunol.* **2020**, *11*, 684. [CrossRef]
29. Shing, C.M.; Peake, J.M.; Suzuki, K.; Jenkins, D.G.; Coombes, J.S. Bovine Colostrum Modulates Cytokine Production in Human Peripheral Blood Mononuclear Cells Stimulated with Lipopolysaccharide and Phytohemagglutinin. *J. Interferon Cytokine Res.* **2008**, *29*, 37–44. [CrossRef]
30. Watson, H. Biological Membranes. *Essays Biochem.* **2015**, *59*, 43–69. [CrossRef] [PubMed]
31. Pietzner, M.; Kaul, A.; Henning, A.-K.; Kastenmüller, G.; Artati, A.; Lerch, M.M.; Adamski, J.; Nauck, M.; Friedrich, N. Comprehensive Metabolic Profiling of Chronic Low-Grade Inflammation among Generally Healthy Individuals. *BMC Med.* **2017**, *15*, 210. [CrossRef] [PubMed]
32. Yu, E.A.; He, S.; Jones, D.P.; Sun, Y.V.; Ramirez-Zea, M.; Stein, A.D. Metabolomic Profiling Demonstrates Postprandial Changes in Fatty Acids and Glycerophospholipids Are Associated with Fasting Inflammation in Guatemalan Adults. *J. Nutr.* **2021**, *151*, 2564–2573. [CrossRef]
33. Yamaguchi, A.; Botta, E.; Holinstat, M. Eicosanoids in Inflammation in the Blood and the Vessel. *Front. Pharmacol.* **2022**, *13*, 997403. [CrossRef] [PubMed]
34. Lone, A.; Taskén, K. Pro-inflammatory and Immunoregulatory Roles of Eicosanoids in T Cells. *Front. Immunol.* **2013**, *4*, 130. [CrossRef]
35. Tan, W.; Zhang, Q.; Dong, Z.; Yan, Y.; Fu, Y.; Liu, X.; Zhao, B.; Duan, X. Phosphatidylcholine Ameliorates LPS-Induced Systemic Inflammation and Cognitive Impairments via Mediating the Gut–Brain Axis Balance. *J. Agric. Food Chem.* **2020**, *68*, 14884–14895. [CrossRef]
36. Choudhary, V.; Uaratanawong, R.; Patel, R.R.; Patel, H.; Bao, W.; Hartney, B.; Cohen, E.; Chen, X.; Zhong, Q.; Isales, C.M.; et al. Phosphatidylglycerol Inhibits Toll-Like Receptor–Mediated Inflammation by Danger-Associated Molecular Patterns. *J. Investig. Dermatol.* **2019**, *139*, 868–877. [CrossRef] [PubMed]
37. Khan, S.A.; Ilies, M.A. The Phospholipase A2 Superfamily: Structure, Isozymes, Catalysis, Physiologic and Pathologic Roles. *Int. J. Mol. Sci.* **2023**, *24*, 1353. [CrossRef] [PubMed]
38. Tallima, H.; El Ridi, R. Arachidonic Acid: Physiological Roles and Potential Health Benefits—A Review. *J. Adv. Res.* **2018**, *11*, 33–41. [CrossRef]
39. Mendes-Frias, A.; Santos-Lima, B.; Furtado, D.Z.S.; Ruperez, F.J.; Assunção, N.A.; Matias, M.J.; Gomes, V.; Gaifem, J.; Barbas, C.; Castro, A.G.; et al. Dysregulation of Glycerophospholipid Metabolism during Behçet's Disease Contributes to a pro-Inflammatory Phenotype of Circulating Monocytes. *J. Transl. Autoimmun.* **2020**, *3*, 100056. [CrossRef] [PubMed]

40. Sevastou, I.; Kaffe, E.; Mouratis, M.-A.; Aidinis, V. Lysoglycerophospholipids in Chronic Inflammatory Disorders: The PLA2/LPC and ATX/LPA Axes. *Biochim. Biophys. Acta Mol. Cell Res.* **2013**, *1831*, 42–60. [CrossRef] [PubMed]
41. Bansal, P.; Gaur, S.N.; Arora, N. Lysophosphatidylcholine Plays Critical Role in Allergic Airway Disease Manifestation. *Sci. Rep.* **2016**, *6*, 27430. [CrossRef]
42. Zhu, Q.; Wu, Y.; Mai, J.; Guo, G.; Meng, J.; Fang, X.; Chen, X.; Liu, C.; Zhong, S. Comprehensive Metabolic Profiling of Inflammation Indicated Key Roles of Glycerophospholipid and Arginine Metabolism in Coronary Artery Disease. *Front. Immunol.* **2022**, *13*, 829425. [CrossRef] [PubMed]
43. Klein Geltink, R.I.; Pearce, E.L. The Importance of Methionine Metabolism. *eLife* **2019**, *8*, e47221. [CrossRef] [PubMed]
44. Brosnan, J.T.; Brosnan, M.E. The Sulfur-Containing Amino Acids: An Overview. *J. Nutr.* **2006**, *136*, 1636S–1640S. [CrossRef] [PubMed]
45. Kumar, A.; Palfrey, H.A.; Pathak, R.; Kadowitz, P.J.; Gettys, T.W.; Murthy, S.N. The Metabolism and Significance of Homocysteine in Nutrition and Health. *Nutr. Metab.* **2017**, *14*, 78. [CrossRef]
46. Esse, R.; Barroso, M.; de Almeida, I.; Castro, R. The Contribution of Homocysteine Metabolism Disruption to Endothelial Dysfunction: State-of-the-Art. *Int. J. Mol. Sci.* **2019**, *20*, 867. [CrossRef]
47. Li, J.-J.; Li, Q.; Du, H.-P.; Wang, Y.-L.; You, S.-J.; Wang, F.; Xu, X.-S.; Cheng, J.; Cao, Y.-J.; Liu, C.-F.; et al. Homocysteine Triggers Inflammatory Responses in Macrophages through Inhibiting CSE-H2S Signaling via DNA Hypermethylation of CSE Promoter. *Int. J. Mol. Sci.* **2015**, *16*, 12560–12577. [CrossRef]
48. Ji, J.; Xu, Y.; Zheng, M.; Luo, C.; Lei, H.; Qu, H.; Shu, D. Methionine Attenuates Lipopolysaccharide-Induced Inflammatory Responses via DNA Methylation in Macrophages. *ACS Omega* **2019**, *4*, 2331–2336. [CrossRef]
49. Sharma, S.; Dixon, T.; Jung, S.; Graff, E.C.; Forney, L.A.; Gettys, T.W.; Wanders, D. Dietary Methionine Restriction Reduces Inflammation Independent of FGF21 Action. *Obesity* **2019**, *27*, 1305–1313. [CrossRef]

Disclaimer/Publisher's Note: The statements, opinions and data contained in all publications are solely those of the individual author(s) and contributor(s) and not of MDPI and/or the editor(s). MDPI and/or the editor(s) disclaim responsibility for any injury to people or property resulting from any ideas, methods, instructions or products referred to in the content.

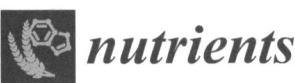

Review

Urolithins: A Prospective Alternative against Brain Aging

Lei An [1], Qiu Lu [1], Ke Wang [1,2,3] and Yousheng Wang [2,*]

[1] Key Laboratory of Geriatric Nutrition and Health, Ministry of Education, Beijing Technology and Business University, Beijing 100048, China; andijia1@126.com (L.A.); echo6939@163.com (Q.L.); wangke9509@163.com (K.W.)
[2] College of Light Industry and Food Engineering, Guangxi University, Nanning 530004, China
[3] Rizhao Huawei Institute of Comprehensive Health Industries, Shandong Keepfit Biotech. Co., Ltd., Rizhao 276800, China
* Correspondence: wangys@gxu.edu.cn

Abstract: The impact of host–microbiome interactions on cognitive health and disease has received increasing attention. Microbial-derived metabolites produced in the gut are one of crucial mechanisms of the gut–brain axis interaction, showing attractive perspectives. Urolithins (Uros) are gut microbial-derived metabolites of ellagitannins and ellagic acid, whose biotransformation varies considerably between individuals and decreases greatly with age. Recently, accumulating evidence has suggested that Uros may have specific advantages in preventing brain aging including favorable blood–brain barrier permeability, selective brain distribution, and increasingly supporting data from preclinical and clinical studies. However, the usability of Uros in diagnosis, prevention, and treatment of neurodegenerative diseases remains elusive. In this review, we aim to present the comprehensive achievements of Uros in age-related brain dysfunctions and neurodegenerative diseases and discuss their prospects and knowledge gaps as functional food, drugs, or biomarkers against brain aging.

Keywords: urolithin; brain; aging; neurodegenerative diseases; microbial-derived; metabolites

1. Introduction

To date, the population of dementia is approximately 45 million worldwide (this number will double if mild cognitive impairment (MCI) is included), and this population is expected to triple (approximately 130 million) by 2050 [1]. As the population of older adults is increasing, interest in the aging brain and the quest for "healthy brain aging" is growing. Modern medicine and nutrition evidence has confirmed that polyphenol consumption is an effective strategy in delaying brain aging [2]. However, the poor bioavailability of dietary polyphenols in vivo is contradictory to their health benefits [3,4]. Recently, there has been increasing evidence suggesting that the health benefits of polyphenols are mainly based on: (1) Polyphenols being either directly absorbed or in most cases converted into bioactive metabolites by gut microbiota and then get to the target tissues; (2) Polyphenols reshaping the gut microbiome during their bidirectional interaction. In addition, microbial-derived metabolites of polyphenols can be used as biomarkers to predict individual health status or even the efficacy of some drugs in vivo [5]. Over the past decade, research on gut microbiota and the gut–brain axis has brought increasingly new insights into humans [6]. Several pathways have been confirmed in the communication of the gut microbiota and the brain: (1) neuroendocrinology: the gut cells secrete a large amount of the signaling molecules in neuroendocrinology which can be influenced by gut microbiota; (2) neuroimmunity: the GI tract itself is the largest immune organ to stress response and the gut microbiota can promote immune cells to produce cytokines that can affect the brain; (3) neurotransmitters: the gut microbiota can affect the neurotransmitter secretion directly (several neurotransmitters, including acetylcholine, dopamine, noradrenaline, and serotonin can be synthesized by gut bacteria) and indirectly; and (4) microbial-derived

Citation: An, L.; Lu, Q.; Wang, K.; Wang, Y. Urolithins: A Prospective Alternative against Brain Aging. *Nutrients* **2023**, *15*, 3884. https://doi.org/10.3390/nu15183884

Academic Editors: Moustapha Dramé and Lidvine Godaert

Received: 13 August 2023
Revised: 1 September 2023
Accepted: 2 September 2023
Published: 6 September 2023

Copyright: © 2023 by the authors. Licensee MDPI, Basel, Switzerland. This article is an open access article distributed under the terms and conditions of the Creative Commons Attribution (CC BY) license (https://creativecommons.org/licenses/by/4.0/).

metabolites: neuroactive metabolites mediate bidirectional interactions between the gut, gut microbiome, and the brain to modulate host neurophysiology and behavior [7–9].

As many of the host–microorganism interactions pertaining to human health are mediated by metabolites, interest in the microbial-derived metabolites has been increasing [10–12]. Among these active metabolites, urolithins (Uros), the gut bacterial metabolites of ellagitannins (ETs) and ellagic acid (EA), have shown to be beneficial in delaying many age-related diseases such as cancer (especially prostate, breast, and colorectal cancers), cardiovascular diseases, and chronic metabolic disorders (diabetes and hyperuricemia) [13–18]. Recently, growing evidence has supported the multiple health benefits of Uros against brain aging and the therapeutic potential for neurodegenerative diseases [17,19–22]. Moreover, Uros have been proposed as biomarkers of gut dysbiosis and disease stage in Parkinson's patients [23]. Herein, we aim to review the recent achievements of Uros in brain aging and neurodegenerative diseases, with a particular emphasis on their therapeutic targets and mechanisms and discuss their prospects and knowledge gaps.

2. Overview and Advantage of Uros

Uros are gut metabolites derived from ETs and EA, which are richly available in many fruits (pomegranates, berries), nuts (walnuts), wood-aged wine, and some medicinal plants (galla chinensis, chebulae fructus, and seabuckthorn leaf) [12]. ETs and EA have very poor bioavailability in vivo and are converted into Uros by intestinal microbes in the colon, which are believed to be responsible for their biological activities [24,25]. ETs are a group of important dietary polyphenols and hydrolysable tannins that share a common core, hexahydroxydiphenoyl (HHDP), and differ in the number of monomer residues. ETs are mainly hydrolyzed to EA in the upper GI tract (stomach and small intestine), and most of the EA is converted to Uros in the lower GI tract (mainly in the colon) [25–27]. Uros are 6H-dibenzo [b, d] pyran-6-one derivatives which differ in their hydroxyl groups. The family includes the main end metabolites, dihydroxy derivatives UroA, Iso-UroA and monohydroxy derivative UroB, and other intermediates UroC, UroD, UroE, UroM-5, UroM-6, and UroM-7. Overall, UroA is the main metabolite produced in humans, which demonstrates the highest concentrations in plasma and urine, and remains high for days after the consumption of ET-rich food [28–30].

The bioconversion of Uros from ETs and EA varies considerably between individuals. Some individuals can produce high plasma concentrations of Uros (high Uro producers), while others cannot produce significant levels of Uros (low Uro producers). Additionally, Uro producers can also be classified into "metabotype A" (only high concentration of UroA is produced), and "metabotype B" (more Iso-UroA and/or UroB in comparison to UroA is produced) [31]. Therefore, the consumption of dietary ETs will produce different health benefits in high or low Uro producers, and those with different metabolic phenotypes. The different capacities for excreting Uros are mainly attributed to the variability of gut microbiota ecology, and vary with age, health status, dietary intake, obesity, and digestive organ surgery [32,33]. Notably, age is a key factor that affects the bioconversion of Uros. The bioconversion of Uros significantly decreases with aging. According to clinical observations, approximately 10% of individuals (aged 5–90) are non-Uro producers, and only 40% of elderly people (>60) can produce meaningful levels of Uros from dietary precursors [34]. Therefore, Uro supplementation may be a good alternative for certain individuals (e.g., elderly people) to meet the required healthy Uro level [35].

In comparison to precursors and live bacteria, Uros possess clear chemical structure, good bioavailability, and high safety in animals and humans [36,37]. Recently, two multi-center clinical trials showed that long-term (4-month) oral administration of UroA is safe and well tolerated [38,39]. Moreover, UroA is considered as GRAS (generally recognized as safe) for its use in food products by the Food and Drug Administration (FDA) [40]. Notably, Uros can also pass through the blood–brain barrier (BBB) and distribute in a brain-targeted manner after absorption [17,41,42], which may greatly facilitate their activities in the central nervous system (CNS), while other ET derivatives cannot cross the BBB. Additionally, as increasing evidence supporting the involvement of the gut metabolites in human health and diseases, metabolite-based treatment has been considered as a novel and promising therapeutic approach. It can overcome limitations and deficiencies of microbiome-based treatment (probiotics and prebiotics supplementation or fecal microbiome transplantation), such as colonization resistance and inter-individual variation in microbial composition [43]. Microbial-derived metabolites may be able to provide an improved efficacy (safety, stability, and individual variation) by exerting a beneficial host effect downstream of the microbiome. Collectively, these findings highlight the advantages of Uros in developing into functional food or drugs.

Many studies have investigated the biotransformations of ETs and EA to Uros. ETs are first converted into EA, facilitated by physiological pH and/or microbial enzymes such as tannin–hydrolase and lactonase. EA is then catalyzed by several microbial enzymes, including lactonase, decarboxylase, dehydroxylases, methyl esterases, and hydrolases, to produce Uros in the colon [25]. The metabolic pathways associated with these enzymes have been elucidated. Recently, several Uro-producing gut bacteria have been identified that can facilitate the conversion of EA to Uros in vitro [44–46]. Therefore, in addition to the chemical synthesis of Uros, the biotransformation of Uros with bacteria or enzymes in vitro in the near future can be expected [28,47].

As previously described, the consumption of dietary polyphenols is highly correlated with human health and the risk of neurodegenerative diseases [12]. Dynamic two-way communications between the gut, gut microbiome, and the CNS have been considered an increasingly vital factor for cognitive health and disease. Novel perspectives suggest that microbial-derived metabolites of polyphenols can be used as biomarkers to predict the risk of neurodegenerative diseases [48]. Therefore, in addition to the potential as functional food or drugs, Uros may be potential biomarkers of age-related cognitive decline and related disorders, which is mainly based on the following: (1) As bioactive metabolites, they exert multiple health benefits against brain aging and related diseases (which we will discuss below in detail); (2) the level of Uros in baseline is an indicator of personalized nutrition status (the consumption of dietary polyphenols in individuals, particularly for ETs and EA consumption), which is highly correlated with the risk of neurodegenerative diseases; (3) the level of Uros after consuming ET- or EA-rich food is an indicator of individual metabotypes associated with specific gut microbial ecologies (gut microbiota composition and functionality), which is tightly involved in neurodegenerative diseases. A recent study based on 52 patients and 117 healthy individuals showed that gut dysbiosis occurred during the onset and progression of Parkinson's disease (PD) and the concentration of Uros in urine was highly associated with the severity of gut dysbiosis and PD in elderly people [23].

3. Preclinical and Clinical Studies

As UroA and UroB are the most abundant final metabolites in vivo, they are the most widely studied Uros across species, particularly UroA. Accumulating preclinical studies have demonstrated the beneficial effects of UroA and UroB on age-related brain dysfunctions. The cell studies in vitro are summarized in Table 1. Although these studies all demonstrated the neuroprotective effect of Uros in aging conditions such as oxidative stress, inflammation, and high concentrations of glucose, the treatment conditions in different laboratories and the sensitivity of different cells to Uros varied considerably. The animal studies in vivo are summarized in Table 2. Uros administration has been shown significantly improve cognition, learning, and memory in aged animals and animal models of neurodegenerative diseases.

It has been reported that ET- or EA-rich food consumption improve cognition and memory in the elderly (summarized in Table 3), whereas the effect of Uros supplementation in the elderly is still unknown. Two sequential randomized, double-blind, placebo-controlled trials in middle-aged and older adults (aged 50–75 years) with MCI showed that drinking 8 ounces (237 mL) of pomegranate juice every day for short-term 4 weeks or long-term 12 months significantly improved performance in the Brief Visuospatial Memory Test–Revised and Buschke Selective Reminding Test, and increased functional brain activation during verbal and visual memory tasks (ClinicalTrials.gov Identifier: NCT02093130) [42,49]. Moreover, cognition and memory improvement by pomegranate juice consumption is in line with the concentration of UroA–glucuronide in plasma and the plasma Trolox-equivalent antioxidant capacity. Additionally, berry and walnut consumption are related to better cognitive function and memory performance in the elderly with normal cognition or MCI [50–53]. Recently, several clinical trials have shown that UroA administration improves skeletal muscle function and mitochondrial health in elderly and middle-aged adults (ClinicalTrials.gov Identifier: NCT02655393, NCT03464500, and NCT03283462) [37–39]. In summary, evidence supporting the role of Uros in preventing the degeneration of brain during aging is accumulating, whereas clinical study in humans is lacking and needs further investigation.

Table 1. Preclinical studies of Uros on brain aging in vitro cell models.

Uros	Cells	Pharmacological or Genetic Interventions	Treatment (Dosage and Time)	Effects	Findings	Refs.
UroA	Neuro-2a cells	H_2O_2 (250 μM) for 45 min	0.5 μM, 1 μM, 2 μM, 4 μM pretreatment for 24 h	antioxidation	↑ cells viability, ↓ MAO-A and Tyrosinase, ↑ free radical (O^{2-} and DPPH), ↓ ROS, lipid peroxidation, ↑ peroxiredoxins expression, ↑ CAT, SOD, GR, GSH-Px,	[54]
UroA	PC12 cells	H_2O_2 (100 μM) for 2 h	10 μg/mL, 30 μg/mL, and 50 μg/mL pretreatment for 24 h	antioxidation	↑ cells viability, ↓ LDH release, ↓ apoptosis, ↓ caspase 3 and Bcl-2	[17]
UroA	SK-N-MC cells	H_2O_2 (300 μM) for 18 h	1.25 μM, 2.5 μM, and 5 μM pretreatment for 6 h	antioxidation	↑ cells viability, ↓ apoptosis, ↓ ROS, Bax/Bcl-2, PARP, cytochrome c, caspase 3/9, p38 MAPK	[55]
UroA	SH-SY5Y cells	H_2O_2 (100 μM) for 24 h	10 μM treatment for 2 h, 6 h or 24 h	antioxidation	↑ REDOX activity, ↓ cytotoxicity, ↓ ROS, ↓ apoptosis, ↓ caspase 3/8 and 9	[20]
UroA	SH-SY5Y cells	H_2O_2 (200 μM) for 6 h	5 μM, 7.5 μM, 10 μM, 15 μM pretreatment for 12 h	antioxidation	↑ cells viability, ↓ ROS, ↑ SOD, CAT, ↑ PKA/CREB/BDNF	[56]
UroB	Neuro-2a cells	H_2O_2 (250 μM) for 2 h	20 μg/mL, 40 μg/mL, and 60 μg/mL pretreatment for 24 h	antioxidation	↑ cells viability, ↓ ROS, ↓ apoptosis, cytotoxicity, ↓ caspase 3, ↑ Bcl-2	[57]
UroB	BV-2 cells	LPS (100 ng/mL) or LTA (10 μg/mL) or poly(I:C) (25 μg/mL) for 16 h	30 μM, 50 μM, or 100 μM pretreatment for 1 h	antioxidation, anti-inflamation	↓ NO, ROS, TNF-α, IL-6, IL-1β, iNOS, COX-2, ↓ NF-κB, p-JNK, p-ERK, p-Akt, AP-1, ↑ IL-10, pAMPK, p47^{phox}, gp91^{phox}	[58]
UroA mUroA UroB mUrOA	BV-2 cells, SH-SY5Y cells	H_2O_2 (100 μM) for 6 h; LPS (1 μg/mL) for 24 h	0.1 μM, 0.5 μM, 5 μM, 10 μM pretreatment for 1 h, 24 h, or 48 h	antioxidation, anti-inflammation	↓ apoptosis, ↓ NO, TNF-α,NO, COX-2, IL-1, IL-6, PGE2, ↓ caspase 3/7 and 9, ↓ oxidative stress	[19]
UroA	BV-2 cells	LPS (500 ng/mL) for 3 h, 12 h, 24 h; IL-4 (100 ng/mL), IL-13 (10 ng/mL) for 24 h	10 μM pretreatment for 12 h	anti-inflammation	↓ IL-6, IL-1β, TNF-α, ↓ NOS, ↓ JNK/c-Jun, ↑ M2 microglia polarization	[59]

Table 1. Cont.

Uros	Cells	Pharmacological or Genetic Interventions	Treatment (Dosage and Time)	Effects	Findings	Refs.
UroA	BV-2 cells	LPS (1 µg/mL) for 6 h, 12 h or 24 h	2.5 µM, 5 µM, and 10µM pretreatment for 2 h	anti-inflammation improved mitochondrial function	↓ IL-1β, iNOS, COX-2, ↓ ROS, ↑ MMP, ↑ p62, ↓ LC3-II, ↑ Parkin, PINK, ↓ caspase 1, NLRP3, ↓ TOM20, Tim23, ↑ mitophagy, ↑ OXPHOS	[14]
UroA, UroB, UroC, mUroA dmUroC	BV-2 cells	LPS (100 ng/mL) for 30 min, 16 h or 24 h	3 µM, 10 µM, 30 µM treatment for 30 min, 1 h, 16 h or 24 h	anti-inflammation	↓ NO, TNF-α, IL-6, IL-1β, iNOS, COX-2, ↓ pAkt, ↓ pERK1/2, p38 MAPK, ↓ NF-κB	[60]
UroA	BV-2 cells, ReNcell VM cells	LPS (100 ng/mL) for 1 h, 24 h, or transfected with APPSwe	2 µM, 5 µM, 10 µM treatment for 30 min, 6 h or 48 h	anti-inflammation, anti-Aβ	↑ cells viability, ↓ NO, TNFα, IL-6, ↓ Aβ, ↑ SIRT1, ↓ NF-Kb, ↑ induction of autophagic flux	[21]
UroA	SH-SY5Y cells, iPSC-ND cells	D-glucose 25 mM for 24 h, 48 h, and 72 h, Aβ$_{(1-42)}$ for 24 h, 48 h, and 72 h	100 nM pretreatment for 30 min	anti-Aβ, improved mitochondrial function	↓ APP, BACE1, TGM2, Aβ$_{(1-42)}$, mitochondrial calcium influx, AhR, mtROS, ↓ LDH release	[61]
UroA	SH-SY5Y cells	transfected with the APP 695	1 µM, 10 µM treatment for 1 h or 24 h	improved mitochondrial function	↑ MMP, ATP, ROS, OXPHOS, mitochondrial biogenesis	[62]
UroA	PC12 cells	6-OHDA (150 µM) for 18 h or 24 h	2.5 µM, 5 µM, 10 mM treatment for 2 h	improved mitochondrial function	↑ cells viability, MPP PGC-1α, SIRT1, TFAM, ↓ apoptosis, ↑ APP, ↓ ROS, ↓ mitochondria damage	[63]
UroA DHA+ LUT+ UroA	BE(2)-M17 cells	oligomeric Aβ$_{1-42}$ (20 µM) for 72 h	5 µM to 40 µM pretreatment for 24 h, 5 µM (combination) pretreatment for 24 h	anti-Aβ	↑ cells viability, ↓ LDH release	[64]
UroA, UroA+ EGCG	HT22 cells	transfected with APP cDNA for 24 h	no concentration mentioned, treatment for 24 h	improved mitochondrial function	↑ mitochondrial respiration	[65]
UroA, UroA+ EGCG	HT22 cells	transfected with Tau cDNA for 24 h	1 µM or 10 mM treatment for 24 h	improved mitochondrial function	↓ Drp1 and Fis1, ↑ PGC-1α, Nrf1, Nrf2, ↑ TFAM, PINK1, Parkin, ↑ Mfn1, Mfn2, and Opa1	[66]
UroA	HT22 cells	transfected with APP cDNA for 24 h	1 µM, 2 µM, 5 µM, 10 mM treatment for 24 h	improved mitochondrial function	↓ Drp1 and Fis1, ↑ PGC-1α, Nrf1, Nrf2, ↑ TFAM, PINK1, Parkin, ↑ Mfn1, Mfn2, and Opa1	[67]

Abbreviations: dmUroC: 8,9-dimethyl-O-Urolithin C, MAO: monoamine oxidase, DPPH: 1,1-diphenyl-2-picrylhydrazyl, ROS: reactive oxygen species, CAT: catalase, GR: glutathione reductase, GSH-Px: glutathione peroxidase, LDH: Lactic dehydrogenase, Bcl-2: B-cell lymphoma-2, Bax: Bcl-2-associated X, TNF-α: tumor necrosis factor-α, iNOS: inducible nitric oxide synthase, IL-6: interleukin-6, IL-1β: interleukin-1β, IL-1: interleukin-1, COX-2: cyclooxygenase-2, PARP: poly ADP-ribose polymerase, MAPK: mitogen-activated protein kinase, REDOX: mitochondrial oxidation-reduction, PKA: protein kinase A, CREB: cAMP-response element binding protein, BDNF: brain derived neurotrophic factor, NLRP3: negative regulation of NLR family pyrin domain containing 3, PGE2: prostaglandin E2, JNK: c-Jun N-terminal kinase, LC3-II: protein light chain 3-II, PINK1: PTEN induced kinase 1, MMP: mitochondrial membrane potential, OXPHOS: oxidative phosphorylation, APP: amyloid precursor protein, TGM2: transglutaminase type 2, PGC-1α: peroxisome proliferator-activated receptor-gamma coactivator-1-alpha, AhR: aryl hydrocarbon receptor, TFAM: transcription factor A, ERK1/2: extracellular signal-regulated kinase 1/2, SIRT1: silent information regulator of transcription 1, BACE1: β-site APP cleaving enzyme-1, poly(I:C): polyinosinic-polycytidylic acid, Drp1: dynamin-related protein 1, Fis1: fission mitochondrial 1; Nrf1: nuclear respiratory factor 1, Nrf2: nuclear respiratory factor 2, Mfn1: mitofusin, Mfn2: mitofusin 2, Opa1: optic atrophy 1.

Table 2. Preclinical studies of Uros on brain aging in vivo animal models.

Uros	Animal	Pharmacological or Genetic Interventions	Route of Administration	Treatment (Dosage and Time)	Effects	Findings	Refs.
UroA	male ICR mice (4–6 weeks, 18–22 g)	D-gal 150 mg/kg/d s.c. for 8 weeks	i.g.	50, 100, 150 mg/kg b.w./day for 8 weeks	anti-brain aging, anti-inflammation, antioxidation	↑spontaneous locomotion, object recognition learning, ↓AchE, MAO, ↑SOD, CAT, GSH-Px, ↓p53/p21, TEAC, SIRT1, ↓TNF-α, IL-1β, and IL-6, ↑Bcl-2, ↓caspase 3, mTOR, ↓dysfunctional autophagy, astrocyte activation, ↓apoptosis	[17]
UroB	male C57BL/6 mice (6–8 weeks, 18–22 g)	D-gal 150 mg/kg/d s.c. for 8 weeks	i.g.	50, 100, 150 mg/kg b.w./day for 8 weeks	anti-brain aging, anti-inflammation, antioxidation	↓cognitive deficits, ↑pAkt, ↑hippocampal LTP, ↑CAT, GSH-Px, TEAC, SOD, ↓MDA, ↓TNF-α, IL-6, IL-1β, AGEs, cytotoxicity, ↓the activation of microglia and astrocytes, ↓AchE, ↑number of neuron, ↓MAO	[57]
UroA	female APP/PS1 transgenic mice (28 weeks)	transgenic AD mice	i.g.	300 mg/kg b.w./day for 14 days	anti-inflammation	↓spatial learning deficits, ↑neurogenesis, ↓neuronal apoptosis, ↓reactive gliosis, ↓Aβ, IL-1β, TNF-α, ↑AMPK, ↓p-P65, NF-κB, p-P38, MAPK, BACE1	[22]
UroA	APP/PS1 transgenic mice (13 months) C.elegans	transgenic AD mice	i.g.	200 mg/kg b.w./day for 1 month or 0.1 mM (C.elegans)	anti-inflammation	↑learning and memory retention, ↑OCR, ↓ROS, ↓Aβ$_{1-40}$, Aβ$_{1-42}$, ↑IL-10, ↓autophagy, ↓IL-6, TNF-α, ↓NLRP3, IL-1β, ↓p-tau, caspase 1	[68]
UroA	CX3CR1-Cre mice	MPTP 15 mg/kg/d, i.p. 4 times a day every 2 h	i.g.	20 mg/kg b.w./day for 7 days	anti-inflammation	↓motor deficits, ↑TH, ↓caspase 1, NLRP3, ↓astrogliosis	[14]

Table 2. Cont.

Uros	Animal	Pharmacological or Genetic Interventions	Route of Administration	Treatment (Dosage and Time)	Effects	Findings	Refs.
UroB	Male ICR mice (7 weeks, 2–37 g)	LPS 5 mg/kg/d, i.p.	i.p.	50 mg/kg b.w./day for 4 days	anti-inflammation	↓ microglia activation, ↓ NADPH, Akt, JNK, ERK, ↑ AMPK, HO-1	[58]
UroA	male C57BL/6J mice (8–10 weeks)	6-OHDA 9 μg	i.p.	10 mg/kg b.w./day for 7 days	improved mitochondria function	↓ neurotoxicity, mitochondria damage, OXPHOS, ↑ PGC-1α, TFAM, ↑ SIRT1	[63]
UroA	mice	STZ 75 mg/kg/d i.p. for 3 days	i.p.	2.5 mg/kg b.w./day for 8 weeks	anti-Aβ, improved mitochondria function	↓ APP, BACE1, p-tau, Aβ$_{(1-42)}$, TGM2	[61]
UroA UroB mUroA mUroB	C. elegans	transgenic AD C. elegans (CL4176)	feeding	10 μg/mL pretreatment for 20 h	anti-Aβ	↑ C. elegans survival and mobility	[69]
UroA UroA + EGCG	hAbKI mice (3 months)	humanized homozygous Aβ knockin (hAbKI) AD mice	i.p.	UroA 2.5 mg/kg b.w., EGCG 25 mg/kg b.w., 3 times per week for 4 months	anti-Aβ, improved mitochondria function	↑ mitochondrial fusion, synaptic, ↓ Aβ$_{(1-40)}$ and Aβ$_{(1-42)}$, ↑ mitophagy, autophagy genes, ↓ mitochondrial fission genes, mitochondrial dysfunction, ↓ fragmented dendritic spines, ↓ mitochondria number, ↑ mitochondrial length, mitophagosomal formations	[65]
UroA	male C57BL/6J mice (5 weeks, 18–22 g)	STZ 30 mg/kg b.w./day i.p. for 4 days	i.g.	200 mg/kg b.w.	anti-brain aging, anti-inflammation	↓ hyperglycemia, ↑ learning and memory, ↓ IL-6, IL-1β, TNF-α, IL-1β, COX-2, iNOS-2, ↑ IL-10, ↓ NLRP3	[70]

Abbreviations: i.p.: intraperitoneal, s.c.: subcuta, i.g.: intragastrical, b.w.: body weight, AchE: acetylcholinesterase, MAO: monoamine oxidase, SOD: superoxide dismutase, CAT: catalase, GSH-Px: glutathione peroxidase, AGEs: advanced glycation end products, NADPH: triphosphopyridine nucleotide, TEAC: Trolox-equivalent antioxidant capacity, SIRT1: silent information regulator of transcription 1, TNF-α: tumor necrosis factor-α, iNOS: inducible nitric oxide synthase, IL-6: interleukin-6, IL-1β: interleukin-1β, IL-1: interleukin-1, COX-2: cyclooxygenase-2, Bcl-2: B-cell lymphoma-2, LTP: long-term potentiation, NLRP3: negative regulation of NLR family pyrin domain containing 3, MDA: malondialdehyde, BACE1: β-site APP cleaving enzyme-1, OCR: oxygen consumption rate, TH: tyrosine hydroxylase, HO-1: heme oxygenase 1, TFAM: transcription factor A, STZ: streptozotocin, TGM2: transglutaminase type 2.

Table 3. Clinical studies of Uro precursors on brain aging.

Source	Subjects	Clinical Trial Procedure	Treatment (Dosage and Time)	Effects	Fundings	Refs
Pomegranate juice	Age: 54–72 years; Cognition and memory: age-related memory decline; Other heath state: no neurological, psychiatric and major medical conditions	Randomized, placebo controlled, double blind trial	Dosage: 240 mL/day of pomegranate juice ($n = 15$) or placebo drink ($n = 13$) Time: 4 weeks	anti-age-related memory decline	↑fMRI activity during verbal and visual memory tasks, ↑memory ability, ↑plasma antioxidant status	[42]
Pomegranate juice	Age: 50–75 years; Cognition and memory: age-related memory decline; other heath state: no cerebrovascular disease, neurological or physical illnesses associated with cognitive deterioration	Randomized, placebo controlled, double blind trial	Dosage: 236.5 mL/day of pomegranate juice ($n = 98$) or placebo drink ($n = 102$) Time: 48 weeks	anti-age-related memory decline	↑visual memory, ↑visual learning and recall, ↑verbal memory, words recall	[49]
Nuts	Age: 55–80 years; Cognition and memory: healthy; other heath state: no diabetes, smoking, hypertension, dyslipidemia, overweight and cardiovascular disease	Randomized, placebo controlled trial	Dosage: MedDiet + EVOO 1 L/week ($n = 224$); MedDiet + nuts 30 g/day ($n = 166$; or low-fat diet ($n = 132$) Time: 6.5 years	anti-age-related memory decline	↑orientation to time and place, ↑registration, attention and calculation, ↑recall, language, and visual construction, ↑visuospatial abilities, working memory, attention, ↑abstract thinking, language comprehension	[71]
Walnuts	Age: 63–79 years; Cognition and memory: healthy; other heath state: no neurodegenerative disease, stroke, head trauma, brain surgery, psychiatric illness, depression, obesity, diabetes, hypertension and chemotherapy	Randomized controlled trial	Dosage: Walnuts 30–60 g/day ($n = 336$) or control diet (abstention from walnuts) ($n = 321$) Time: 2 years	anti-age-related memory decline	↑global cognition and perception	[51]
Strawberry	Age: 60–75 years; Cognition and memory: age-related motor and cognitive decline; other heath state: BMI (18.5–29.9), no psychological or psychiatric disorders and chronic disease	Randomized, placebo controlled, double blind trial	Dosage: Strawberry 24 g/day ($n = 18$) or placebo ($n = 19$) Time: 45 or 90 days	anti-age-related memory decline	↑words recalled, verbal learning	[72]

Table 3. Cont.

Source	Subjects	Clinical Trial Procedure	Treatment (Dosage and Time)	Effects	Fundings	Refs
Mixture of berries	Age: 50–70 years; Cognition and memory: healthy; other heath state: no metabolic disorders, food allergies and, gastrointestinal disorder	Randomized cross-over trial	Dosage: mixture of berries (150 g blueberries, 50 g blackcurrant, 50 g elderberry, 50 g lingonberries, 50 g strawberry, and 100 g tomatoes/day) (n = 20); or placebo drink (n = 21) Time: 5 weeks	anti-age-related memory decline	↑verbal working memory, ↑ selective attention, ↓total- and LDL cholesterol, ↑insulin concentrations	[73]
Grape and blueberry extract	Age: 60–70 years; Cognition and memory: age-related memory decline; other heath state: no metabolic disorders and diabetes BMI (20–30)	Randomized, placebo controlled, double blind trial	Dosage: grape and blueberry extract 600 mg/day (n = 91) or placebo (n = 98) Time: 6 months	anti-age-related memory decline	↑verbal episodic, ↑recognition memory, ↑working memory	[74]
Blueberry and blueberry extract	Age: 65–80 years; Cognition and memory: age-related memory decline; other heath state: no metabolic disorders and diabetes	Randomized, placebo controlled, double blind trial	Dosage: blueberry 500 mg/day (n = 28); blueberry 1000 mg/day (n = 29); blueberry extract 111 mg/day (n = 28); or placebo (n = 27) Time: 6 months	anti-age-related memory decline	↑word recognition, ↑total number of sequences correctly recalled, ↓ systolic blood pressure	[75]
Blueberry	Age: >65 years; Cognition and memory: age-related memory decline other heath state: healthy	Pilot, single-blind, one-arm trial	Dosage: blueberry 444 mL/day (weighing 54–64 kg); 532 mL/day (weighing 54–64 kg); 621 mL/day (weighing 77–91 kg); (n = 9) Time: 12 weeks	anti-age-related memory decline; antidepressant	↑paired associate learning, ↑word list recall, ↓depressive symptoms, ↓ fasting glucose levels	[50]

Table 3. Cont.

Source	Subjects	Clinical Trial Procedure	Treatment (Dosage and Time)	Effects	Fundings	Refs
Blueberry	Age: <65 years; Cognition and memory: healthy other heath state: no contraindications to fMRI	Randomized, placebo controlled, double blind trial	Dosage: blueberry 30 mL/day ($n = 12$) or placebo drink ($n = 14$) Time: 12 weeks	anti-age-related memory decline	↑ brain perfusion and activation, ↑ psychomotor function, visual processing, executive function, verbal and spatial memory	[52]
Blueberry	Age: 62–80 years; Cognition and memory: age-related memory decline; other heath state: no diabetes, kidney disease, liver disease, hematological coagulation disorder	Randomized, parallel groups, placebo controlled, double blind trial	Dosage: fish oil (1.6 g EPA + 0.8 g DHA/day) ($n = 15$); blueberry 25 g/day ($n = 16$); fish oil + blueberry 24 g/day ($n = 17$); or placebo ($n = 17$) Time: 24 weeks	anti-age-related memory decline	↑ psychomotor speed, working memory, ↑ lexical access, ↑ long-term memory	[53]
Frozen blueberry	Age: 60–75 years; Cognition and memory: healthy; other heath state: BMI (18.5–29.9), no smoking or use of medications	Randomized, placebo controlled, double blind trial	Dosage: frozen blueberry 24 g/day ($n = 19$) or placebo ($n = 19$) Time: 90 days	anti-age-related memory decline	↑ executive function, ↑ long-term memory, short term memory, ↑ spatial cognition, and attention	[76]
Frozen blueberry	Age: 68–92 years; Cognition and memory: age-related memory decline; other heath state: no serious psychiatric disorder, substance abuse, and claustrophobia	Randomized, placebo controlled, double blind trial	Dosage: frozen blueberry 25 g/day ($n = 8$) or placebo ($n = 8$) Time: 16 weeks	anti-age-related memory decline	↑ working memory, accuracy, ↑ blood oxygen level dependent activation	[77]
Frozen blueberry	Age: >68 years; Cognition and memory: age-related memory decline; other heath state: no dementia, serious psychiatric condition, substance abuse	Randomized, placebo controlled, double blind trial	Dosage: frozen blueberry 24 g/day ($n = 16$) or placebo 20 g/day ($n = 21$) Time: 16 weeks	anti-age-related memory decline	↑ lexical access for semantic information, ↑ speed of processing and working memory, ↑ verbal and nonverbal long-term memory	[78]

Abbreviations: fMRI: functional magnetic resonance imaging, BMI: body mass index, EVOO: extra-virgin olive oil, MedDiet: Mediterranean diet, LDL: low-density lipoprotein, EPA: eicosapentaenoic acid, DHA: docosahexaenoic acid.

4. Mechanisms of Action

The beneficial effects of Uros on brain function during aging are associated with multi-target actions that involve relieving chronic oxidative stress and inflammation, promoting mitophagy and mitochondrial function, inhibiting amyloid-β (Aβ) and tau pathology, and regulating tryptophan (Trp) metabolism. The mechanisms are summarized in Figure 1.

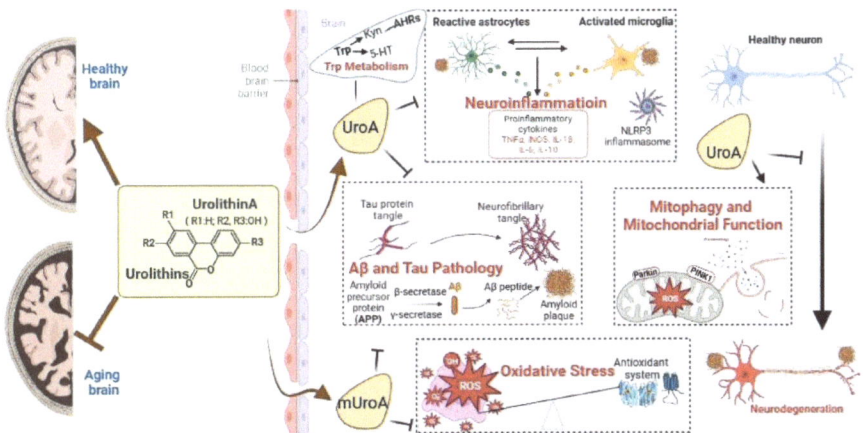

Figure 1. Outline of effects of UroA on brain aging (actions and mechanisms). The mechanisms of UroA on aging brain mainly focus on promoting mitophagy and mitochondrial function and relieving neuroinflammation. Other mechanisms include mitigating oxidative stress, inhibiting Aβ and tau pathology, and regulating Trp metabolism. Although UroA has been shown to activate anti-aging signaling pathways such as AMPK, SIRTs, and mTOR in vivo, the direct or key targets of UroA have not been fully elucidated.

4.1. Antioxidant Activity in CNS

As the brain consumes more than one-fifth of the total oxygen, the oxidative stress exerted by reactive oxygen species (ROS) and related degeneration is particularly severe in the brain owing to aging. Damage to neural cells occurs when ROS production overwhelms the antioxidant defense mechanisms. Endogenous antioxidant defenses in the brain are relatively low compared to those in other vital organs [79,80]. This makes the protection of antioxidants, which can pass through the BBB, particularly important for the progression of brain aging. Although ETs and EA cannot cross the BBB, Uros are potent antioxidants with good BBB permeability [36,69].

First, UroA and UroB are evidenced as direct radical scavengers (details listed in Table 4) [54,57]. Furthermore, cell models have shown that UroA and UroB protected neuron-like cells from direct H_2O_2-induced damage, including PC12 cells, SK-N-MC cells, SH-SY5Y cells, and Neuro-2a cells, in which they effectively inhibited ROS formation and lipid peroxidation [17,20,54,55,57,81]. Moreover, Uros can boost endogenous antioxidant defenses in neuronal cells and brains of aged mice. Data from an array of studies have shown that UroA and UroB increased the activity of antioxidant enzymes, including catalase, superoxide dismutase, glutathione reductase, and glutathione peroxidase [58,82]. UroA increases the expression of cytoprotective peroxiredoxins 1 and 3 in Neuro-2a cells [54]. A study on UroB demonstrated that pretreatment with UroB significantly decreased the mRNA expression of nicotinamide adenine dinucleotide phosphate oxidase subunits ($p47^{phox}$ and $gp91^{phox}$) and increased the antioxidant hemeoxygenase-1 expression via nuclear factor erythroid-2 related factor 2/antioxidant response element signaling in lipopolysaccharide (LPS)-treated BV2 cells [58].

Table 4. IC$_{50}$ of Uros and corresponding references on synthetic and oxygen free radicals.

Sample	Superoxide Radical [1]	DPPH Radical	Peroxyl Radicals [2]	ABTS Radical	Hydroxyl Radical
UroA	5.01 ± 5.01 µM	152.66 ± 35.01 µM	13.1 µM	---	---
Gallic acid	0.26 ± 0.21 µM	3.10 ± 3.11 µM	---	---	---
Ascorbic acid	---	14.81 ± 14.90 µM	---	---	---
Pomegranate extracts	---	---	0.49 µM	---	---
UroB	495.32 ± 3.28 mM	295.41 ± 2.36 mM	---	316.18 ± 1.85 mM	306.28 ± 4.61 mM
Ascorbic acid	874.39 ± 1.48 mM	446.25 ± 1.78 mM	---	526.24 ± 3.18 mM	540.16 ± 2.52 mM

IC$_{50}$ is expressed as mean ± SD, and data for peroxyl radicals are expressed as µmol Trolox equivalents per mg of sample. [1] UroA scavenges superoxide radicals generated by the xanthine/xanthine oxidase system. [2] The capacity of UroA to scavenge peroxyl radicals was measured by the oxygen radical antioxidant capacity (ORAC).

Additionally, Uros are inhibitors of several oxidases (pro-oxidant enzymes) that can promote ROS formation. It is shown that Uros inhibited the activity of monoamine oxidase (MAO), which is responsible for the metabolism of monoamine neurotransmitters such as serotonin and dopamine [54,57,83]. A recent study demonstrated that Uros (A, B, and C) were selective inhibitors of human MAO-A (rather than MAO-B), and UroB was the strongest inhibitor with the IC$_{50}$ of 0.88 ± 0.24 µM (the IC$_{50}$ of UroA and UroC was 5.88 ± 0.69 µM and 29.6 ± 1.8 µM, respectively), whereas EA had no effect on MAO-A [83]. Clinically, MAO inhibitors may alleviate the symptoms of depression and Parkinson's disease (PD). Therefore, these findings may suggest the potential benefits of Uros for related disorders. Saha et al. reported that UroA significantly inhibited heme peroxidase activity, including myeloperoxidase and lactoperoxidase in in vitro and in vivo models [84], which may provide a better understanding of the peroxidase inhibitory and anti-inflammatory activities of UroA.

The antioxidant effects of Uros are beyond the traditional antioxidant activities of their precursors. ETs and EA are typical antioxidants, which are mainly attributed to their potent free radical scavenging activity, including a wide variety of ROS and reactive nitrogen species [85,86]. As the bioavailability of ETs and EA is poor, the high antioxidant capacity of dietary ETs and EA may be important and restricted mostly to local actions in the GI tract [25,87]. González-Sarrías et al. suggested a lower neuroprotective activity of Uros against oxidative stress-induced cell death than that of their precursors [20,59]. It appears that Uros are not as potent antioxidants as their precursors, at least in vitro, and may systemically exert their antioxidant activity. Recently, we found that UroA (5, 10 µM) treatment significantly increased protein kinase A (PKA)/cAMP-response element binding protein (CREB)/brain derived neurotrophic factor (BDNF) neurotrophic signaling pathway in H$_2$O$_2$-treated SH-SY5Y cells, and pretreatment with PKA inhibitor H89 abolished the protective effects of UroA in H$_2$O$_2$-treated SH-SY5Y cells [56]. These results indicated that PKA/CREB/BDNF neurotrophic signaling pathway might involve the neuroprotective effect of UroA against oxidative stress.

4.2. Mitigation of Neuroinflammatioin

Chronic inflammation caused by innate immune cells such as glia is thought to play a key role in brain aging and related diseases. Glial activation and the release of inflammatory molecules such as proinflammatory cytokines are hallmarks of chronic inflammation in the brain. Mitigating neuroinflammation is one of the most important mechanisms underlying the health benefits of Uros.

It has been well documented that UroA and UroB significantly attenuated the inflammation induced by LPS in mouse microglia BV2 cells, including inhibiting the production of NO and the expression of inducible nitric oxide synthase (iNOS) and cyclo-oxygenase-2 (COX-2), regulating the levels of proinflammatory cytokines such as interleukin (IL)-6, IL-1β, tumor necrosis factor-α (TNF-α), and anti-inflammatory cytokines such as IL-10 [19,21,58,60,88]. In addition to LPS, Lee et al. reported that UroB significantly inhibited lipoteichoic acid (LTA)- and polyinosinic-polycytidylic acid (poly(I:C))-induced inflammation in BV2 cells, which are known as toll-like receptor (TLR) 2 and TLR3 agonists, respectively [58]. These results suggested that the anti-inflammatory effect of UroB is not confined to LPS stimulation. Moreover, UroA can induce M2 polarization from the M1 state in microglia and other macrophage-like cells which can subsequently inhibit pro-inflammatory cytokines generation and promote neuroprotection [59,89]. Animal studies have shown that the administration of UroA and UroB could significantly improve behavioral deficits and neuroinflammation in D-galactose-induced aged mice, transgenic APP/PS1 mice, LPS-brain-injected mice, and 1-methyl-4-phenyl-1,2,3,6-tetrahydropyridine (MPTP)-induced PD mice, including decreasing the level of pro-inflammatory cytokines in the brain and inhibiting the activation of microglia and astrocytes in the hippocampus and cortex [14,17,22,57,58]. In addition, UroA was evidenced to reduce the expression and activity of the NACHT, LRR, and PYD domains-containing protein 3 (NLRP3) inflammasome in LPS-treated BV2 cells and mouse models (APP/PS1 mice and MPTP-treated mice) [30,68].

Multiple proteins and signaling pathways such as adenosine monophosphate (AMP)-dependent kinase (AMPK), mitogen-activated protein kinase (MAPK), nuclear factor-κB (NF-κB), and silent information regulator of transcription 1 (SIRT1) are considered to participate in the anti-inflammatory effects of Uros [58,68,88–94]. The NF-κB pathway is the best-studied inflammatory signaling pathway and is thought to be critical for the synthesis and effects of pro-inflammatory cytokines. An experiment in LPS-induced BV2 cells showed that UroA and UroB significantly inhibited NF-κB p65 expression and nuclear translocation in a dose-dependent manner and that UroB displayed more potent inhibitory activity than UroA [60]. AMPK, a central regulator of energy and metabolism involved in the pathophysiology of aging and age-related diseases, plays an important role in chronic inflammation. AMPK activation exerts anti-inflammatory effects by regulating cytokine synthesis and multiple inflammatory signaling pathways, such as NF-κB and MAPK pathways [95–97]. Moreover, AMPK signaling regulates NLRP3 inflammasome formation and activation during aging [98]. In addition to its established role in inflammation, AMPK activation has recently been implicated in promoting microglial M2 polarization, thereby relieving brain inflammation [99]. Experiments in cell and animal models have indicated that AMPK activation is tightly involved in the anti-inflammatory effects of Uros. In LPS-treated BV2 cells, UroB increases AMPK phosphorylation and decreases the phosphorylation of its downstream molecules Akt, JNK, and ERK [58,60]. In APP/PS1 mice, Zhuo et al. found that UroA treatment significantly upregulated AMPK signaling and downregulated NF-κB and MAPK signaling in the cortex and hippocampus, which was responsible for the improvement of memory and neuroinflammation [22]. SIRT1, a histone deacetylase, plays a key role in regulating neuroinflammation and the release of pro-inflammatory cytokines [100–103]. SIRT1 activation inhibits NF-κB signaling by involving deacetylation of the p65 subunit [104]. A study on UroA showed that treatment with UroA (5 and 10 μM) significantly increased the level (nuclear) and the activity (cell) of SIRT1 in BV2 cells, and the anti-inflammatory effect of UroA was abolished in the presence of EX527, a SIRT1 inhibitor, suggesting that the activation of SIRT1 is required for the anti-inflammatory effect of UroA [21].

Additionally, to compare the anti-inflammatory effect of UroA and its precursors, Ashley et al. investigated the difference between whole red raspberry polyphenols (RRW) and UroA in BV-2 cells under 3 h, 12 h, and 24 h inflammatory conditions (LPS and ATP treatment). The results demonstrated that RRW only inhibited the inflammation induced by 3 h of LPS stimulation, whereas UroA inhibited the inflammation caused by LPS treatments (3, 12, and 24 h). Moreover, the anti-inflammatory effects of RRW and UroA were both mediated by downregulation of the JNK/c-Jun pathway [59].

4.3. Promotion of Mitophagy and Mitochondrial Function

The brain possesses high mitochondrial activity to meet its relatively high energy demands. Mitochondrial dysfunction, including the abnormalities of mitochondrial bioenergetics, mitochondrial biogenesis, and autophagy in neurons, accumulate during aging. An increasing number of studies have indicated that the maintenance of mitochondrial homeostasis is particularly important for brain function in the elderly and may be a potential therapeutic strategy for age-related neurodegenerative diseases. Accumulating evidence suggests that UroA is an important regulator of mitochondrial homeostasis, particularly a robust mitophagy inducer, which seems to be one of the crucial mechanisms underlying its health benefits against aging [61,105]. Ryu et al. were the first to report that UroA extended the lifespan of *C. elegans* and improved muscle function in mice through mitophagy activation [106]. Recently, an increasing number of clinical trials have confirmed the impact of UroA on mitophagy in humans. Results from two clinical trials in elderly individuals demonstrated that supplementation with UroA at doses of 500 mg and 1000 mg daily for 4 weeks or 4 months significantly improved mitophagy and mitochondrial biogenesis in skeletal muscles [37]. Moreover, another recent clinical trial in middle-aged adults showed that supplementation with UroA increased mitophagy proteins and reduced inflammation [38]. Fang et al. conducted a systematic study on the promotion of mitophagy by UroA and found that mitophagy induction underlies the multiple actions of UroA in the brain, including the improvement of cognition and memory deficits, the alleviation of chronic neuroinflammation, and the inhibition of Aβ and tau pathology [68,107]. In vitro study demonstrated that UroA increased the levels of a series of mitophagy-related proteins, including phosphatase and tensin homolog deleted on chromosome ten induced kinase 1 (PINK1), Parkinson's disease-related-1, beclin-1, Bcl-2-like protein 13, activating molecule in BECN1-regulated autophagy protein 1, and serine/threonine-protein kinase ULK1 (ULK1) in human neuronal SH-SY5Y cells. Moreover, UroA inhibited the phosphorylation of tau (p-tau) in a mitophagy-dependent manner, and the inhibitory effect was diminished in PINK1 or ULK1 knockdown cells. Consistently, in vivo studies showed that UroA activated neuronal mitophagy and reduced mtROS levels and mitochondrial damage in the hippocampus and prefrontal cortex of APP/PS1 mice, and mitophagy induction was also required for memory improvement of UroA in tau transgenic *C. elegans* and mice [68]. More recently, a study in humanized homozygous Aβ knockin (hAbKI) mice of late-onset AD demonstrated that UroA administration for 4 months significantly improved phenotypic behavior changes and mitochondrial dysfunction, including mitochondrial bioenergetics, biogenesis, and mitophagy [65].

Similar to neuronal cells, UroA promotes mitophagy and improves mitochondrial dysfunction in microglial cells. Treatment with the autophagy inhibitor 3-methyladenine abolished the effect of UroA on mitochondrial dysfunction and inflammation in LPS-treated BV2 cells [14,21]. Studies in animals demonstrated that mitophagy in microglial cells decreased by 60% in the hippocampus of AD mice, whereas UroA treatment normalized the decreased mitophagy, thereby increasing the phagocytic efficiency of microglia and the removal of Aβ plaques [68]. Similarly, UroA reduced the elevated expression and activity of NLRP3 and related neuroinflammation in AD mice by inducing mitophagy in the microglia. Moreover, using Atg5flox/flox:CX3CR1-Cre mice to block microglial mitophagy in vivo, the improvement in behavioral deficits and neuroinflammation induced by UroA in PD mice was diminished [14].

However, studies on the autophagy and mitophagy of UroA have also yielded conflicting results. Research conducted by Esselun et al. revealed that UroA did not affect mitophagy in SH-SY5Y-APP695 cells but moderately promoted mitochondrial biogenesis [62]. Another recent study indicated UroA induced robust neuronal mitophagy but did not increase neuronal macroautophagy in transgenic nematodes [68]. Additionally, Ahsan et al. demonstrated that UroA activated autophagy but not mitophagy in ischemia/reperfusion injured neuronal cells and mice [108].

Studies have indicated that UroA activated autophagy and mitophagy by regulating several key signaling molecules, including AMPK, peroxisome proliferator-activated receptor-gamma coactivator-1-alpha (PGC-1α), and SIRT, and inhibition of the mammalian target of rapamycin (mTOR). These signaling pathways stimulate mitophagy and mitochondrial biogenesis and are regulated by Uros. As discussed in the anti-inflammatory section, AMPK is one of the most important targets in aging and has been well documented in age-related mitochondrial dysfunction [109–111]. The downregulation of AMPK activity during aging impairs metabolic regulation, increases oxidative stress, and reduces autophagic clearance [98]. Activated AMPK increases PGC-1α level, which directly increases mitochondrial biogenesis [112]. The key autophagy/mitophagy effectors, such as SIRT, mTOR, and ULK1, are all downstream molecules of AMPK signaling [113–115]. Moreover, SIRT can deacetylate and activate liver kinase B1 (LKB1), an upstream kinase that activates AMPK [116]. Recent studies have demonstrated that Uros activate AMPK activity in a variety of cell types in vitro, including microglia, macrophages, and nucleus pulposus cells [22,58,117], as well as in multiple tissues in vivo, including the brain, muscle, and pancreas [92,118,119], indicating that Uros may be an AMPK activator. Therefore, AMPK may be a crucial target underlying the beneficial effects of Uros on aging, which requires further investigation.

Additionally, UroA activates SIRT1 and SIRT3. UroA stimulates SIRT3 promoter activity in Caco-2 cells [120] and increases ATP and NAD+ levels, leading to activation of the SIRT1-PGC-1α pathway in murine muscle [121]. Moreover, Chen et al. reported that UroA improved impaired autophagy in D-galactose-induced mice by upregulating SIRT1 signaling and downregulating mTOR signaling, and these effects appear to be mediated by the activation of miR-34a [17]. Treatment with both SIRT1 inhibitor EX527 and autophagy inhibitor chloroquine abolished the neuroprotective effect of UroA in APPSwe-transfected ReNcell VM human neural cells, as well as the anti-inflammatory effect of UroA in LPS-treated BV2 cells [21]. SIRT1 increases mitofusin 2 (Mfn2) and Parkin levels during mitophagy activation [122,123], and UroA has been shown to increase Mfn2 and Parkin expression in humans after 4 weeks of administration [37]. In addition, UroA activates autophagy by inhibiting endoplasmic reticulum (ER) stress in cell and mouse models of ischemic neuronal injury [62]. In summary, mitophagy deficiency and subsequent mitochondrial dysfunctions are early and pivotal events in brain aging and neurodegenerative diseases, and mitophagy or autophagy induction seems to be a crucial mechanism in the effects of Uros.

4.4. Inhibition of Aβ and Tau Pathology

Abnormal accumulation of Aβ and neurofibrillary tangles of p-tau protein are hallmark features of AD. It has been well documented that Aβ deposition in the brain occurs approximately two decades before the onset of the disease. Several studies have shown that Uros inhibited Aβ deposition and p-tau generation during brain aging [22,61,68,69]. The thioflavin T (ThT) binding assay in vitro showed that UroA, UroB, methyl-UroA (mUroA), and mUroB inhibited Aβ fibrillation including Aβ fibril content, β-sheet formation, and peptide oligomerization, whereas only mUroB reversed the neurotoxicity and muscular paralysis in the $Aβ_{1-42}$-induced *C. elegans* model of AD [69]. A more recent study in vitro demonstrated that UroA inhibited $Aβ_{1-42}$-induced toxicity in human neuroblastoma BE(2)-M17 cells [64]. In transgenic APP/PS1 AD mice, immunohistochemistry and ELIAS results demonstrated that UroA treatment significantly decreased $Aβ_{1-40}$ and $Aβ_{1-42}$ plaques in the cortex and hippocampus [22]. Moreover, UroA administration for 4 months significantly reduced the levels of $Aβ_{1-40}$ and $Aβ_{1-42}$, and improved inflammation, synaptic structure, and function in the brain of hAbKI AD mice [65]. In a further study conducted by Fang et al., UroA treatment restored memory impairment in both Aβ nematodes expressing pan-neuronal human $Aβ_{1-42}$ (CL2355) protein and tau nematodes expressing pan-neuronal tau fragments (BR5270) [68]. Aβ plaque formation is a result of imbalance between Aβ clearance and its production from amyloid precursor protein (APP), and cleavage of APP by β-site APP cleaving enzyme-1 (BACE-1) is responsible for Aβ production. Although the precursors of Uros, such as EA and punicalagin, have been reported to inhibit the activity of BACE1 [124,125], UroA was shown to decrease only the expression of BACE1 in mice, and the effects of UroA on APP expression are inconsistent [61,62]. Additionally, microglia play a crucial role in the clearance of extracellular Aβ plaques [126,127]. In a study by Fang, UroA administration enhanced the removal of insoluble $Aβ_{1-42}$ and $Aβ_{1-40}$ proteins in the hippocampus of APP/PS1 mice by increasing the phagocytic efficiency of microglia, whereas no significant effect on the levels of APP cleavage intermediates was observed, suggesting that APP proteolysis may not be the target of UroA. Furthermore, the study also revealed that UroA treatment inhibited the phosphorylation of tau at Thr181, Ser202/Thr205, and Ser262 in tau-overexpressing human SH-SY5Y cells. Consistently, UroA administration inhibited p-tau and improved memory impairment in the 3×Tg AD mice [68]. More recently, Tu et al. showed that dual-specific tyrosine phosphorylation-regulated kinase 1A (DYRK1A) is the main target of UroA in its anti-AD effect. UroA significantly inhibited the activity of DYRK1A, which led to the de-phosphorylation of tau and further stabilized microtubule polymerization [128].

Hyperglycemia and diabetes are risk factors for neurodegeneration and critical contributors to amyloidogenesis. Uros were shown to improve diabetes-associated neurodegeneration. Lee et al. systematically studied and reported that UroA attenuated the amyloidogenesis and neurodegeneration in a diabetes model. Their experiments in vitro showed that pretreatment with UroA significantly decreased high glucose-induced $Aβ_{1-42}$ formation, as well as APP and BACE1 expression in both SH-SY5Y cells and human iPSC-derived neuronal differentiated cells. Furthermore, the experiments in vivo showed that UroA injection at dose of 2.5 mg/kg for 8 weeks improved cognitive impairment in streptozotocin-induced diabetic mice and decreased the levels of $Aβ_{1-42}$, APP, BACE1, and p-tau (Ser262 and Ser396) in the prefrontal cortex and hippocampus [61]. In addition, Chen et al. reported that UroB supplementation improved learning and memory impairment by inhibiting the accumulation of advanced glycation end products in the brain of aged mice [57]. Xiao et al. found that UroA relieved diabetes-associated cognitive impairment and neuroinflammation by alleviating intestinal barrier dysfunction via N-glycan biosynthesis pathway [70].

4.5. Regulation of Trp Metabolism

Recent studies have indicated that the regulation of Trp metabolism may be a novel mechanism underlying the health benefits of UroA against brain aging. Trp metabolism is an important communication strategy in the "microbiome–gut–brain" axis, in which both host and gut microbiota are involved. Trp metabolites can serve as neurotransmitters and signaling molecules in CNS. Although it is well known that Trp is used for the synthesis of serotonin, a large majority of Trp (>95%) is metabolized by the kynurenine (Kyn) pathway, thus producing bioactive metabolites with distinct activities in CNS. In humans, the activity of Kyn pathway increases with age [129]. Several lines of evidence suggest that the imbalance in Trp metabolism is associated with various neurodegenerative and neurological diseases [130,131]. Trp metabolites can control the pathogenic activities of microglia and astrocytes via aryl hydrocarbon receptors (AhRs), and further inhibit neuroinflammation and neurodegeneration [132,133]. A recent study showed that oral administration of EA and UroA for 8 weeks significantly regulated the microbial composition and Trp metabolism in DBA/2J mice fed with a high-fat and high-sucrose diet. Both UroA and EA supplementation reduced the Kyn pathway, and UroA significantly decreased the level of indole sulfate in serum [134]. Additionally, UroA elevated Trp hydroxylase-2 transcription, the rate-limiting enzyme in Trp metabolism to serotonin, and subsequently increased serotonin production in differentiated rat serotonergic raphe cells [135]. Therefore, the regulation of UroA on Trp metabolism may be an important mechanism underlying its beneficial effect, but this has not been clarified and deserves further research.

4.6. Others

Uros have been evidenced to exert neuroprotection by direct action on estrogen receptors (ERs) [136,137] and AhRs [138] in the brain. They are considered as "enterophytoestrogens", which are microflora-derived metabolites with estrogenic and/or antiestrogenic activities [139,140]. Furthermore, UroA has demonstrated high selectivity on ERα and has recently been reported to regulate ERα-dependent gene expression in endometrial cancer cells [141]. AhRs are ligand-activated transcription factors involved in multiple physiological and pathological processes. In addition to indirectly regulating AhRs through Trp metabolites, UroA has been evidenced as a human-selective AhR antagonist [142,143], which is considered to mediate its anti-inflammatory activity. Additionally, UroA can alleviate BBB dysfunction [144].

Although these studies have clarified the effects of Uros from different aspects, they are relatively isolated from each other. The key targets and intracellular signaling pathways underlying the effects of Uros on aging brain remain to be elucidated. Recently, pharmaceutical studies have been conducted on Uros. Several natural and synthetic Uro analogs exhibit inhibitory effects on various enzymes, including cholinesterases, MAO-B, and cyclooxygenases [145,146]. Therefore, Uros may be multi-target agents against neurodegenerative and neurological diseases.

5. Knowledge Gaps

First, clinical evidence for Uros or UroA on age-related cognitive decline or neurodegenerative diseases is still unclear. UroA has been designated as GRAS by FDA in 2018 and sold as an ingredient of anti-aging products in USA. Growing clinical evidence has demonstrated that precursors of Uros including pomegranate, blueberry, and walnut supplementation significantly improved age-related brain dysfunctions (Table 3). The specific advantages of UroA in preventing brain aging is mainly based on (i) good safety and tolerance, (ii) favorable blood–brain barrier permeability and selective brain distribution, (iii) the accumulating evidence from preclinical studies, (iv) the different capacities for producing Uros between individuals and the decreased capacities in the elderly, and (v) overcoming limitations and deficiencies of microbiome-based treatment. Therefore, clinical trials of UroA supplementation on cognitive and memory decline in the elderly should be carried out as soon as possible, which seem to be the crucial obstacle on the way to its application.

Second, the pharmacokinetic features of UroA (pharmacokinetic research of Uros is mainly focused on UroA) in the brain have not been clarified. UroA is easily absorbed after oral administration and mainly metabolized to UroA glucuronide, UroA sulfate, and mUroA. Studies in rodents have shown that UroA and mUroA are detectable in the brain after administration of UroA or pomegranate juice [147]. The Uro metabolites identified in the brain are summarized in Table 5. A recent study depicted a more detailed profile of UroA in the brain, in which the concentration of UroA increased slowly after 0–3 h of oral administration (UroA, 200 mg/kg) and reached the maximum concentration (Cmax) at approximately 28 ng/g and 35 ng/g in the cortex and hippocampus, respectively, after 4 h (Tmax) of oral administration. In contrast, the Cmax and Tmax of UroA in plasma were 15 ng/mL and 2 h, respectively [148]. This study is the first to report that UroA was detectable in the specific brain regions (cortex and hippocampus) and remained at high levels for hours after a single oral administration. However, more detailed pharmacokinetic parameters should be determined and investigated.

Third, the therapeutic targets and molecular mechanisms underlying the effects of UroA against brain aging remain to be elucidated. Although UroA has been found to activate anti-aging signaling pathways such as AMPK, SIRTs, and mTOR in vivo, the direct actions of UroA on these targets are currently unclear.

Table 5. Summary of Uros metabolites identified in the brain.

Animals	Route of Administration	Treatment	Brain Tissue	Identified Metabolites in Brain	Plasma Concentratio	Refs
male C57BL/6 mice (7 months, 25–30 g)	i.g.	UroA 0.3 mg/mouse, single administration	brain tissues	mUroA: 8 ng/g	---	[147]
male C57BL/6 mice (6 weeks)	i.g.	UroA 200 mg/kg b.w., single administration	cortex hippocampus	UroA: 28 ng/g UroA: 35 ng/g	15 ng/mL	[148]
male rats (12 weeks, 288 ± 20 g)	i.v.	Polyphenol metabolites (12.5 μg UroA + 5.3 μgUroB) 2.7 μmol/rat/day for 2 days	brain tissues	UroA: 2.2 ng/g UroB: 0.5 ng/g	---	[41]
male albino Wistar rats (6 weeks, 250–300 g)	i.g.	Pomegranate juice 500 mg/kg b.w./day for 10 days	brain tissues	UroA: 1.68 ± 0.25 ng/g	18.75 ± 3.21 ng/mL	[36]
male albino Wistar rats (6 weeks, 250–300 g)	i.g.	Pomegranate juice 500 mg/kg b.w./day for 45 days	brain tissues	UroA: 2.068 ± 0.274 ng/g	---	[149]

Abbreviations: i.v.: intravenous, i.g.: intragastrical, b.w.: body weight.

Fourth, the biotransformation of Uros in vitro is essential for their further application. Although there are anti-aging products containing high purity UroA of chemical synthesis on sale, biotransformation may greatly improve producing efficiency. This process is a two-step bioconversion. In the first step, the conversion of ETs to EA has been clarified and achieved in vitro [150]. Elucidating the second step and achieving the transformation of EA into Uros in vitro could yield promising application.

Fifth, it has been reported that UroA can attenuate diabetes-associated cognitive impairment by ameliorating intestinal barrier dysfunction [70]. However, the impact of UroA supplementation on gut microbiota ecology is unclear. The role of UroA supplementation on the gut microbiota composition and other neuroactive metabolites, e.g., SCFAs need further investigation.

Last, recent studies in animals and cells indicated that the combination of UroA with other food functional factors such as docosahexaenoic acid (DHA) and egpigallocatechin gallate (EGCG) produced significantly synergistic effects against brain aging and AD [64,65]. The combined treatments may have referential value for UroA to develop into related functional food and drugs. However, the synergistic efficacy and mechanisms warrant further elaboration.

Author Contributions: Conceptualization: L.A.; Investigation: L.A. and Q.L.; Formal analysis: L.A.; Writing original draft: L.A.; Review and editing: L.A., Q.L. and K.W.; Visualization: L.A.; Supervision: Y.W.; Project administration: Y.W.; Funding acquisition: Y.W. All authors have read and agreed to the published version of the manuscript.

Funding: This work was supported by the National Natural Science Foundation of China (31972127; 31471626), the Science and Technology Program of the Beijing Municipal Education Commission (KZ201910011013), and the Natural Science Foundation of Rizhao (202117).

Institutional Review Board Statement: Not applicable.

Informed Consent Statement: Not applicable.

Data Availability Statement: No new data were created.

Acknowledgments: We would like to show our deepest gratitude to all persons who have made substantial contributions to the work reported in the manuscript.

Conflicts of Interest: The authors declare no conflict of interest.

References

1. Livingston, G.; Huntley, J.; Sommerlad, A.; Ames, D.; Ballard, C.; Banerjee, S.; Brayne, C.; Burns, A.; Cohen-Mansfield, J.; Cooper, C.; et al. Dementia prevention, intervention, and care: 2020 report of the Lancet Commission. *Lancet* **2020**, *396*, 413–446. [CrossRef] [PubMed]
2. Wahl, D.; Cogger, V.C.; Solon-Biet, S.M.; Waern, R.V.; Gokarn, R.; Pulpitel, T.; Cabo, R.; Mattson, M.P.; Raubenheimer, D.; Simpson, S.J.; et al. Nutritional strategies to optimise cognitive function in the aging brain. *Ageing Res. Rev.* **2016**, *31*, 80–92. [CrossRef]
3. D'Archivio, M.; Filesi, C.; Varì, R.; Scazzocchio, B.; Masella, R. Bioavailability of the polyphenols: Status and controversies. *Int. J. Mol. Sci.* **2010**, *11*, 1321–1342. [CrossRef] [PubMed]
4. Walle, T.; Hsieh, F.; DeLegge, M.H.; Oatis, J.E., Jr.; Walle, U.K. High absorption but very low bioavailability of oral resveratrol in humans. *Drug Metab. Dispos. Biol. Fate Chem.* **2004**, *32*, 1377–1382. [CrossRef] [PubMed]
5. Gentile, C.L.; Weir, T.L. The gut microbiota at the intersection of diet and human health. *Science* **2018**, *362*, 776–780. [CrossRef]
6. Pistollato, F.; Cano, S.S.; Elio, I.; Vergara, M.M.; Giampieri, F.; Battino, M. Role of gut microbiota and nutrients in amyloid formation and pathogenesis of Alzheimer disease. *Nutr. Rev.* **2016**, *74*, 624–634. [CrossRef] [PubMed]
7. Cryan, J.F.; O'Riordan, K.J.; Cowan, C.S.M.; Sandhu, K.V.; Bastiaanssen, T.F.S.; Boehme, M.; Codagnone, M.G.; Cussotto, S.; Fulling, C.; Golubeva, A.V.; et al. The Microbiota-Gut-Brain Axis. *Physiol. Rev.* **2019**, *99*, 1877–2013. [CrossRef] [PubMed]
8. Megur, A.; Baltriukienė, D.; Bukelskienė, V.; Burokas, A. The Microbiota-Gut-Brain Axis and Alzheimer's Disease: Neuroinflammation Is to Blame? *Nutrients* **2020**, *13*, 37. [CrossRef]
9. Jie, Z.; Xia, H.; Zhong, S.L.; Feng, Q.; Li, S.; Liang, S.; Zhong, H.; Liu, Z.; Gao, Y.; Zhao, H.; et al. The gut microbiome in atherosclerotic cardiovascular disease. *Nat. Commun.* **2017**, *8*, 845. [CrossRef]
10. Luca, S.V.; Macovei, I.; Bujor, A.; Miron, A.; Skalicka-Woźniak, K.; Aprotosoaie, A.C.; Trifan, A. Bioactivity of dietary polyphenols: The role of metabolites. *Crit. Rev. Food Sci. Nutr.* **2020**, *60*, 626–659. [CrossRef]
11. Reddy, V.P.; Aryal, P.; Robinson, S.; Rafiu, R.; Obrenovich, M.; Perry, G. Polyphenols in Alzheimer's Disease and in the Gut-Brain Axis. *Microorganisms* **2020**, *8*, 199. [CrossRef]
12. Aravind, S.M.; Wichienchot, S.; Tsao, R.; Ramakrishnan, S.; Chakkaravarthi, S. Role of dietary polyphenols on gut microbiota, their metabolites and health benefits. *Food Res. Int.* **2021**, *142*, 110189. [CrossRef]
13. Hasheminezhad, S.H.; Boozari, M.; Iranshahi, M.; Yazarlu, O.; Sahebkar, A.; Hasanpour, M.; Iranshahy, M. A mechanistic insight into the biological activities of urolithins as gut microbial metabolites of ellagitannins. *Phytother. Res.* **2022**, *36*, 112–146. [CrossRef]
14. Qiu, J.; Chen, Y.; Zhuo, J.; Zhang, L.; Liu, J.; Wang, B.; Sun, D.; Yu, S.; Lou, H. Urolithin A promotes mitophagy and suppresses NLRP3 inflammasome activation in lipopolysaccharide-induced BV2 microglial cells and MPTP-induced Parkinson's disease model. *Neuropharmacology* **2022**, *207*, 108963. [CrossRef]
15. D'Amico, D.; Andreux, P.A.; Valdes, P.; Singh, A.; Rinsch, C.; Auwerx, J. Impact of the Natural Compound Urolithin A on Health, Disease, and Aging. *Trends Mol. Med.* **2021**, *27*, 687–699. [CrossRef]
16. Adachi, S.-i.; Sasaki, K.; Kondo, S.; Komatsu, W.; Yoshizawa, F.; Isoda, H.; Yagasaki, K. Antihyperuricemic Effect of Urolithin A in Cultured Hepatocytes and Model Mice. *Molecules* **2020**, *25*, 5136. [CrossRef]
17. Chen, P.; Chen, F.; Lei, J.; Li, Q.; Zhou, B. Activation of the miR-34a-Mediated SIRT1/mTOR Signaling Pathway by Urolithin A Attenuates d-Galactose-Induced Brain Aging in Mice. *Neurotherapeutics* **2019**, *16*, 1269–1282. [CrossRef]
18. Lv, M.Y.; Shi, C.J.; Pan, F.F.; Shao, J.; Feng, L.; Chen, G.; Ou, C.; Zhang, J.F.; Fu, W.M. Urolithin B suppresses tumor growth in hepatocellular carcinoma through inducing the inactivation of Wnt/β-catenin signaling. *J. Cell. Biochem.* **2019**, *120*, 17273–17282. [CrossRef]
19. DaSilva, N.A.; Nahar, P.P.; Ma, H.; Eid, A.; Wei, Z.; Meschwitz, S.; Zawia, N.H.; Slitt, A.L.; Seeram, N.P. Pomegranate ellagitannin-gut microbial-derived metabolites, urolithins, inhibit neuroinflammation in vitro. *Nutr. Neurosci.* **2019**, *22*, 185–195. [CrossRef]
20. Gonzalez-Sarrias, A.; Angeles Nunez-Sanchez, M.; Tomas-Barberan, F.A.; Carlos Espin, J. Neuroprotective Effects of Bioavailable Polyphenol-Derived Metabolites against Oxidative Stress-Induced Cytotoxicity in Human Neuroblastoma SH-SY5Y Cells. *J. Agric. Food Chem.* **2017**, *65*, 752–758. [CrossRef]
21. Velagapudi, R.; Lepiarz, I.; El-Bakoush, A.; Katola, F.O.; Bhatia, H.; Fiebich, B.L.; Olajide, O.A. Induction of autophagy and activation of SIRT-1 deacetylation mechanisms mediate neuroprotection by the pomegranate metabolite urolithin A in BV2 microglia and differentiated 3D human neural progenitor cells. *Mol. Nutr. Food Res.* **2019**, *63*, 1801237. [CrossRef]
22. Gong, Z.; Huang, J.; Xu, B.; Ou, Z.; Zhang, L.; Lin, X.; Ye, X.; Kong, X.; Long, D.; Sun, X.; et al. Urolithin A attenuates memory impairment and neuroinflammation in APP/PS1 mice. *J. Neuroinflammation* **2019**, *16*, 62. [CrossRef]
23. Romo-Vaquero, M.; Fernández-Villalba, E.; Gil-Martinez, A.L.; Cuenca-Bermejo, L.; Espín, J.C.; Herrero, M.T.; Selma, M.V. Urolithins: Potential biomarkers of gut dysbiosis and disease stage in Parkinson's patients. *Food Funct.* **2022**, *13*, 6306–6316. [CrossRef]
24. Sanchez-Gonzalez, C.; Ciudad, C.J.; Noe, V.; Izquierdo-Pulido, M. Health benefits of walnut polyphenols: An exploration beyond their lipid profile. *Crit. Rev. Food Sci. Nutr.* **2017**, *57*, 3373–3383. [CrossRef]
25. Garcia-Munoz, C.; Vaillant, F. Metabolic Fate of Ellagitannins: Implications for Health, and Research Perspectives for Innovative Functional Foods. *Crit. Rev. Food Sci. Nutr.* **2014**, *54*, 1584–1598. [CrossRef]
26. Gonzalez-Barrio, R.; Edwards, C.A.; Crozier, A. Colonic Catabolism of Ellagitannins, Ellagic Acid, and Raspberry Anthocyanins: In Vivo and In Vitro Studies. *Drug Metab. Dispos.* **2011**, *39*, 1680–1688. [CrossRef]

27. Tomas-Barberan, F.A.; Garcia-Villalba, R.; Gonzalez-Sarrias, A.; Selma, M.V.; Espin, J.C. Ellagic Acid Metabolism by Human Gut Microbiota: Consistent Observation of Three Urolithin Phenotypes in Intervention Trials, Independent of Food Source, Age, and Health Status. *J. Agric. Food Chem.* 2014, *62*, 6535–6538. [CrossRef]
28. Piwowarski, J.P.; Granica, S.; Stefanska, J.; Kisst, A.K. Differences in Metabolism of Ellagitannins by Human Gut Microbiota Ex Vivo Cultures. *J. Nat. Prod.* 2016, *79*, 3022–3030. [CrossRef]
29. Nunez-Sanchez, M.A.; Garcia-Villalba, R.; Monedero-Saiz, T.; Garcia-Talavera, N.V.; Gomez-Sanchez, M.B.; Sanchez-Alvarez, C.; Garcia-Albert, A.M.; Rodriguez-Gil, F.J.; Ruiz-Marin, M.; Pastor-Quirante, F.A.; et al. Targeted metabolic profiling of pomegranate polyphenols and urolithins in plasma, urine and colon tissues from colorectal cancer patients. *Mol. Nutr. Food Res.* 2014, *58*, 1199–1211. [CrossRef]
30. Cerdá, B.; Espín, J.C.; Parra, S.; Martínez, P.; Tomás-Barberán, F.A. The potent in vitro antioxidant ellagitannins from pomegranate juice are metabolised into bioavailable but poor antioxidant hydroxy-6H-dibenzopyran-6-one derivatives by the colonic microflora of healthy humans. *Eur. J. Nutr.* 2004, *43*, 205–220. [CrossRef]
31. Tomas-Barberan, F.A.; Gonzalez-Sarrias, A.; Garcia-Villalba, R.; Nunez-Sanchez, M.A.; Selma, M.V.; Garcia-Conesa, M.T.; Espin, J.C. Urolithins, the rescue of "old" metabolites to understand a "new" concept: Metabotypes as a nexus among phenolic metabolism, microbiota dysbiosis, and host health status. *Mol. Nutr. Food Res.* 2017, *61*. [CrossRef] [PubMed]
32. Selma, M.V.; Gonzalez-Sarrias, A.; Salas-Salvado, J.; Andres-Lacueva, C.; Alasalvar, C.; Orem, A.; Tomas-Barberan, F.A.; Espin, J.C. The gut microbiota metabolism of pomegranate or walnut ellagitannins yields two urolithin-metabotypes that correlate with cardiometabolic risk biomarkers: Comparison between normoweight, overweight-obesity and metabolic syndrome. *Clin. Nutr.* 2018, *37*, 897–905. [CrossRef] [PubMed]
33. Zhang, M.; Cui, S.; Mao, B.; Zhang, Q.; Zhao, J.; Zhang, H.; Tang, X.; Chen, W. Ellagic acid and intestinal microflora metabolite urolithin A: A review on its sources, metabolic distribution, health benefits, and biotransformation. *Crit. Rev. Food Sci. Nutr.* 2022; online ahead of print. [CrossRef]
34. Cortes-Martin, A.; Garcia-Villalba, R.; Gonzalez-Sarrias, A.; Romo-Vaquero, M.; Loria-Kohen, V.; Ramirez-de-Molina, A.; Tomas-Barberan, F.A.; Selma, M.V.; Espin, J.C. The gut microbiota urolithin metabotypes revisited: The human metabolism of ellagic acid is mainly determined by aging. *Food Funct.* 2018, *9*, 4100–4106. [CrossRef] [PubMed]
35. Singh, A.; D'Amico, D.; Andreux, P.A.; Dunngalvin, G.; Kern, T.; Blanco-Bose, W.; Auwerx, J.; Aebischer, P.; Rinsch, C. Direct supplementation with Urolithin A overcomes limitations of dietary exposure and gut microbiome variability in healthy adults to achieve consistent levels across the population. *Eur. J. Clin. Nutr.* 2022, *76*, 297–308. [CrossRef] [PubMed]
36. Kujawska, M.; Jourdes, M.; Kurpik, M.; Szulc, H.; Szaefer, H.; Chmielarz, P.; Kreiner, G.; Krajka-Kuzniak, V.; Mikolajczak, P.L.; Teissedre, P.-L.; et al. Neuroprotective Effects of Pomegranate Juice against Parkinson's Disease and Presence of Ellagitannins-Derived Metabolite-Urolithin A-In the Brain. *Int. J. Mol. Sci.* 2020, *21*, 202. [CrossRef] [PubMed]
37. Andreux, P.A.; Blanco-Bose, W.; Ryu, D.; Burdet, F.; Ibberson, M.; Aebischer, P.; Auwerx, J.; Singh, A.; Rinsch, C. The mitophagy activator urolithin A is safe and induces a molecular signature of improved mitochondrial and cellular health in humans. *Nat. Metab.* 2019, *1*, 595–603. [CrossRef]
38. Singh, A.; D'Amico, D.; Andreux, P.A.; Fouassier, A.M.; Blanco-Bose, W.; Evans, M.; Aebischer, P.; Auwerx, J.; Rinsch, C. Urolithin A improves muscle strength, exercise performance, and biomarkers of mitochondrial health in a randomized trial in middle-aged adults. *Cell Rep. Med.* 2022, *3*, 100633. [CrossRef]
39. Liu, S.; D'Amico, D.; Shankland, E.; Bhayana, S.; Garcia, J.M.; Aebischer, P.; Rinsch, C.; Singh, A.; Marcinek, D.J. Effect of Urolithin A Supplementation on Muscle Endurance and Mitochondrial Health in Older Adults A Randomized Clinical Trial. *JAMA Netw. Open* 2022, *5*, e2144279. [CrossRef]
40. García-Villalba, R.; Giménez-Bastida, J.A.; Cortés-Martín, A.; Ávila-Gálvez, M.; Tomás-Barberán, F.A.; Selma, M.V.; Espín, J.C.; González-Sarrías, A. Urolithins: A Comprehensive Update on their Metabolism, Bioactivity, and Associated Gut Microbiota. *Mol. Nutr. Food Res.* 2022, *66*, e2101019. [CrossRef]
41. Gasperotti, M.; Passamonti, S.; Tramer, F.; Masuero, D.; Guella, G.; Mattivi, F.; Vrhovsek, U. Fate of microbial metabolites of dietary polyphenols in rats: Is the brain their target destination? *ACS Chem. Neurosci.* 2015, *6*, 1341–1352. [CrossRef]
42. Bookheimer, S.Y.; Renner, B.A.; Ekstrom, A.; Li, Z.; Henning, S.M.; Brown, J.A.; Jones, M.; Moody, T.; Small, G.W. Pomegranate juice augments memory and FMRI activity in middle-aged and older adults with mild memory complaints. *Evid.-Based Complement. Altern. Med.* 2013, *2013*, 946298. [CrossRef] [PubMed]
43. Suez, J.; Elinav, E. The path towards microbiome-based metabolite treatment. *Nat. Microbiol.* 2017, *2*, 17075. [CrossRef]
44. Gaya, P.; Peiroten, A.; Medina, M.; Alvarez, I.; Landete, J.M. Bifidobacterium pseudocatenulatum INIA P815: The first bacterium able to produce urolithins A and B from ellagic acid. *J. Funct. Foods* 2018, *45*, 95–99. [CrossRef]
45. Selma, M.V.; Beltran, D.; Garcia-Villalba, R.; Espin, J.C.; Tomas-Barberan, F.A. Description of urolithin production capacity from ellagic acid of two human intestinal Gordonibacter species. *Food Funct.* 2014, *5*, 1779–1784. [CrossRef] [PubMed]
46. Selma, M.V.; Beltran, D.; Luna, M.C.; Romo-Vaquero, M.; Garcia-Villalba, R.; Mira, A.; Espin, J.C.; Tomas-Barberan, F.A. Isolation of Human Intestinal Bacteria Capable of Producing the Bioactive Metabolite Isourolithin A from Ellagic Acid. *Front. Microbiol.* 2017, *8*, 1521. [CrossRef] [PubMed]
47. Watanabe, H.; Kishino, S.; Kudoh, M.; Yamamoto, H.; Ogawa, J. Evaluation of electron-transferring cofactor mediating enzyme systems involved in urolithin dehydroxylation in Gordonibacter urolithinfaciens DSM 27213. *J. Biosci. Bioeng.* 2020, *129*, 552–557. [CrossRef]

48. Connell, E.; Le Gall, G.; Pontifex, M.G.; Sami, S.; Cryan, J.F.; Clarke, G.; Müller, M.; Vauzour, D. Microbial-derived metabolites as a risk factor of age-related cognitive decline and dementia. *Mol. Neurodegen.* **2022**, *17*, 43. [CrossRef]
49. Siddarth, P.; Li, Z.; Miller, K.J.; Ercoli, L.M.; Merril, D.A.; Henning, S.M.; Heber, D.; Small, G.W. Randomized placebo-controlled study of the memory effects of pomegranate juice in middle-aged and older adults. *Am. J. Clin. Nutr.* **2020**, *111*, 170–177. [CrossRef] [PubMed]
50. Krikorian, R.; Shidler, M.D.; Nash, T.A.; Kalt, W.; Vinqvist-Tymchuk, M.R.; Shukitt-Hale, B.; Joseph, J.A. Blueberry supplementation improves memory in older adults. *J. Agric. Food Chem.* **2010**, *58*, 3996–4000. [CrossRef] [PubMed]
51. Sala-Vila, A.; Valls-Pedret, C.; Rajaram, S.; Coll-Padrós, N.; Cofán, M.; Serra-Mir, M.; Pérez-Heras, A.M.; Roth, I.; Freitas-Simoes, T.M.; Doménech, M.; et al. Effect of a 2-year diet intervention with walnuts on cognitive decline. The Walnuts And Healthy Aging (WAHA) study: A randomized controlled trial. *Am. J. Clin. Nutr.* **2020**, *111*, 590–600. [CrossRef]
52. Bowtell, J.L.; Aboo-Bakkar, Z.; Conway, M.E.; Adlam, A.R.; Fulford, J. Enhanced task-related brain activation and resting perfusion in healthy older adults after chronic blueberry supplementation. *Appl. Physiol. Nutr. Metab.* **2017**, *42*, 773–779. [CrossRef]
53. McNamara, R.K.; Kalt, W.; Shidler, M.D.; McDonald, J.; Summer, S.S.; Stein, A.L.; Stover, A.N.; Krikorian, R. Cognitive response to fish oil, blueberry, and combined supplementation in older adults with subjective cognitive impairment. *Neurobiol. Aging* **2018**, *64*, 147–156. [CrossRef]
54. Cásedas, G.; Les, F.; Choya-Foces, C.; Hugo, M.; López, V. The Metabolite Urolithin-A Ameliorates Oxidative Stress in Neuro-2a Cells, Becoming a Potential Neuroprotective Agent. *Antioxidants* **2020**, *9*, 177. [CrossRef]
55. Kim, K.B.; Lee, S.; Kim, J.H. Neuroprotective effects of urolithin A on H_2O_2-induced oxidative stress-mediated apoptosis in SK-N-MC cells. *Nutr Res Prac.* **2020**, *14*, 3–11. [CrossRef]
56. An, L.; Li, M.; Zou, C.; Wang, K.; Zhang, W.; Huang, X.; Wang, Y. Walnut polyphenols and the active metabolite urolithin A improve oxidative damage in SH-SY5Y cells by up-regulating PKA/CREB/BDNF signaling. *Food Funct.* **2023**, *14*, 2698–2709. [CrossRef]
57. Chen, P.; Chen, F.; Lei, J.; Wang, G.; Zhou, B. The Gut Microbiota Metabolite Urolithin B Improves Cognitive Deficits by Inhibiting Cyt C-Mediated Apoptosis and Promoting the Survival of Neurons through the PI3K Pathway in Aging Mice. *Front. Pharmacol.* **2021**, *12*, 768097. [CrossRef]
58. Lee, G.; Park, J.S.; Lee, E.J.; Ahn, J.H.; Kim, H.S. Anti-inflammatory and antioxidant mechanisms of urolithin B in activated microglia. *Phytomedicine Int. J. Phytother. Phytopharm.* **2019**, *55*, 50–57. [CrossRef]
59. Toney, A.M.; Albusharif, M.; Works, D.; Polenz, L.; Schlange, S.; Chaidez, V.; Ramer-Tait, A.E.; Chung, S. Differential Effects of Whole Red Raspberry Polyphenols and Their Gut Metabolite Urolithin A on Neuroinflammation in BV-2 Microglia. *Int. J. Environ. Res. Public Health* **2020**, *18*, 68. [CrossRef]
60. Xu, J.; Yuan, C.; Wang, G.; Luo, J.; Ma, H.; Xu, L.; Mu, Y.; Li, Y.; Seeram, N.P.; Huang, X.; et al. Urolithins Attenuate LPS-Induced Neuroinflammation in BV2Microglia via MAPK, Akt, and NF-κB Signaling Pathways. *J. Agric. Food Chem.* **2018**, *66*, 571–580. [CrossRef]
61. Lee, H.J.; Jung, Y.H.; Choi, G.E.; Kim, J.S.; Chae, C.W.; Lim, J.R.; Kim, S.Y.; Yoon, J.H.; Cho, J.H.; Lee, S.-J.; et al. Urolithin A suppresses high glucose-induced neuronal amyloidogenesis by modulating TGM2-dependent ER-mitochondria contacts and calcium homeostasis. *Cell Death Differ.* **2021**, *28*, 184–202. [CrossRef]
62. Esselun, C.; Theyssen, E.; Eckert, G.P. Effects of Urolithin A on Mitochondrial Parameters in a Cellular Model of Early Alzheimer Disease. *Int. J. Mol. Sci.* **2021**, *22*, 8333. [CrossRef] [PubMed]
63. Liu, J.; Jiang, J.; Qiu, J.; Wang, L.; Zhuo, J.; Wang, B.; Sun, D.; Yu, S.; Lou, H. Urolithin A protects dopaminergic neurons in experimental models of Parkinson's disease by promoting mitochondrial biogenesis through the SIRT1/PGC-1 alpha signaling pathway. *Food Funct.* **2022**, *13*, 375–385. [CrossRef] [PubMed]
64. Jayatunga, D.P.W.; Hone, E.; Fernando, W.M.A.D.B.; Garg, M.L.; Verdile, G.; Martins, R.N. A Synergistic Combination of DHA, Luteolin, and Urolithin A Against Alzheimer's Disease. *Front. Aging Neurosci.* **2022**, *14*, 780602. [CrossRef]
65. Kshirsagar, S.; Alvir, R.V.; Pradeepkiran, J.A.; Hindle, A.; Vijayan, M.; Ramasubramaniam, B.; Kumar, S.; Reddy, A.P.; Reddy, P.H. A Combination Therapy of Urolithin A plus EGCG Has Stronger Protective Effects than Single Drug Urolithin A in a Humanized Amyloid Beta Knockin Mice for Late-Onset Alzheimer's Disease. *Cells* **2022**, *11*, 2660. [CrossRef]
66. Kshirsagar, S.; Sawant, N.; Morton, H.; Reddy, A.P.; Reddy, P.H. Mitophagy enhancers against phosphorylated Tau-induced mitochondrial and synaptic toxicities in Alzheimer disease. *Pharmacol. Res.* **2021**, *174*, 105973. [CrossRef] [PubMed]
67. Kshirsagar, S.; Sawant, N.; Morton, H.; Reddy, A.P.; Reddy, P.H. Protective effects of mitophagy enhancers against amyloid beta-induced mitochondrial and synaptic toxicities in Alzheimer disease. *Hum. Mol. Genet.* **2022**, *31*, 423–439. [CrossRef]
68. Fang, E.F.; Hou, Y.; Palikaras, K.; Adriaanse, B.A.; Kerr, J.S.; Yang, B.; Lautrup, S.; Hasan-Olive, M.M.; Caponio, D.; Dan, X.; et al. Mitophagy inhibits amyloid-β and tau pathology and reverses cognitive deficits in models of Alzheimer's disease. *Nat. Neurosci.* **2019**, *22*, 401–412. [CrossRef]
69. Yuan, T.; Ma, H.; Liu, W.; Niesen, D.B.; Shah, N.; Crews, R.; Rose, K.N.; Vattem, D.A.; Seeram, N.P. Pomegranate's Neuroprotective Effects against Alzheimer's Disease Are Mediated by Urolithins, Its Ellagitannin-Gut Microbial Derived Metabolites. *ACS Chem. Neurosci.* **2016**, *7*, 26–33. [CrossRef]
70. Yao, X.; Kailin, L.; Ji, B.; Hang, L.; Xiaotong, Z.; El-Omar, E.; Lin, H.; Lan, G.; Min, W. Urolithin a attenuates diabetes-associated cognitive impairment by ameliorating intestinal barrier dysfunction via n-glycan biosynthesis pathway. *Mol. Nutr. Food Res.* **2022**, *66*, 2100863. [CrossRef]

71. Martínez-Lapiscina, E.H.; Clavero, P.; Toledo, E.; Estruch, R.; Salas-Salvadó, J.; San Julián, B.; Sanchez-Tainta, A.; Ros, E.; Valls-Pedret, C.; Martinez-Gonzalez, M. Mediterranean diet improves cognition: The PREDIMED-NAVARRA randomised trial. *J. Neurol. Neurosurg. Psychiatry* **2013**, *84*, 1318–1325. [CrossRef]
72. Miller, M.G.; Thangthaeng, N.; Rutledge, G.A.; Scott, T.M.; Shukitt-Hale, B. Dietary strawberry improves cognition in a randomised, double-blind, placebo-controlled trial in older adults. *Br. J. Nutr.* **2021**, *126*, 253–263. [CrossRef] [PubMed]
73. Nilsson, A.; Salo, I.; Plaza, M.; Björck, I. Effects of a mixed berry beverage on cognitive functions and cardiometabolic risk markers; A randomized cross-over study in healthy older adults. *PLoS ONE* **2017**, *12*, e0188173. [CrossRef] [PubMed]
74. Bensalem, J.; Dudonné, S.; Etchamendy, N.; Pellay, H.; Amadieu, C.; Gaudout, D.; Dubreuil, S.; Paradis, M.E.; Pomerleau, S.; Capuron, L.; et al. Polyphenols From Grape and Blueberry Improve Episodic Memory in Healthy Elderly with Lower Level of Memory Performance: A Bicentric Double-Blind, Randomized, Placebo-Controlled Clinical Study. *J. Gerontol. Ser. A Biol. Sci. Med. Sci.* **2019**, *74*, 996–1007. [CrossRef]
75. Whyte, A.R.; Cheng, N.; Fromentin, E.; Williams, C.M. A Randomized, Double-Blinded, Placebo-Controlled Study to Compare the Safety and Efficacy of Low Dose Enhanced Wild Blueberry Powder and Wild Blueberry Extract (ThinkBlue™) in Maintenance of Episodic and Working Memory in Older Adults. *Nutrients* **2018**, *10*, 660. [CrossRef] [PubMed]
76. Miller, M.G.; Hamilton, D.A.; Joseph, J.A.; Shukitt-Hale, B. Dietary blueberry improves cognition among older adults in a randomized, double-blind, placebo-controlled trial. *Eur. J. Nutr.* **2018**, *57*, 1169–1180. [CrossRef]
77. Boespflug, E.L.; Eliassen, J.C.; Dudley, J.A.; Shidler, M.D.; Kalt, W.; Summer, S.S.; Stein, A.L.; Stover, A.N.; Krikorian, R. Enhanced neural activation with blueberry supplementation in mild cognitive impairment. *Nutr. Neurosci.* **2018**, *21*, 297–305. [CrossRef]
78. Krikorian, R.; Kalt, W.; McDonald, J.E.; Shidler, M.D.; Summer, S.S.; Stein, A.L. Cognitive performance in relation to urinary anthocyanins and their flavonoid-based products following blueberry supplementation in older adults at risk for dementia. *J. Funct. Foods* **2020**, *64*, 103667. [CrossRef]
79. Halliwell, B. Reactive oxygen species and the central nervous system. *J. Neurochem.* **1992**, *59*, 1609–1623. [CrossRef]
80. Shohami, E.; Beit-Yannai, E.; Horowitz, M.; Kohen, R. Oxidative stress in closed-head injury: Brain antioxidant capacity as an indicator of functional outcome. *J. Cereb. Blood Flow Metab.* **1997**, *17*, 1007–1019. [CrossRef]
81. Shi, P.Z.; Wang, J.W.; Wang, P.C.; Han, B.; Lu, X.H.; Ren, Y.X.; Feng, X.M.; Cheng, X.F.; Zhang, L. Urolithin a alleviates oxidative stress-induced senescence in nucleus pulposus-derived mesenchymal stem cells through SIRT1/PGC-1α pathway. *World J. Stem Cells* **2021**, *13*, 1928–1946. [CrossRef]
82. Mazumder, M.K.; Choudhury, S.; Borah, A. An in silico investigation on the inhibitory potential of the constituents of Pomegranate juice on antioxidant defense mechanism: Relevance to neurodegenerative diseases. *IBRO Rep.* **2019**, *6*. [CrossRef]
83. Singh, R.; Chandrashekharappa, S.; Vemula, P.K.; Haribabu, B.; Jala, V.R. Microbial Metabolite Urolithin B Inhibits Recombinant Human Monoamine Oxidase A Enzyme. *Metabolites* **2020**, *10*, 258. [CrossRef] [PubMed]
84. Saha, P.; Yeoh, B.S.; Singh, R.; Chandrasekar, B.; Vemula, P.K.; Haribabu, B.; Vijay-Kumar, M.; Jala, V.R. Gut Microbiota Conversion of Dietary Ellagic Acid into Bioactive Phytoceutical Urolithin A Inhibits Heme Peroxidases. *PLoS ONE* **2016**, *11*, e0156811. [CrossRef] [PubMed]
85. Priyadarsini, K.I.; Khopde, S.M.; Kumar, S.S.; Mohan, H. Free radical studies of ellagic acid, a natural phenolic antioxidant. *J. Agric. Food Chem.* **2002**, *50*, 2200–2206. [CrossRef] [PubMed]
86. Galano, A.; Francisco Marquez, M.; Pérez-González, A. Ellagic acid: An unusually versatile protector against oxidative stress. *Chem. Res. Toxicol.* **2014**, *27*, 904–918. [CrossRef] [PubMed]
87. Ríos, J.L.; Giner, R.M.; Marín, M.; Recio, M.C. A Pharmacological Update of Ellagic Acid. *Planta Medica* **2018**, *84*, 1068–1093. [CrossRef] [PubMed]
88. Fu, X.; Gong, L.F.; Wu, Y.F.; Lin, Z.; Jiang, B.J.; Wu, L.; Yu, K.H. Urolithin A targets the PI3K/Akt/NF-κB pathways and prevents IL-1β-induced inflammatory response in human osteoarthritis: In vitro and in vivo studies. *Food Funct.* **2019**, *10*, 6135–6146. [CrossRef]
89. Yan, C.; Ma, Z.; Ma, H.; Li, Q.; Zhai, Q.; Jiang, T.; Zhang, Z.; Wang, Q. Mitochondrial Transplantation Attenuates Brain Dysfunction in Sepsis by Driving Microglial M2 Polarization. *Mol. Neurobiol.* **2020**, *57*, 3875–3890. [CrossRef]
90. Lin, X.H.; Ye, X.J.; Li, Q.F.; Gong, Z.; Cao, X.; Li, J.H.; Zhao, S.T.; Sun, X.D.; He, X.S.; Xuan, A.G. Urolithin A Prevents Focal Cerebral Ischemic Injury via Attenuating Apoptosis and Neuroinflammation in Mice. *Neuroscience* **2020**, *448*, 94–106. [CrossRef]
91. Komatsu, W.; Kishi, H.; Yagasaki, K.; Ohhira, S. Urolithin A attenuates pro-inflammatory mediator production by suppressing PI3-K/Akt/NF-κB and JNK/AP-1 signaling pathways in lipopolysaccharide-stimulated RAW264 macrophages: Possible involvement of NADPH oxidase-derived reactive oxygen species. *Eur. J. Pharmacol.* **2018**, *833*, 411–424. [CrossRef]
92. Zhang, Y.; Aisker, G.; Dong, H.; Halemahebai, G.; Zhang, Y.; Tian, L. Urolithin A suppresses glucolipotoxicity-induced ER stress and TXNIP/NLRP3/IL-1β inflammation signal in pancreatic β cells by regulating AMPK and autophagy. *Phytomed. Int. J. Phytother. Phytopharm.* **2021**, *93*, 153741. [CrossRef]
93. Ding, S.L.; Pang, Z.Y.; Chen, X.M.; Li, Z.; Liu, X.X.; Zhai, Q.L.; Huang, J.M.; Ruan, Z.Y. Urolithin a attenuates IL-1β-induced inflammatory responses and cartilage degradation via inhibiting the MAPK/NF-κB signaling pathways in rat articular chondrocytes. *J. Inflamm.* **2020**, *17*, 13. [CrossRef] [PubMed]
94. Toney, A.M.; Fan, R.; Xian, Y.; Chaidez, V.; Ramer-Tait, A.E.; Chung, S. Urolithin A, a Gut Metabolite, Improves Insulin Sensitivity Through Augmentation of Mitochondrial Function and Biogenesis. *Obesity* **2019**, *27*, 612–620. [CrossRef] [PubMed]

95. Cordero, M.D.; Williams, M.R.; Ryffel, B. AMP-Activated Protein Kinase Regulation of the NLRP3 Inflammasome during Aging. *Trends Endocrinol. Metab. TEM* **2018**, *29*, 8–17. [CrossRef] [PubMed]
96. Salt, I.P.; Palmer, T.M. Exploiting the anti-inflammatory effects of AMP-activated protein kinase activation. *Expert Opin. Investig. Drugs* **2012**, *21*, 1155–1167. [CrossRef]
97. Carling, D. AMPK signalling in health and disease. *Curr. Opin. Cell Biol.* **2017**, *45*, 31–37. [CrossRef] [PubMed]
98. Salminen, A.; Kaarniranta, K. AMP-activated protein kinase (AMPK) controls the aging process via an integrated signaling network. *Ageing Res. Rev.* **2012**, *11*, 230–241. [CrossRef]
99. Wang, Y.; Huang, Y.; Xu, Y.; Ruan, W.; Wang, H.; Zhang, Y.; Saavedra, J.M.; Zhang, L.; Huang, Z.; Pang, T. A Dual AMPK/Nrf2 Activator Reduces Brain Inflammation After Stroke by Enhancing Microglia M2 Polarization. *Antioxid. Redox Signal.* **2018**, *28*, 141–163. [CrossRef]
100. Jęśko, H.; Wencel, P.; Strosznajder, R.P.; Strosznajder, J.B. Sirtuins and Their Roles in Brain Aging and Neurodegenerative Disorders. *Neurochem. Res.* **2017**, *42*, 876–890. [CrossRef]
101. Cho, S.H.; Chen, J.A.; Sayed, F.; Ward, M.E.; Gao, F.; Nguyen, T.A.; Krabbe, G.; Sohn, P.D.; Lo, I.; Minami, S.; et al. SIRT1 deficiency in microglia contributes to cognitive decline in aging and neurodegeneration via epigenetic regulation of IL-1β. *J. Neurosci.* **2015**, *35*, 807–818. [CrossRef]
102. Ye, J.; Liu, Z.; Wei, J.; Lu, L.; Huang, Y.; Luo, L.; Xie, H. Protective effect of SIRT1 on toxicity of microglial-derived factors induced by LPS to PC12 cells via the p53-caspase-3-dependent apoptotic pathway. *Neurosci. Lett.* **2013**, *553*, 72–77. [CrossRef] [PubMed]
103. Rizzi, L.; Roriz-Cruz, M. Sirtuin 1 and Alzheimer's disease: An up-to-date review. *Neuropeptides* **2018**, *71*, 54–60. [CrossRef] [PubMed]
104. Yang, L.; Zhang, J.; Yan, C.; Zhou, J.; Lin, R.; Lin, Q.; Wang, W.; Zhang, K.; Yang, G.; Bian, X.; et al. SIRT1 regulates CD40 expression induced by TNF-α via NF-κB pathway in endothelial cells. *Cell. Physiol. Biochem.* **2012**, *30*, 1287–1298. [CrossRef] [PubMed]
105. Fonseca, É.; Marques, C.C.; Pimenta, J.; Jorge, J.; Baptista, M.C.; Gonçalves, A.C.; Pereira, R. Anti-Aging Effect of Urolithin A on Bovine Oocytes In Vitro. *Animals* **2021**, *11*, 2048. [CrossRef] [PubMed]
106. Ryu, D.; Mouchiroud, L.; Andreux, P.A.; Katsyuba, E.; Moullan, N.; Nicolet-Dit-Félix, A.A.; Williams, E.G.; Jha, P.; Lo Sasso, G.; Huzard, D.; et al. Urolithin A induces mitophagy and prolongs lifespan in C. elegans and increases muscle function in rodents. *Nat. Med.* **2016**, *22*, 879–888. [CrossRef]
107. Fivenson, E.M.; Lautrup, S.; Sun, N.; Scheibye-Knudsen, M.; Stevnsner, T.; Nilsen, H.; Bohr, V.A.; Fang, E.F. Mitophagy in neurodegeneration and aging. *Neurochem. Int.* **2017**, *109*, 202–209. [CrossRef]
108. Ahsan, A.; Zheng, Y.R.; Wu, X.L.; Tang, W.D.; Liu, M.R.; Ma, S.J.; Jiang, L.; Hu, W.W.; Zhang, X.N.; Chen, Z. Urolithin A-activated autophagy but not mitophagy protects against ischemic neuronal injury by inhibiting ER stress in vitro and in vivo. *CNS Neurosci. Ther.* **2019**, *25*, 976–986. [CrossRef]
109. Iorio, R.; Celenza, G.; Petricca, S. Mitophagy: Molecular Mechanisms, New Concepts on Parkin Activation and the Emerging Role of AMPK/ULK1 Axis. *Cells* **2022**, *11*, 30. [CrossRef]
110. Wang, Y.; Xu, E.; Musich, P.R.; Lin, F. Mitochondrial dysfunction in neurodegenerative diseases and the potential countermeasure. *CNS Neurosci. Ther.* **2019**, *25*, 816–824. [CrossRef]
111. Wang, S.; Kandadi, M.R.; Ren, J. Double knockout of Akt2 and AMPK predisposes cardiac aging without affecting lifespan: Role of autophagy and mitophagy. *Biochim. Biophys. Acta. Mol. Basis Dis.* **2019**, *1865*, 1865–1875. [CrossRef]
112. Atherton, P.J.; Babraj, J.A.; Smith, K.; Singh, J.; Rennie, M.J.; Wackerhage, H. Selective activation of AMPK-PGC-1 alpha or PKB-TSC2-mTOR signaling can explain specific adaptive responses to endurance or resistance training-like electrical muscle stimulation. *FASEB J.* **2005**, *19*, 786–788. [CrossRef] [PubMed]
113. Laker, R.C.; Drake, J.C.; Wilson, R.J.; Lira, V.A.; Lewellen, B.M.; Ryall, K.A.; Fisher, C.C.; Zhang, M.; Saucerman, J.J.; Goodyear, L.J.; et al. Ampk phosphorylation of Ulk1 is required for targeting of mitochondria to lysosomes in exercise-induced mitophagy. *Nat. Commun.* **2017**, *8*, 548. [CrossRef] [PubMed]
114. Egan, D.F.; Shackelford, D.B.; Mihaylova, M.M.; Gelino, S.; Kohnz, R.A.; Mair, W.; Vasquez, D.S.; Joshi, A.; Gwinn, D.M.; Taylor, R.; et al. Phosphorylation of ULK1 (hATG1) by AMP-Activated Protein Kinase Connects Energy Sensing to Mitophagy. *Science* **2011**, *331*, 456–461. [CrossRef] [PubMed]
115. Kim, J.; Kundu, M.; Viollet, B.; Guan, K.-L. AMPK and mTOR regulate autophagy through direct phosphorylation of Ulk1. *Nat. Cell Biol.* **2011**, *13*, 132–141. [CrossRef] [PubMed]
116. Pillai, V.B.; Sundaresan, N.R.; Kim, G.; Gupta, M.; Rajamohan, S.B.; Pillai, J.B.; Samant, S.; Ravindra, P.V.; Isbatan, A.; Gupta, M.P. Exogenous NAD Blocks Cardiac Hypertrophic Response via Activation of the SIRT3-LKB1-AMP-activated Kinase Pathway. *J. Biol. Chem.* **2010**, *285*, 3133–3144. [CrossRef]
117. Lin, J.; Zhuge, J.; Zheng, X.; Wu, Y.; Zhang, Z.; Xu, T.; Meftah, Z.; Xu, H.; Wu, Y.; Tian, N.; et al. Urolithin A-induced mitophagy suppresses apoptosis and attenuates intervertebral disc degeneration via the AMPK signaling pathway. *Free Radic. Biol. Med.* **2020**, *150*, 109–119. [CrossRef]
118. Han, Q.-a.; Su, D.; Shi, C.; Liu, P.; Wang, Y.; Zhu, B.; Xia, X. Urolithin A attenuated ox-LDL-induced cholesterol accumulation in macrophages partly through regulating miR-33a and ERK/AMPK/SREBP1 signaling pathways. *Food Funct.* **2020**, *11*, 3432–3440. [CrossRef]

119. Rodriguez, J.; Pierre, N.; Naslain, D.; Bontemps, F.; Ferreira, D.; Priem, F.; Deldicque, L.; Francaux, M. Urolithin B, a newly identified regulator of skeletal muscle mass. *J. Cachexia Sarcopenia Muscle* **2017**, *8*, 583–597. [CrossRef]
120. Zhao, C.; Sakaguchi, T.; Fujita, K.; Ito, H.; Nishida, N.; Nagatomo, A.; Tanaka-Azuma, Y.; Katakura, Y. Pomegranate-Derived Polyphenols Reduce Reactive Oxygen Species Production via SIRT3-Mediated SOD2 Activation. *Oxidative Med. Cell. Longev.* **2016**, *2016*, 2927131. [CrossRef]
121. Ghosh, N.; Das, A.; Biswas, N.; Gnyawali, S.; Singh, K.; Gorain, M.; Polcyn, C.; Khanna, S.; Roy, S.; Sen, C.K. Urolithin A augments angiogenic pathways in skeletal muscle by bolstering NAD$^+$ and SIRT1. *Sci. Rep.* **2020**, *10*, 20184. [CrossRef]
122. Sebastián, D.; Sorianello, E.; Segalés, J.; Irazoki, A.; Ruiz-Bonilla, V.; Sala, D.; Planet, E.; Berenguer-Llergo, A.; Muñoz, J.P.; Sánchez-Feutrie, M.; et al. Mfn2 deficiency links age-related sarcopenia and impaired autophagy to activation of an adaptive mitophagy pathway. *EMBO J.* **2016**, *35*, 1677–1693. [CrossRef] [PubMed]
123. Qiao, H.; Ren, H.; Du, H.; Zhang, M.; Xiong, X.; Lv, R. Liraglutide repairs the infarcted heart: The role of the SIRT1/Parkin/mitophagy pathway. *Mol. Med. Rep.* **2018**, *17*, 3722–3734. [CrossRef] [PubMed]
124. Kwak, H.M.; Jeon, S.Y.; Sohng, B.H.; Kim, J.G.; Lee, J.M.; Lee, K.B.; Jeong, H.H.; Hur, J.M.; Kang, Y.H.; Song, K.S. Beta-Secretase (BACE1) inhibitors from pomegranate (*Punica granatum*) husk. *Arch. Pharmacal Res.* **2005**, *28*, 1328–1332. [CrossRef] [PubMed]
125. Youn, K.; Jun, M. In Vitro BACE1 inhibitory activity of geraniin and corilagin from Geranium thunbergii. *Planta Medica* **2013**, *79*, 1038–1042. [CrossRef]
126. Iaccarino, H.F.; Singer, A.C.; Martorell, A.J.; Rudenko, A.; Gao, F.; Gillingham, T.Z.; Mathys, H.; Seo, J.; Kritskiy, O.; Abdurrob, F.; et al. Gamma frequency entrainment attenuates amyloid load and modifies microglia. *Nature* **2016**, *540*, 230–235. [CrossRef]
127. Keren-Shaul, H.; Spinrad, A.; Weiner, A.; Matcovitch-Natan, O.; Dvir-Szternfeld, R.; Ulland, T.K.; David, E.; Baruch, K.; Lara-Astaiso, D.; Toth, B.; et al. A Unique Microglia Type Associated with Restricting Development of Alzheimer's Disease. *Cell* **2017**, *169*, 1276–1290.e1217. [CrossRef]
128. Tu, H.J.; Su, C.J.; Peng, C.S.; Lin, T.E.; HuangFu, W.C.; Hsu, K.C.; Hwang, T.L.; Pan, S.L. Urolithin A exhibits a neuroprotective effect against Alzheimer's disease by inhibiting DYRK1A activity. *J. Food Drug Anal.* **2023**, *31*, 358–370. [CrossRef]
129. Frick, B.; Schroecksnadel, K.; Neurauter, G.; Leblhuber, F.; Fuchs, D. Increasing production of homocysteine and neopterin and degradation of tryptophan with older age. *Clin. Biochem.* **2004**, *37*, 684–687. [CrossRef]
130. Platten, M.; Nollen, E.A.A.; Röhrig, U.F.; Fallarino, F.; Opitz, C.A. Tryptophan metabolism as a common therapeutic target in cancer, neurodegeneration and beyond. *Nat. Rev. Drug Discov.* **2019**, *18*, 379–401. [CrossRef]
131. Roager, H.M.; Licht, T.R. Microbial tryptophan catabolites in health and disease. *Nat. Commun.* **2018**, *9*, 3294. [CrossRef]
132. Rothhammer, V.; Mascanfroni, I.D.; Bunse, L.; Takenaka, M.C.; Kenison, J.E.; Mayo, L.; Chao, C.C.; Patel, B.; Yan, R.; Blain, M.; et al. Type I interferons and microbial metabolites of tryptophan modulate astrocyte activity and central nervous system inflammation via the aryl hydrocarbon receptor. *Nat. Med.* **2016**, *22*, 586–597. [CrossRef] [PubMed]
133. Rothhammer, V.; Borucki, D.M.; Tjon, E.C.; Takenaka, M.C.; Chao, C.C.; Ardura-Fabregat, A.; de Lima, K.A.; Gutiérrez-Vázquez, C.; Hewson, P.; Staszewski, O.; et al. Microglial control of astrocytes in response to microbial metabolites. *Nature* **2018**, *557*, 724–728. [CrossRef]
134. Yang, J.; Guo, Y.; Lee, R.; Henning, S.M.; Wang, J.; Pan, Y.; Qing, T.; Hsu, M.; Nguyen, A.; Prabha, S.; et al. Pomegranate Metabolites Impact Tryptophan Metabolism in Humans and Mice. *Curr. Dev. Nutr.* **2020**, *4*, nzaa165. [CrossRef] [PubMed]
135. Livingston, S.; Mallick, S.; Lucas, D.A.; Sabir, M.S.; Sabir, Z.L.; Purdin, H.; Nidamanuri, S.; Haussler, C.A.; Haussler, M.R.; Jurutka, P.W. Pomegranate derivative urolithin A enhances vitamin D receptor signaling to amplify serotonin-related gene induction by 1,25-dihydroxyvitamin D. *Biochem. Biophys. Rep.* **2020**, *24*, 100825. [CrossRef] [PubMed]
136. Green, P.S.; Simpkins, J.W. Neuroprotective effects of estrogens: Potential mechanisms of action. *Int. J. Dev. Neurosci.* **2000**, *18*, 347–358. [CrossRef] [PubMed]
137. Brann, D.W.; Dhandapani, K.; Wakade, C.; Mahesh, V.B.; Khan, M.M. Neurotrophic and neuroprotective actions of estrogen: Basic mechanisms and clinical implications. *Steroids* **2007**, *72*, 381–405. [CrossRef]
138. Barroso, A.; Mahler, J.V.; Fonseca-Castro, P.H.; Quintana, F.J. The aryl hydrocarbon receptor and the gut-brain axis. *Cell. Mol. Immunol.* **2021**, *18*, 259–268. [CrossRef]
139. Larrosa, M.; Gonzalez-Sarrias, A.; Garcia-Conesa, M.T.; Tomas-Barberan, F.A.; Espin, J.C. Urolithins, ellagic acid-derived metabolites produced by human colonic microflora, exhibit estrogenic and antiestrogenic activities. *J. Agric. Food Chem.* **2006**, *54*, 1611–1620. [CrossRef]
140. Skledar, D.G.; Tomasic, T.; Dolenc, M.S.; Masic, L.P.; Zega, A. Evaluation of endocrine activities of ellagic acid and urolithins using reporter gene assays. *Chemosphere* **2019**, *220*, 706–713. [CrossRef]
141. Zhang, W.; Chen, J.-H.; Aguilera-Barrantes, I.; Shiau, C.-W.; Sheng, X.; Wang, L.-S.; Stoner, G.D.; Huang, Y.-W. Urolithin A suppresses the proliferation of endometrial cancer cells by mediating estrogen receptor-alpha-dependent gene expression. *Mol. Nutr. Food Res.* **2016**, *60*, 2387–2395. [CrossRef]
142. Shen, P.-X.; Li, X.; Deng, S.-Y.; Zhao, L.; Zhang, Y.-Y.; Deng, X.; Han, B.; Yu, J.; Li, Y.; Wang, Z.-Z.; et al. Urolithin A ameliorates experimental autoimmune encephalomyelitis by targeting aryl hydrocarbon receptor. *Ebiomedicine* **2021**, *64*, 103227. [CrossRef] [PubMed]
143. Muku, G.E.; Murray, I.A.; Espín, J.C.; Perdew, G.H. Urolithin A Is a Dietary Microbiota-Derived Human Aryl Hydrocarbon Receptor Antagonist. *Metabolites* **2018**, *8*, 86. [CrossRef] [PubMed]

144. Gong, Q.-Y.; Cai, L.; Jing, Y.; Wang, W.; Yang, D.-X.; Chen, S.-W.; Tian, H.-L. Urolithin A alleviates blood-brain barrier disruption and attenuates neuronal apoptosis following traumatic brain injury in mice. *Neural Regen. Res.* **2022**, *17*, 2007–2013. [CrossRef]
145. Shukur, K.T.; Ercetin, T.; Luise, C.; Sippl, W.; Sirkecioglu, O.; Ulgen, M.; Coskun, G.P.; Yarim, M.; Gazi, M.; Gulcan, H.O. Design, synthesis, and biological evaluation of new urolithin amides as multitarget agents against Alzheimer's disease. *Arch. Pharm.* **2021**, *354*, e2000467. [CrossRef] [PubMed]
146. Noshadi, B.; Ercetin, T.; Luise, C.; Yuksel, M.Y.; Sippl, W.; Sahin, M.F.; Gazi, M.; Gulcan, H.O. Synthesis, Characterization, Molecular Docking, and Biological Activities of Some Natural and Synthetic Urolithin Analogs. *Chem. Biodivers.* **2020**, *17*, e2000197. [CrossRef]
147. Seeram, N.P.; Aronson, W.J.; Zhang, Y.; Henning, S.M.; Moro, A.; Lee, R.-P.; Sartippour, N.; Harris, D.M.; Rettig, M.; Suchard, M.A.; et al. Pomegranate ellagitannin-derived metabolites inhibit prostate cancer growth and localize to the mouse prostate gland. *J. Agric. Food Chem.* **2007**, *55*, 7732–7737. [CrossRef]
148. Yao, X.; Kailin, L.; Haiyan, Z.; Yunlong, L.; Lin, H.; Hang, L.; Min, W. The profile of buckwheat tannins based on widely targeted metabolome analysis and pharmacokinetic study of ellagitannin metabolite urolithin A. *LWT Food Sci. Technol.* **2022**, *156*, 113069. [CrossRef]
149. Kujawska, M.; Jourdes, M.; Witucki, Ł.; Karaźniewicz-Łada, M.; Szulc, M.; Górska, A.; Mikołajczak, P.; Teissedre, P.L.; Jodynis-Liebert, J. Pomegranate Juice Ameliorates Dopamine Release and Behavioral Deficits in a Rat Model of Parkinson's Disease. *Brain Sci.* **2021**, *11*, 1127. [CrossRef]
150. Aguilera-Carbo, A.; Augur, C.; Prado-Barragan, L.A.; Favela-Torres, E.; Aguilar, C.N. Microbial production of ellagic acid and biodegradation of ellagitannins. *Appl. Microbiol. Biotechnol.* **2008**, *78*, 189–199. [CrossRef]

Disclaimer/Publisher's Note: The statements, opinions and data contained in all publications are solely those of the individual author(s) and contributor(s) and not of MDPI and/or the editor(s). MDPI and/or the editor(s) disclaim responsibility for any injury to people or property resulting from any ideas, methods, instructions or products referred to in the content.

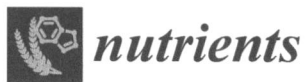

Review

The Role of One-Carbon Metabolism in Healthy Brain Aging

Sapna Virdi [1,2], Abbey M. McKee [1,2], Manogna Nuthi [1,2] and Nafisa M. Jadavji [1,2,3,4,5,*]

1. Department of Biomedical Sciences, Midwestern University, Glendale, AZ 85308, USA; svirdi89@midwestern.edu (S.V.); amckee92@midwestern.edu (A.M.M.); manogna.nuthi@midwestern.edu (M.N.)
2. College of Osteopathic Medicine, Midwestern University, Glendale, AZ 85308, USA
3. College of Veterinary Medicine, Midwestern University, Glendale, AZ 85308, USA
4. Department of Child Health, College of Medicine Phoenix, University of Arizona, Phoenix, AZ 85308, USA
5. Department of Neuroscience, Carleton University, Ottawa, ON K1S 5B6, Canada
* Correspondence: nafisa.jadavji@mail.mcgill.ca

Abstract: Aging results in more health challenges, including neurodegeneration. Healthy aging is possible through nutrition as well as other lifestyle changes. One-carbon (1C) metabolism is a key metabolic network that integrates nutritional signals with several processes in the human body. Dietary supplementation of 1C components, such as folic acid, vitamin B12, and choline are reported to have beneficial effects on normal and diseased brain function. The aim of this review is to summarize the current clinical studies investigating dietary supplementation of 1C, specifically folic acid, choline, and vitamin B12, and its effects on healthy aging. Preclinical studies using model systems have been included to discuss supplementation mechanisms of action. This article will also discuss future steps to consider for supplementation. Dietary supplementation of folic acid, vitamin B12, or choline has positive effects on normal and diseased brain function. Considerations for dietary supplementation to promote healthy aging include using precision medicine for individualized plans, avoiding over-supplementation, and combining therapies.

Keywords: neurodegeneration; healthy aging; one-carbon metabolism; folic acid; vitamin B12; choline

Citation: Virdi, S.; McKee, A.M.; Nuthi, M.; Jadavji, N.M. The Role of One-Carbon Metabolism in Healthy Brain Aging. Nutrients 2023, 15, 3891. https://doi.org/10.3390/nu15183891

Academic Editors: Moustapha Dramé and Lidvine Godaert

Received: 3 August 2023
Revised: 3 September 2023
Accepted: 5 September 2023
Published: 7 September 2023

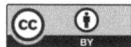

Copyright: © 2023 by the authors. Licensee MDPI, Basel, Switzerland. This article is an open access article distributed under the terms and conditions of the Creative Commons Attribution (CC BY) license (https://creativecommons.org/licenses/by/4.0/).

1. Introduction

The world's population is aging, and the number of age-related diseases is on the rise [1]. Healthy aging is possible through nutrition as well as other lifestyle changes [2]. One-carbon (1C) metabolism is a key metabolic network that integrates nutritional signals with biosynthesis, redox homeostasis, and epigenetics. One-carbon metabolism plays an essential role in the regulation of cell proliferation, stress resistance, and embryo development [3,4]. In the brain, 1C plays an important role in methylation, lipid metabolism, DNA repair, and purine synthesis (Figure 1).

B-vitamins such as vitamin B9 (folic acid) and vitamin B12, as well as the nutrient choline, play important roles in 1C (Figure 1). For example, they are all involved in the methylation of a non-protein amino acid called homocysteine. Increased levels of homocysteine indicate deficiencies, genetic or nutritional, within the 1C pathway. Some clinical studies have demonstrated that increased levels of homocysteine have been associated with negative outcomes for brain health, such as Alzheimer's disease [5], stroke [6], vascular dementia [7], as well as neural tube defects [8] in developing babies. However, the link between elevated levels of homocysteine and neurodegeneration are not clear [9].

Deficiencies in 1C can arise through either genetic changes or reduced intake from diet. As individuals age, there are changes in physiology which can lead to deficiencies in 1C components. For example, changes in stomach acid pH and reduced levels of intrinsic factor led to less vitamin B12 absorption from the diet resulting in a deficiency [10]. Reduced levels of vitamin B12 have been linked to increased risk of stroke and worse outcomes [11].

In terms of healthy aging, dietary supplementation of 1C may be a prudent step to take prior to the onset of neurodegeneration [9,12]. The aim of this review is to summarize the current clinical studies investigating dietary supplementation of 1C, specifically folic acid, choline, and vitamin B12, and its effects on healthy aging. We have also included a preclinical study section that provides details on the mechanisms through which supplementation may be changing brain function to promote healthy aging. This article will also discuss future steps to consider for the dietary supplementation of folic acid, choline, and vitamin B12.

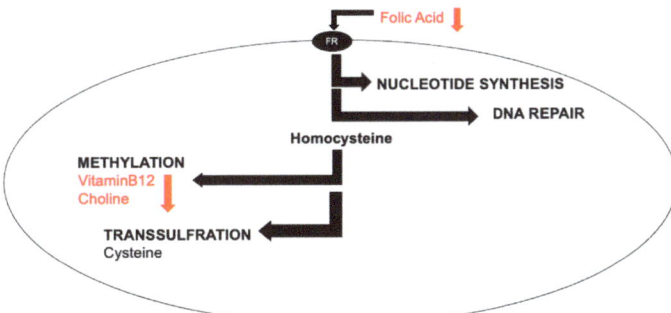

Figure 1. Simplified cellular one-carbon (1C) metabolism. B-vitamins are pleiotropic molecules, as they are involved in nucleotide synthesis, DNA repair, methylation, and transsulfuration. In this review, we focus on the impact of increasing dietary levels of folic acid, vitamin B12, and choline (red text). A control diet with adequate levels will also be used. Abbreviations: folate receptor, FR.

2. Folic Acid

2.1. Functional Role of Folic Acid

Homocysteine plays an important role in methylation reactions in the body and is dependent on folic acid, as well as vitamins B6 and B12, for synthesis [13]. Folic acid deficiency results in elevated homocysteine levels, and hyperhomocysteinemia has been identified as a risk factor for various diseases, such as vascular disease. In patients with hypertension, the role of folic acid supplementation on SAH (S-adenosylhomocysteine) levels was measured [14]. This study also investigated the effect of the 5,10-methylenetetrahydrofolate reductase (MTHFR) C677T gene polymorphism on SAH levels. MTHFR is another enzyme that plays a role in folate metabolism. The patients recruited for this study were aged 45–75 years old with a history of primary hypertension and were grouped based on their MTHFR C677T polymorphism (CC, CT, or TT). The treatment groups included a daily oral dose of 10 mg enalapril with either 0.4, 0.6, 0.8, 1.2, 1.6, 2.0, or 2.4 mg of folic acid. Treatment groups administered 10 mg of enalapril with 0.4–2.0 mg of folic acid did not have altered S-adenosylhomocysteine (SAH) levels, but supplementation with 2.4 mg increased SAH levels. Patients with the MTHFR C677T genotype CT and TT supplemented with 2.4 mg of folic acid had increased SAH levels. The CC genotype did not show an increase in SAH levels with the supplementation of 2.4 mg of folic acid. These findings indicated that the MTHFR genotypes affected by folic acid supplementation were both CT and TT. Additionally, higher levels of folic acid supplementation (2.4 mg) resulted in increased homocysteine levels like what is reported during folate deficiency. This suggests that higher levels of folic acid supplementation could be harmful, which was confirmed by two other studies [15,16]. Low and high serum folate concentrations were associated with increased risk of mortality related to cardiovascular disease.

Telomere attrition or shortening is a key finding in many age-related disorders. The role of folic acid in telomere shortening was investigated, noting that folic acid had been implicated in astrocyte (glial cell) apoptosis and in aging disorders, but its role in telomere attrition was unknown [17]. Four-month-old male mice were fed diets with varying folic acid concentrations, including 0.1 (folic acid deficient diet), 2.0 (folic acid normal diet), 2.5

(low folic acid supplemented diet), and 3.0 mg (high folic acid supplemented) of folic acid per kg of diet for six months. The mice were euthanized when they were 10 months old, and astrocytes in the hippocampal and cerebral cortex tissue were analyzed, along with telomere length and telomerase activity. Folic acid supplementation prevented astrocyte apoptosis, telomere shortening and apoptosis, and degeneration in both the hippocampus and cortex. Telomerase activity was also shown to increase with folic acid supplementation, which is likely what prevented telomere attrition.

2.2. Folic Acid's Implications in Neurodegeneration

The role of 1C metabolism in cognitive health has been explored [18,19]. Altered 1C metabolism through dietary deficiencies in B-vitamins may have a role in cognitive decline resulting from changes in DNA methylation [18], increased homocysteine levels [19], and decreased levels of neurotransmitters, as well as nucleotides [20]. Inflammation has been implicated in cognitive impairment and conditions such as Alzheimer's disease [21]. The link between inflammation and folate status is also being studied, specifically the role of folic acid supplementation in inflammation and cognition in patients with Alzheimer's disease. The participants for this study were patients aged 40–90 years old with new diagnoses of mild to moderate Alzheimer's disease who were being treated with Donepezil. The control group included patients taking just the Donepezil, and the treatment group included patients taking Donepezil with 1.25 mg of oral folic acid daily for six months with assessment every six weeks. Inflammation levels were determined through the measurement of IL-6 and TNFα mRNA. The effect of folic acid supplementation on present Alzheimer's disease pathology was determined through measurements of serum Aβ (amyloid beta) 40, Aβ 42, Aβ 42/Aβ 40, APP (amyloid precursor protein) mRNA, PS1 (presenilin 1) mRNA, and PS2 mRNA. Cognition was studied through Mini-Mental State Examination (MMSE) score and Activities of Daily Living (ADL) score. Participants in the treatment group had higher levels in the MMSE compared to the control group indicating improved cognition with folate supplementation. However, levels of Aβ 40 decreased after folic acid supplementation leading to a higher Aβ 42/Aβ 40 ratio which is typically the case in familial Alzheimer's disease. SAM (S-adenosylmethionine) increased post-treatment, and TNFα mRNA decreased indicating lower levels of inflammation. Prior studies have demonstrated a relationship between increasing SAM levels and decreasing TNFα. It was concluded that folic acid supplementation along with Donepezil treatment improved cognition, as well as inflammation in patients with Alzheimer's disease.

Another study investigated folic acid and vitamin B12 supplementation on inflammation and cognitive health in Alzheimer's disease patients [22]. The patients for this study had a diagnosis of "stable" Alzheimer's disease with a Montreal Cognitive Assessment score of less than 22 and were taking medication individually prescribed to them for their diagnosis. The treatment group was administered 1.2 mg of folic acid and 50 µg of vitamin B12 orally per day for six months, while the control or placebo group was administered the equivalent number of starch tablets resembling both folic acid and vitamin B12. Blood samples were analyzed for folate, vitamin B12, SAM, and SAH levels. There was also quantification of Aβ 40, Aβ 42, and the following inflammatory markers: IL2, IL6, IL10, MCP1, and TNF-α. Cognitive health was tested through neuropsychological testing including the Montreal Cognitive Assessment and the Alzheimer's Disease Assessment Scale-Cognitive subscale. Supplementation of both folic acid and vitamin B12 resulted in higher total, naming, and orientation scores of the Montreal Cognitive Assessment. Scoring for attention improved for the Alzheimer's Disease Assessment Scale-Cognitive subscale. The results of this neuropsychiatric testing indicated that the combined supplementation improved cognition in these patients. Combined supplementation also increased SAM and SAM/SAH levels and decreased homocysteine levels. Levels of inflammatory marker TNFα also decreased indicating a decrease in inflammation with combined folic acid and vitamin B12 supplementation.

A similar study aimed to determine the effect of folic acid and vitamin B12 (separately and combined) on patients with mild cognitive impairment (MCI) [9]. Participants were divided into four groups, including the control group that was not administered treatment, folic acid alone with 400 μg of folic acid daily, vitamin B12 alone with 25 μg daily, and combined treatment with 400 μg of folic acid and 25 μg of vitamin B12 daily for 6 months. Blood analysis was completed for the quantification of inflammatory cytokines: IL2, IL6, IL10, TNFα, IFN-y, and MCP-1. Cognitive testing was completed through the Wechsler Adult Intelligence Scale-Revised (WAIS-RC). Findings revealed that combined treatment decreased inflammatory cytokines IL6, TNFα, and MCP-1 while improving cognitive testing (WAIS-RC) scores.

Another example of the positive effects of dietary supplementation with folic acid, vitamin B6, and vitamin B12 is that they reduce the risk of age-related macular degeneration (AMD), which is the leading cause of severe irreversible vision loss in the elderly [23]. The study supplemented female participants that had a preexisting cardiovascular disease with 2.5 mg/day, vitamin B6 50 mg/day, and vitamin B12 1.0 mg/day for 7.3 years; there were 55 cases of AMD in the treated group, and 82 in the placebo group. Other studies investigating 1C supplementation have also reported that dietary supplementation is beneficial for people at high risk of AMD [23,24].

2.3. Folic Acid Interactions with Vitamin B12

The effect of high serum folate was studied in elderly individuals with a history of diabetes and vitamin B12 deficiency [25]. Prior studies have shown that high folate supplementation can result in increased cognitive impairment [26]. There is also evidence that folate supplementation in individuals with vitamin B12 deficiency can result in cognitive impairment [27]. The goal of this study was to determine if there was a correlation between high levels of folate supplementation and cognitive impairment in individuals with vitamin B12 deficiency. The participants for this study were recruited from an established study of vitamin B12 supplementation in elderly Chinese individuals (average of 75 years old) with a history of diabetes. Serum methylmalonic acid and folate levels were assessed in these individuals, and those with high methylmalonic acid with a concentration greater than 0.3 μmol and high serum folate with a concentration greater than 31.4 nmol/L were chosen for this study. Magnetic resonance imaging was used to analyze brain structure in relation to methylmalonic and folate levels in these individuals. Imaging revealed atrophy of the gray matter in the right middle occipital gyrus, as well as the inferior frontal gyrus, in individuals with high folate concentrations and vitamin B12 deficiency. This led to the conclusion that high folate concentrations could be harmful to neuronal structure resulting in degeneration in the setting of vitamin B12 deficiency.

3. Vitamin B12

Data suggest that as healthy humans age, both males and females exhibit a decrease in plasma concentrations of vitamin B12 as the body ages and metabolism changes [10]. Vitamin B12 deficiency has been linked to cognitive and memory impairment in some individuals, as shown with inverse correlations between methyl malonic acid (MMA) and global cognition and executive function tests [28–31]. Research also suggests that in addition to decreased levels of B12 in healthy individuals, the brain atrophies at a slow, steady rate, decreasing in volume over time, but this is exacerbated when deficient in vitamin B12 [29]. Very few studies deny that B12 supplementation shows significant reduction in total plasma homocysteine in patients, and multiple studies have demonstrated that B12 supplementation may somehow be linked to decreasing rates of brain atrophy and volume loss, primarily in patients with high concentrations of homocysteine at baseline.

In a study performed in 2020, 92 amnesic mild cognitive impairment (aMCI) patients were split into two groups, control (46 cases) or treatment (46 cases), to assess whether folate and vitamin B12 supplementation would decrease total serum homocysteine and improve cognitive function [32]. Both study groups received routine treatment, but the treatment group received an additional 5.0 mg/day folate + 500 μg × 3/day vitamin B12. The groups were assessed prior to treatment, and at 4, 12, and 24 weeks of treatment. As anticipated, participants in the treatment group demonstrated significant and steady increased concentrations of total serum folate and vitamin B12, with inversely related concentrations of homocysteine, at weeks 4, 12, and 24. This suggests that supplementation of folate and vitamin B12 sufficiently serves in decreasing total homocysteine. As intervention time increased, the Montreal Cognitive Assessment Scale score improved significantly by the 24th week compared to before treatment, and with respect to the control group at the same time point. These data show that, with respect to intervention duration, neurocognition function increased with decreased levels of total homocysteine. Additionally, the intervention group exhibited a significantly shorter P300 latency at 24 weeks compared to before treatment, intra-group latency at 12 weeks, and the control group at 24 weeks, despite a lack of significant change in amplitude for either group at all time points. P300 potential is an assessment of cognitive function by using the Oxford Multimedia Electromyography (EMG) system to assess response times to an electrical stimulus. This further supports that with decreased concentrations of total homocysteine at 24 weeks of treatment, the neurocognitive function of aMCI patients improved. It is important to keep in mind that the results of this study were based on a small sample of amnesic MCI patients.

Where the literature demonstrates the most inconsistency is regarding whether vitamin B12 supplementation also affects cognitive function, for example, episodic and spatial memory. Vitamin B12 supplementation in participants diagnosed with dementia and B12 deficiency, without folate deficiency, was responsible for significant increases in the Mini Mental State Exam (MMSE) scores, decreased hippocampus atrophy, decreased homocysteine, and increased vitamin B12 levels in plasma [33]. Another randomized, double-blinded study suggests that patients diagnosed with mild cognitive impairment (MCI), and especially in patients with hyperhomocysteinemia, demonstrate an impeded regression in neurocognition when supplemented with vitamin B12 [34]. However, other studies suggest that, despite vitamin B12 supplementation, cognitive and memory impairment persist despite biochemical restorations to healthy concentrations [35]. In patients that have a history of hypertension, anemia, or are healthy without MCI, several studies suggest the sole benefit of vitamin B12 supplementation is to decrease plasma homocysteine concentrations [36,37]. These studies suggest a lack of long-term benefits in immediate recall or attention, or cognitive function in general [38].

4. Choline

In healthy elderly populations, choline supplementation has an overall positive effect on cognition [39]. In a cross-sectional study, it was reported that choline supplementation had a neuroprotective effect on the elderly [40]. Specifically, in the 187.60 to 399.0 mg/day intake range, there was a significantly lower risk of cognitive impairment of 50%, as assessed by the CERAD (Consortium to Establish a Registry for Alzheimer's Disease), AF (Animal Fluency), and DSST (Digital Symbol Substitution) tests of cognitive function [40]. Another study further supported this positive correlation by looking at the four neuropsychological factors of verbal memory, visual memory, verbal learning, and executive function along with white matter hyperintensity [39]. Higher choline intake was associated with better performance in the four factors, and there was a significant inverse relationship to white matter hyperintensity in a non-demented healthy population of elderly adults [39]. Another form of choline, known as citicoline or CDP-choline, was measured for its effects on elderly populations with age-associated memory impairment. This form of choline also showed significant improvements in overall memory, especially episodic memory, compared to the placebo group [41].

Contrary to the elderly populations, a double blind, placebo controlled cross-over experiment that assessed choline bitartrate supplementation showed no significant improvement in acute memory performance in young adults [42]. However, this study did not look at long-term effects for comparison, and the rapid turnaround from supplementation to memory testing may have limited the results.

5. Preclinical Studies of Folic, Choline, and Vitamin B12 Supplementation Using Model Systems

In an effort to understand the mechanisms through which the supplementation of folic acid, vitamin B12, and choline impacts brain function, we have reviewed model system studies. These studies have an important role in our understanding of mechanisms. It is important to note that some of the preclinical studies we have included in this review article were not conducted in aged model systems. There are several challenges involved when using aged animals such as increased costs and translation to humans [43,44].

5.1. Brain Metabolism Is Affected by Folate and Vitamin B12 Status

As the brain ages, total volume decreases [45], as well as glucose metabolism [46] in the brain. Folic acid supplementation can prevent cognitive impairment, but its role in glucose metabolism is unknown. Researchers aimed to identify if folic acid status resulted in structural or metabolic changes in the brain [47]. Three-month-old male rats were administered diets containing either 0.1 (folic acid deficient), 2.0 (folic acid normal), 4.0 (low folic acid supplementation), or 8.0 mg (high folic acid supplementation) per kg diet for 22 months. Magnetic resonance imaging (MRI) and diffusion tensor imaging was completed to determine changes in brain structure. Folic acid supplementation reduced age-induced atrophy in the hippocampus. Brain positron emission tomography (PET) for glucose distribution in the brain revealed that folic acid supplementation resulted in increased glucose uptake in the brain. Behavioral testing was carried out using the Morris Water Maze test and the Open Field test. Testing revealed that folic acid supplementation altered age-related cognitive impairment. Overall, folic acid supplementation resulted in improved glucose brain metabolism and decreased age-related structural changes in the hippocampus and age-related cognitive decline.

S-adenosylmethionine (SAM) plays a direct role in methylation reactions, and folate deficiency results in a decline in SAM [48]. SAM also controls neurotransmitter levels, and thus a decline in folate levels may result in altered cognition, as is seen in Alzheimer's disease through altered acetylcholine levels. A 5,10-methylene tetrahydrofolate reductase (MTHFR) deficiency has also been identified to reduce choline levels, which ultimately results in lower acetylcholine. Folic acid deficiency and its role on cognitive health and behavior through SAM and acetylcholine was studied in adult (9- to 12-month-old) and aged (2.0- to 2.5-year-old) mice [49]. In this study, both a dietary folic acid deficiency and oxidative stress-induced folate deficiency were included. There were varying mice strains used, including "normal" adult and aged mice, $Mthfr^{+/+}$ and $Mthfr^{-/-}$ mice, and mice with murine apolipoprotein (ApoE) knocked out, as ApoE4 is a gene predictive for the onset of Alzheimer's disease, and these mice additionally either expressed an empty vector, ApoE2, ApoE3, or ApoE4. The mice were administered two different diets: a diet deplete of folate and vitamin E with iron (to induce oxidative stress), or a diet supplemented with 4mg/kg folic acid and vitamin E for one month. A separate group of mice on the deficient diet were also administered a supplementation of 100 mg/kg SAM for one month. Following this, cognitive testing was carried out via the standard Y maze test, and behavior (aggression) was also observed in the mice at that time. Folate-depleted "normal" and $Mthfr^{+/+}$ mice had cognitive impairment per Y maze testing, but mice expressing ApoE2 and ApoE3 did not. $Mthfr^{+/-}$ mice on a "complete" diet with folate supplementation also showed cognitive impairment compared to the $Mthfr^{+/+}$ mice. However, on the folate-depleted diet, both groups showed increasing cognitive impairment. Mice expressing ApoE3, ApoE4, or MTHFR on a folate-deficient diet showed aggression. The mice were killed, and the cortical and hippocampal areas were assayed to quantify levels of acetylcholine and SAM. The findings revealed that folate deficiency resulted in declined levels of SAM in all mice. Supplementation of SAM in the folate-deficient mice resulted in repleted acetylcholine levels in the mice and improved aggression, as well as cognitive impairment. These results led to the conclusion that SAM supplementation can play a role in the repletion of acetylcholine even in the setting of dietary or stress-induced folate deficiency while also improving cognitive impairment and altered behavior.

Altered 1C metabolism through folate deficiency and its role in neuroprogenitor cell proliferation has not been studied extensively [50]. One study carried out in adult mice revealed that folate deficiency reduced the proliferation of cells in the hippocampal dentate gyrus (in vivo) and reduced the proliferation of embryonic neuroprogenitor cells (in vitro). For one part of the study, mice embryo trunks were dissected and incubated in folate-deficient solution or solution containing methotrexate, which inhibited folate metabolism. Cell counts were performed to quantify neuroprogenitor cells, which revealed that folate deficiency led to decreased proliferation of these cells. For the in vivo study, one-month-old mice were maintained on a standard or folate-deficient diet for 3.5 months and then sacrificed. Similar to the in vitro findings, there was decreased proliferation of progenitor cells in the dentate gyrus, thus producing the conclusion that deficient one-carbon metabolism through decreased folate and elevated homocysteine altered neuroprogenitor cell proliferation.

Using aged rats with hyperhomocysteinemia, researchers assessed folate and B12 supplementation that reduced levels of homocysteinemia-induced tau deposition in the hippocampus, and the reversal of statistically significant spatial memory deficits without any impairment to their learning ability or alterations to the tau biochemical signaling [51]. These results suggest the need to perform clinical tests on whether folic acid and B12 supplementation can reverse, slow, or stop the progression of hyperhomocysteinemia and prevent the deposition of tau aggregates.

5.2. Mechanisms of Choline Supplementation

In a preclinical study on choline supplementation, there was significant improvement in the spatial memory performance of healthy normal rats treated with choline at embryonic ages of 12–17 days and 16–30 days. Dendritic spine branching and spread was higher in CA1 pyramidal and upper and lower limb dorsal ganglion granule cells from control. Supplementation was also correlated with a higher amount of acetylcholine in hippocampal regions as opposed to the control supporting good cognition over time [52]. The potential biochemical pathways driving related behavioral changes such as improved spatial and cued navigational abilities was investigated after choline was supplemented [53]. They found that choline enhanced the phosphorylation of hippocampal MAPK and CREB signaling pathways, whereas deficiency of choline reduced it. Lastly, another perspective was explored on prenatal choline's effect on risk or resilience behavior in the cognition and preservation of hippocampal plasticity in old age [54]. Researchers found that prenatal exposure only attenuated but did not prevent age-related decline in risky behavior. Additionally, these male and female rats showed some preserved hippocampal plasticity with age, indicating some protective effect [54].

Furthermore, looking at diseased models, choline supplementation reduced disease markers in Alzheimer's and hippocampal-dependent memory impairment. In the Alzheimer's model, it was reported that supplementation with choline significantly decreased amyloid-plaque load and improved spatial memory in the APP/PS1 Alzheimer's disease mouse model [51]. The only limitation of this study is that only female mice were studied, so gender-dependent variations could occur and need to be further studied. Similarly, long-term dietary supplementation of CDP-choline could improve hippocampal-dependent memory impairment in rat models raised in food-impoverished conditions versus the control [53]. However, there was no improvement seen in food-enriched rats between the control and CDP-choline supplemented.

In addition to preclinical studies on choline's benefits in normal aging and disease models, there were also studies showing other neuroprotective effects of choline in the brain and its enhancement of sensory modality processing. A study investigated prenatal choline supplementation and nerve growth factor (NGF) levels in the hippocampal and frontal cortex region. Researchers reported that there was significantly increased NGF in choline-supplemented rats. In the 20- and 90-day-old rats, there was a 25–30% NGF increase in the hippocampal region. However, in the frontal cortex, there was only a 16-fold increase in the 20-day-old rats, whereas there was a decrease in NGF in the 90-day-old rats [55]. In relation to the timing of auditory and visual processing, researchers found that there were differences in temporal integration between auditory and visual stimuli in aged rats when supplemented with prenatal choline. The auditory signal had faster duration discrimination than visual stimuli in choline-supplemented rats. They also showed increased attention and memory during adulthood with reduced age-related decline in cognition [56].

6. Future Directions and Conclusions

As humans age, the ability to absorb nutrients from our diet decreases. Reduced levels of 1C can impact brain health by increasing the risk for diseases and worsen outcomes when the brain is stressed by disease. As our review article has demonstrated, supplementation with folic acid, vitamin B12, or choline can have positive effects on normal and diseased brain function.

The clinical trials reviewed in this study lack longevity amongst trials in the elderly population. Rarely do studies surpass 24 months, let alone 5 or 10 years. It also remains increasingly difficult to maintain a properly powered trial due to exclusion criteria like loss of life or failure to comply with the treatment regimen. Additional research needs to be conducted with more participants, including comparable participation amongst both males and females, and a control group properly age matched. Trials that follow these improvements will provide stronger-powered data to contribute to this critical research.

Maintaining adequate levels of 1C can promote healthy aging; this can take place through dietary supplementation. We propose the use of precision medicine to guide healthcare providers in implementing ideal supplementation for patients. This could include genetic testing for polymorphisms of enzymes involved in 1C or blood tests measuring levels of 1C metabolites [57,58] and then customizing supplementation to specific needs. Over-supplementation of 1C, specifically folic acid, has recently become a concern in childbearing women and the elderly. This is something that should be avoided, as the data do not show any positive health outcomes.

Combination therapies have proven to be effective for patients suffering from ischemic stroke [59] as well as other neurological diseases [60]. We propose that nutrition should be added to a therapeutic plan for patients in addition to other interventions. The timing of dietary supplementation with 1C may be something that requires further investigation, since the onset of neurodegeneration is thought to occur well before the onset of symptoms [61–63].

Healthy aging is possible. In this review article, we propose that nutrition, especially 1C, plays an important role in promoting healthy neurological function through the aging process.

Author Contributions: S.V., A.M.M. and M.N.: investigation, writing—review and editing. N.M.J.: conceptualization, investigation, resources, writing—original draft, writing—review and editing, visualization, supervision, project administration, and funding acquisition. All authors have read and agreed to the published version of the manuscript.

Funding: This research received no external funding.

Institutional Review Board Statement: Not applicable.

Informed Consent Statement: Not applicable.

Data Availability Statement: Not applicable.

Conflicts of Interest: The authors declare no conflict of interest.

References

1. Ageing and Health. Available online: https://www.who.int/news-room/fact-sheets/detail/ageing-and-health (accessed on 28 July 2023).
2. Rudnicka, E.; Napierała, P.; Podfigurna, A.; Męczekalski, B.; Smolarczyk, R.; Grymowicz, M. The World Health Organization (WHO) Approach to Healthy Ageing. *Maturitas* **2020**, *139*, 6–11. [CrossRef]
3. Clare, C.E.; Brassington, A.H.; Kwong, W.Y.; Sinclair, K.D. One-Carbon Metabolism: Linking Nutritional Biochemistry to Epigenetic Programming of Long-Term Development. *Annu. Rev. Anim. Biosci.* **2019**, *7*, 263–287. [CrossRef] [PubMed]
4. Shiraki, N.; Shiraki, Y.; Tsuyama, T.; Obata, F.; Miura, M.; Nagae, G.; Aburatani, H.; Kume, K.; Endo, F.; Kume, S. Methionine Metabolism Regulates Maintenance and Differentiation of Human Pluripotent Stem Cells. *Cell Metab.* **2014**, *19*, 780–794. [CrossRef] [PubMed]
5. Seshadri, S. Homocysteine and the Risk of Dementia. *Clin. Chem.* **2012**, *58*, 1059–1060. [CrossRef]
6. Spence, J.D. Nutrition and Risk of Stroke. *Nutrients* **2019**, *11*, 647. [CrossRef]
7. Castro, R.; Rivera, I.; Blom, H.J.; Jakobs, C.; de Almeida, I.T. Homocysteine Metabolism, Hyperhomocysteinaemia and Vascular Disease: An Overview. *J. Inherit. Metab. Dis.* **2006**, *29*, 3–20. [CrossRef]
8. Osterhues, A.; Ali, N.S.; Michels, K.B. The Role of Folic Acid Fortification in Neural Tube Defects: A Review. *Crit. Rev. Food Sci. Nutr.* **2013**, *53*, 1180–1190. [CrossRef]
9. Smith, A.D.; Refsum, H. Homocysteine, B Vitamins, and Cognitive Impairment. *Annu. Rev. Nutr.* **2016**, *36*, 211–239. [CrossRef]
10. Yahn, G.; Abato, J.; Jadavji, N. Role of Vitamin B12 Deficiency in Ischemic Stroke Risk and Outcome. *Neural Regen. Res.* **2021**, *16*, 470. [CrossRef]
11. Ahmed, S.; Bogiatzi, C.; Hackam, D.G.; Rutledge, A.C.; Sposato, L.A.; Khaw, A.; Mandzia, J.; Azarpazhoo, M.R.; Hachinski, V.; Spence, J.D. Vitamin B 12 Deficiency and Hyperhomocysteinaemia in Outpatients with Stroke or Transient Ischaemic Attack: A Cohort Study at an Academic Medical Centre. *BMJ Open* **2019**, *9*, e026564. [CrossRef]
12. Smith, A.D.; Refsum, H.; Bottiglieri, T.; Fenech, M.; Hooshmand, B.; McCaddon, A.; Miller, J.W.; Rosenberg, I.H.; Obeid, R. Homocysteine and Dementia: An International Consensus Statement. *J. Alzheimers Dis.* **2018**, *62*, 561–570. [CrossRef] [PubMed]
13. Kaye, A.D.; Jeha, G.M.; Pham, A.D.; Fuller, M.C.; Lerner, Z.I.; Sibley, G.T.; Cornett, E.M.; Urits, I.; Viswanath, O.; Kevil, C.G. Folic Acid Supplementation in Patients with Elevated Homocysteine Levels. *Adv. Ther.* **2020**, *37*, 4149–4164. [CrossRef]
14. Zhang, R.-S.; Tang, L.; Zhang, Y.; Shi, X.-L.; Shu, J.; Wang, L.; Zhang, X.; Xu, Y.-P.; Zou, J.-F.; Wang, R.; et al. Effect of Folic Acid Supplementation on the Change of Plasma S-Adenosylhomocysteine Level in Chinese Hypertensive Patients: A Randomized, Double-Blind, Controlled Clinical Trial. *J. Clin. Biochem. Nutr.* **2022**, *71*, 238–244. [CrossRef] [PubMed]
15. Nkemjika, S.; Ifebi, E.; Cowan, L.T.; Chun-Hai Fung, I.; Twum, F.; Liu, F.; Zhang, J. Association between Serum Folate and Cardiovascular Deaths among Adults with Hypertension. *Eur. J. Clin. Nutr.* **2020**, *74*, 970–978. [CrossRef] [PubMed]
16. Xu, J.; Zhu, X.; Guan, G.; Zhang, Y.; Hui, R.; Xing, Y.; Wang, J.; Zhu, L. Non-Linear Associations of Serum and Red Blood Cell Folate with Risk of Cardiovascular and All-Cause Mortality in Hypertensive Adults. *Hypertens. Res. Off. J. Jpn. Soc. Hypertens.* **2023**, *46*, 1504–1515. [CrossRef] [PubMed]
17. Li, Z.; Zhou, D.; Zhang, D.; Zhao, J.; Li, W.; Sun, Y.; Chen, Y.; Liu, H.; Wilson, J.X.; Qian, Z.; et al. Folic Acid Inhibits Aging-Induced Telomere Attrition and Apoptosis in Astrocytes In Vivo and In Vitro. *Cereb. Cortex* **2022**, *32*, 286–297. [CrossRef]
18. Robinson, N.; Grabowski, P.; Rehman, I. Alzheimer's Disease Pathogenesis: Is There a Role for Folate? *Mech. Ageing Dev.* **2018**, *174*, 86–94. [CrossRef]
19. Smith, A.D. The Worldwide Challenge of the Dementias: A Role for B Vitamins and Homocysteine? *Food Nutr. Bull.* **2008**, *29*, S143–S172. [CrossRef]
20. Locasale, J.W. Serine, Glycine and One-Carbon Units: Cancer Metabolism in Full Circle. *Nat. Rev. Cancer* **2013**, *13*, 572–583. [CrossRef]
21. Chen, H.; Liu, S.; Ji, L.; Wu, T.; Ji, Y.; Zhou, Y.; Zheng, M.; Zhang, M.; Xu, W.; Huang, G. Folic Acid Supplementation Mitigates Alzheimer's Disease by Reducing Inflammation: A Randomized Controlled Trial. *Mediators Inflamm.* **2016**, *2016*, 5912146. [CrossRef]
22. Chen, H.; Liu, S.; Ge, B.; Zhou, D.; Li, M.; Li, W.; Ma, F.; Liu, Z.; Ji, Y.; Huang, G. Effects of Folic Acid and Vitamin B12 Supplementation on Cognitive Impairment and Inflammation in Patients with Alzheimer's Disease: A Randomized, Single-Blinded, Placebo-Controlled Trial. *J. Prev. Alzheimers Dis.* **2021**, *8*, 249–256. [CrossRef]
23. Christen, W.G.; Glynn, R.J.; Chew, E.Y.; Albert, C.M.; Manson, J.E. Folic Acid, Vitamin B6, and Vitamin B12 in Combination and Age-Related Macular Degeneration in a Randomized Trial of Women. *Arch. Intern. Med.* **2009**, *169*, 335–341. [CrossRef] [PubMed]
24. Merle, B.M.J.; Barthes, S.; Féart, C.; Cougnard-Grégoire, A.; Korobelnik, J.-F.; Rougier, M.-B.; Delyfer, M.-N.; Delcourt, C. B Vitamins and Incidence of Advanced Age-Related Macular Degeneration: The Alienor Study. *Nutrients* **2022**, *14*, 2821. [CrossRef]
25. Deng, Y.; Wang, D.; Wang, K.; Kwok, T. High Serum Folate Is Associated with Brain Atrophy in Older Diabetic People with Vitamin B12 Deficiency. *J. Nutr. Health Aging* **2017**, *21*, 1065–1071. [CrossRef] [PubMed]
26. Morris, M.C.; Evans, D.A.; Bienias, J.L.; Tangney, C.C.; Hebert, L.E.; Scherr, P.A.; Schneider, J.A. Dietary Folate and Vitamin B12 Intake and Cognitive Decline among Community-Dwelling Older Persons. *Arch. Neurol.* **2005**, *62*, 641–645. [CrossRef]
27. Mills, J.L.; Molloy, A.M.; Reynolds, E.H. Do the Benefits of Folic Acid Fortification Outweigh the Risk of Masking Vitamin B12 Deficiency? *BMJ* **2018**, *360*, k724. [CrossRef] [PubMed]

28. Vogiatzoglou, A.; Refsum, H.; Johnston, C.; Smith, S.M.; Bradley, K.M.; de Jager, C.; Budge, M.M.; Smith, A.D. Vitamin B12 Status and Rate of Brain Volume Loss in Community-Dwelling Elderly. *Neurology* **2008**, *71*, 826–832. [CrossRef] [PubMed]
29. Douaud, G.; Refsum, H.; de Jager, C.A.; Jacoby, R.; Nichols, T.E.; Smith, S.M.; Smith, A.D. Preventing Alzheimer's Disease-Related Gray Matter Atrophy by B-Vitamin Treatment. *Proc. Natl. Acad. Sci. USA* **2013**, *110*, 9523–9528. [CrossRef]
30. Ueno, A.; Hamano, T.; Enomoto, S.; Shirafuji, N.; Nagata, M.; Kimura, H.; Ikawa, M.; Yamamura, O.; Yamanaka, D.; Ito, T.; et al. Influences of Vitamin B12 Supplementation on Cognition and Homocysteine in Patients with Vitamin B12 Deficiency and Cognitive Impairment. *Nutrients* **2022**, *14*, 1494. [CrossRef]
31. Song, H.; Bharadwaj, P.K.; Raichlen, D.A.; Habeck, C.G.; Huentelman, M.J.; Hishaw, G.A.; Trouard, T.P.; Alexander, G.E. Association of Homocysteine-Related Subcortical Brain Atrophy with White Matter Lesion Volume and Cognition in Healthy Aging. *Neurobiol. Aging* **2023**, *121*, 129–138. [CrossRef]
32. Jiang, B.; Yao, G.; Yao, C.; Zheng, N. The effect of folate and VitB$_{12}$ in the treatment of MCI patients with hyperhomocysteinemia. *J. Clin. Neurosci.* **2020**, *81*, 65–69. [CrossRef] [PubMed]
33. Vogiatzoglou, A.; Smith, A.D.; Nurk, E.; Drevon, C.A.; Ueland, P.M.; Vollset, S.E.; Nygaard, H.A.; Engedal, K.; Tell, G.S.; Refsum, H. Cognitive Function in an Elderly Population: Interaction Between Vitamin B12 Status, Depression, and Apolipoprotein E4: The Hordaland Homocysteine Study. *Psychosom. Med.* **2012**, *75*, 20–29. [CrossRef] [PubMed]
34. de Jager, C.A.; Oulhaj, A.; Jacoby, R.; Refsum, H.; Smith, A.D. Cognitive and Clinical Outcomes of Homocysteine-Lowering B-Vitamin Treatment in Mild Cognitive Impairment: A Randomized Controlled Trial. *Int. J. Geriatr. Psychiatry* **2012**, *27*, 592–600. [CrossRef] [PubMed]
35. Kwok, T.; Wu, Y.; Lee, J.; Lee, R.; Yung, C.Y.; Choi, G.; Lee, V.; Harrison, J.; Lam, L.; Mok, V. A Randomized Placebo-Controlled Trial of Using B Vitamins to Prevent Cognitive Decline in Older Mild Cognitive Impairment Patients. *Clin. Nutr.* **2019**, *39*, 2399–2405. [CrossRef]
36. Aisen, P.S.; Schneider, L.S.; Sano, M.; Diaz-Arrastia, R.; van Dyck, C.H.; Weiner, M.F.; Bottiglieri, T.; Jin, S.; Stokes, K.T.; Thomas, R.G.; et al. High Dose B Vitamin Supplementation and Cognitive Decline in Alzheimer's Disease: A Randomized Controlled Trial. *J. Am. Med. Assoc.* **2008**, *300*, 1774–1783. [CrossRef]
37. Ford, A.H.; Flicker, L.; Alfonso, H.; Thomas, J.; Clarnette, R.; Martins, R.; Almeida, O.P. Vitamins B12, B6, and Folic Acid for Cognition in Older Men. *Neurology* **2010**, *75*, 1540–1547. [CrossRef]
38. Dangour, A.D.; Allen, E.; Clarke, R.; Elbourne, D.; Fletcher, A.E.; Letley, L.; Richards, M.; Whyte, K.; Uauy, R.; Mills, K. Effects of Vitamin B-12 Supplementation on Neurologic and Cognitive Function in Older People: A Randomized Controlled Trial. *Am. J. Clin. Nutr.* **2015**, *102*, 639–647. [CrossRef]
39. Poly, C.; Massaro, J.M.; Seshadri, S.; Wolf, P.A.; Cho, E.; Krall, E.; Jacques, P.F.; Au, R. The Relation of Dietary Choline to Cognitive Performance and White-Matter Hyperintensity in the Framingham Offspring Cohort 1–4. *Am. J. Clin. Nutr.* **2011**, *94*, 1584–1591. [CrossRef]
40. Liu, L.; Qiao, S.; Zhuang, L.; Xu, S.; Chen, L.; Lai, Q.; Wang, W. Choline Intake Correlates with Cognitive Performance among Elder Adults in the United States. *Behav. Neurol.* **2021**, *2021*, 2962245. [CrossRef]
41. Nakazaki, E.; Mah, E.; Sanoshy, K.; Citrolo, D.; Watanabe, F. Citicoline and Memory Function in Healthy Older Adults: A Randomized, Double-Blind, Placebo-Controlled Clinical Trial. *J. Nutr.* **2021**, *151*, 2153–2160. [CrossRef]
42. Lippelt, D.P.; van der Kint, S.; van Herk, K.; Naber, M. No Acute Effects of Choline Bitartrate Food Supplements on Memory in Healthy, Young, Human Adults. *PLoS ONE* **2016**, *11*, e0157714. [CrossRef] [PubMed]
43. Jackson, S.J.; Andrews, N.; Ball, D.; Bellantuono, I.; Gray, J.; Hachoumi, L.; Holmes, A.; Latcham, J.; Petrie, A.; Potter, P.; et al. Does Age Matter? The Impact of Rodent Age on Study Outcomes. *Lab. Anim.* **2017**, *51*, 160–169. [CrossRef] [PubMed]
44. Holtze, S.; Gorshkova, E.; Braude, S.; Cellerino, A.; Dammann, P.; Hildebrandt, T.B.; Hoeflich, A.; Hoffmann, S.; Koch, P.; Terzibasi Tozzini, E.; et al. Alternative Animal Models of Aging Research. *Front. Mol. Biosci.* **2021**, *8*, 660959. [CrossRef] [PubMed]
45. Fotenos, A.F.; Snyder, A.Z.; Girton, L.E.; Morris, J.C.; Buckner, R.L. Normative Estimates of Cross-Sectional and Longitudinal Brain Volume Decline in Aging and AD. *Neurology* **2005**, *64*, 1032–1039. [CrossRef] [PubMed]
46. Deery, H.A.; Di Paolo, R.; Moran, C.; Egan, G.F.; Jamadar, S.D. Lower Brain Glucose Metabolism in Normal Ageing Is Predominantly Frontal and Temporal: A Systematic Review and Pooled Effect Size and Activation Likelihood Estimates Meta-analyses. *Hum. Brain Mapp.* **2022**, *44*, 1251–1277. [CrossRef]
47. Zhou, D.; Sun, Y.; Qian, Z.; Wang, Z.; Zhang, D.; Li, Z.; Zhao, J.; Dong, C.; Li, W.; Huang, G. Long-Term Dietary Folic Acid Supplementation Attenuated Aging-Induced Hippocampus Atrophy and Promoted Glucose Uptake in 25-Month-Old Rats with Cognitive Decline. *J. Nutr. Biochem.* **2023**, *117*, 109328. [CrossRef]
48. Serra, M.; Chan, A.; Dubey, M.; Gilman, V.; Shea, T.B. Folate and S-Adenosylmethionine Modulate Synaptic Activity in Cultured Cortical Neurons: Acute Differential Impact on Normal and Apolipoprotein-Deficient Mice. *Phys. Biol.* **2008**, *5*, 044002. [CrossRef]
49. Chan, A.; Tchantchou, F.; Graves, V.; Rozen, R.; Shea, T.B. Dietary and Genetic Compromise in Folate Availability Reduces Acetylcholine, Cognitive Performance and Increases Aggression: Critical Role of S-Adenosyl Methionine. *J. Nutr. Health Aging* **2008**, *12*, 252–261. [CrossRef]
50. Kruman, I.I.; Mouton, P.R.; Emokpae, R.; Cutler, R.G.; Mattson, M.P. Folate Deficiency Inhibits Proliferation of Adult Hippocampal Progenitors. *Neuroreport* **2005**, *16*, 1055–1059. [CrossRef]

51. Wei, W.; Liu, Y.-H.; Zhang, C.-E.; Qang, Q.; Wei, Z.; Mousseau, D.D.; Wang, J.-Z.; Tian, Q.; Liu, G.-P. Folate/Vitamin-B12 Prevents Chronic Hyperhomocysteinemia-Induced Tau Hyperphosphorylation and Memory Deficits in Aged Rats. *J. Alzheimers Dis.* **2011**, *27*, 639–650. [CrossRef]
52. Bahnfleth, C.L.; Strupp, B.J.; Caudill, M.A.; Canfield, R.L. Prenatal Choline Supplementation Improves Child Sustained Attention: A 7-year Follow-up of a Randomized Controlled Feeding Trial. *FASEB J.* **2022**, *36*, e22054. [CrossRef] [PubMed]
53. Mellott, T.J.; Williams, C.L.; Meck, W.H.; Blusztajn, J.K. Prenatal Choline Supplementation Advances Hippocampal Development and Enhances MAPK and CREB Activation. *FASEB J. Off. Publ. Fed. Am. Soc. Exp. Biol.* **2004**, *18*, 545–547. [CrossRef]
54. Glenn, M.J.; Kirby, E.D.; Gibson, E.M.; Wong-Goodrich, S.J.; Mellott, T.J.; Blusztajn, J.K.; Williams, C.L. Age-Related Declines in Exploratory Behavior and Markers of Hippocampal Plasticity Are Attenuated by Prenatal Choline Supplementation in Rats. *Brain Res.* **2008**, *1237*, 110–123. [CrossRef]
55. Sandstrom, N.J.; Loy, R.; Williams, C.L. Prenatal Choline Supplementation Increases NGF Levels in the Hippocampus and Frontal Cortex of Young and Adult Rats. *Brain Res.* **2002**, *947*, 9–16. [CrossRef] [PubMed]
56. Cheng, R.-K.; Scott, A.C.; Penney, T.B.; Williams, C.L.; Meck, W.H. Prenatal-Choline Supplementation Differentially Modulates Timing of Auditory and Visual Stimuli in Aged Rats. *Brain Res.* **2008**, *1237*, 167–175. [CrossRef]
57. Konno, M.; Asai, A.; Kawamoto, K.; Nishida, N.; Satoh, T.; Doki, Y.; Mori, M.; Ishii, H. The One-Carbon Metabolism Pathway Highlights Therapeutic Targets for Gastrointestinal Cancer (Review). *Int. J. Oncol.* **2017**, *50*, 1057–1063. [CrossRef] [PubMed]
58. Franco, C.N.; Seabrook, L.J.; Nguyen, S.T.; Leonard, J.T.; Albrecht, L.V. Simplifying the B Complex: How Vitamins B6 and B9 Modulate One Carbon Metabolism in Cancer and Beyond. *Metabolites* **2022**, *12*, 961. [CrossRef]
59. Lapchak, P.A.; Araujo, D.M. Advances in Ischemic Stroke Treatment: Neuroprotective and Combination Therapies. *Expert Opin. Emerg. Drugs* **2007**, *12*, 97–112. [CrossRef]
60. Arranz-Romera, A.; Esteban-Pérez, S.; Garcia-Herranz, D.; Aragón-Navas, A.; Bravo-Osuna, I.; Herrero-Vanrell, R. Combination Therapy and Co-Delivery Strategies to Optimize Treatment of Posterior Segment Neurodegenerative Diseases. *Drug Discov. Today* **2019**, *24*, 1644–1653. [CrossRef]
61. Mau, K.J.; Jadavji, N.M. A New Perspective on Parkinson's Disease: Pathology Begins in the Gastrointestinal Tract. *J. Young Investig.* **2017**, *33*, 1–8. [CrossRef]
62. Hörder, H.; Johansson, L.; Guo, X.; Grimby, G.; Kern, S.; Östling, S.; Skoog, I. Midlife Cardiovascular Fitness and Dementia: A 44-Year Longitudinal Population Study in Women. *Neurology* **2018**, *90*, e1298–e1305. [CrossRef] [PubMed]
63. Suvila, K.; Lima, J.A.C.; Yano, Y.; Tan, Z.S.; Cheng, S.; Niiranen, T.J. Early-but Not Late-Onset Hypertension Is Related to Midlife Cognitive Function. *Hypertension* **2021**, *77*, 972–979. [CrossRef] [PubMed]

Disclaimer/Publisher's Note: The statements, opinions and data contained in all publications are solely those of the individual author(s) and contributor(s) and not of MDPI and/or the editor(s). MDPI and/or the editor(s) disclaim responsibility for any injury to people or property resulting from any ideas, methods, instructions or products referred to in the content.

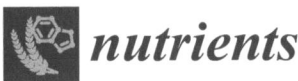

Article

Practicing Interoceptive Sensitivity as a Couple: A Mixed-Methods Acceptance Analysis of a Dyadic vs. Single Pilot Randomized Controlled Trial

Nadja-R. Baer [1,2,*], Noemi Vanessa Grissmer [1,2], Liane Schenk [1,2], Hanna R. Wortmann [1,3], Petra Warschburger [1,3,†] and Ulrike A. Gisch [1,3,4,†]

1 NutriAct—Competence Cluster Nutrition Research Berlin-Potsdam, 14558 Nuthetal, Germany; noemi-vanessa.grissmer@charite.de (N.V.G.); liane.schenk@charite.de (L.S.); hwortman@uni-potsdam.de (H.R.W.); petra.warschburger@uni-potsdam.de (P.W.); ulrike.gisch@ernaehrung.uni-giessen.de (U.A.G.)
2 Institute for Medical Sociology and Rehabilitation Science, Charité—Universitätsmedizin Berlin, Charitéplatz 1, 10117 Berlin, Germany
3 Counseling Psychology, Department of Psychology, University of Potsdam, Karl-Liebknecht-Str. 24-25, 14476 Potsdam, Germany
4 Department of Nutritional Psychology, Institute of Nutritional Science, Justus Liebig University Giessen, Senckenbergstr. 3, 35390 Giessen, Germany
* Correspondence: nadja-raphaela.baer@charite.de; Tel.: +49-30-450-529-118
† These authors contributed equally to this work as last author.

Abstract: Training interoceptive sensitivity (IS) might be a first step in effectively promoting intuitive eating (IE). A dyadic interoception-based pilot randomized controlled trial was conducted to increase IE among couples aged 50+. The training consisted of three exercises, a Body Scan (BS), a hunger exercise (HU), and a satiety (SA) exercise. This study explored how spouses accepted the (dyadic vs. single) training. In a mixed-methods convergence design, the findings of a survey (n = 68 couples) and focus groups (n = 4) were synthesized. Moderate general acceptance (e.g., regarding feasibility and low burden) and a hierarchical gradient in favor of the BS (e.g., pleasantness and improved sleep quality) emerged. Barriers concerned a perceived lack of the exercises' usefulness and a limited understanding of the training purpose. A wish for regular feedback and exchange with the study stuff and other participants was expressed. Spousal training involvement was experienced as being rather beneficial. Previously harmonized dietary practices and daily routines appeared as constructive pre-conditions for the joint training. This study highlights the potential and implications of training couples in IS. Future interventions should involve a regular exchange and closer guidance by study staff to promote a better understanding of the processes and goals of IS and IE.

Keywords: intuitive eating; interoceptive sensitivity; healthy eating practice; interoception-based training; dyadic intervention; couple influence; acceptance; Theoretical Framework of Acceptability (TFA); mixed methods; Pillar Integration Process (PIP)

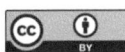

1. Introduction

Dietary behavior, such as food choices, is dynamically shaped by a complex interplay of factors, including an individual's personal state and social as well as (digital) food environments [1,2]. Individual factors comprise biological features, physiological needs (e.g., metabolism, genetic predisposition, and hunger), and psychological components (e.g., personality and emotions), which have been shown to be central for the development of maladaptive eating behavior as restrained or emotional eating [1,3]. On the macro level, socio-cultural factors include normative ideas and discourses (e.g., body image and dieting) and economic as well as political interests (e.g., food marketing and food policy and regulations) [1,4]. In turn, such factors manifest in specific food environments that encompass, for instance, food availability, affordability, and accessibility [4,5]. A prominent food environment, particularly prevalent in high-income countries, is the so-called obesogenic environment, which is characterized by a high density and proximity of (fast) food outlets and easy access to energy-dense, ultra-processed foods [6,7]. Embedded in such external food environments, the individual's immediate social environment also plays a crucial role in shaping their dietary practices—including (mal-)adaptive eating behavior—throughout the entire life course [8]. In (later) adulthood, the couple relationship is a specifically focal socialization context, in which lifestyle behaviors in general and dietary practices in particular are (pre-consciously) shaped, negotiated, and (re-)established [9].

Both the food and social environment may be in tension with a favorable diet, e.g., by constant (over)consumption stimuli. Against this background, the concept of intuitive eating (IE) has gained scientific interest as a critical response to dieting [10]. IE is an adaptive eating behavior characterized by an attunement to one's hunger and satiety signals. IE involves trusting the body's needs, following unconditional permission to eat rather than a restrictive approach to food, and monitoring and reacting to the effects of food on the body (so-called body–food–choice congruence) [10,11]. Hence, the concept of IE emphasizes eating with an intentional focus on internal cues rather than responding to external cues, which may include food availability, sensing food, served portion sizes, or social settings, where eating is encouraged or the norm [12]. Eating in an intuitive manner requires the innate yet often unlearned ability to perceive and process internal bodily signals, which is referred to as interoceptive sensitivity (IS) [13,14]. Previous research suggests a positive association between IS and IE [15,16]. Hence, IS training might be a first step in effectively promoting IE. IS differs considerably among people [17] and was found, for instance, to be lower in individuals with overweight and obesity [18,19] and to decline with increasing age [20].

Previous correlational research suggests substantial associations between IE and various physical and psychological health indicators [21], thereby supporting its adaptive properties [15]. Positive correlations were found, for instance, between IE and life satisfaction, a positive body image, self-esteem, self-efficacy, and health-related quality of life [11]. In addition, IE is negatively associated with maladaptive eating behavior, such as restraint eating, emotional eating, and eating disorder symptomatology, as well as BMI [21,22]. Despite the scarce body of evidence concerning older age groups, one study examined women aged 60–75 years and replicated the positive relationships between IE and psychological health indicators [23].

So far, IE has mainly been researched by observational studies, while only few interventional studies have addressed this topic [24]. Overall, the existing research indicates positive effects of IE on (adaptive) dietary practices and psychological health indicators [25–28]. However, the state of evidence is sparse and rather inconsistent [25,26,29], suggesting further research directions: a systematic review highlights the need for more research on IE with longer follow-up periods to analyze long-term changes in dietary behavior and diet quality after participation in an IE intervention [25]. Moreover, previous research has mostly focused on younger adults [30–32] and the interventive effects of IE in the context of obesity [19], maladaptive eating behavior (e.g., binge eating disorder) [27], or among chronic dieters [33]. Until now, investigating IE in general populations and, more specifically, in middle-aged and older adults and those without diet-related disorders [27,34,35] has been neglected. Along with this, a lack of qualitative explorations of people's attitudes towards and experiences with practicing IE has been stressed. Currently, there are only a few qualitative studies exploring general populations. Findings from Van Dyk et al. [36] and Erhardt et al. [37] both underline the nature of IE as a dynamic learning process. According to their findings, a central barrier for IE lies in the overcoming of dietary habits and the unlearning of the "conditioning" towards pre-established non-IE practices (e.g., stimulated by the food environment). Both requires discipline in resisting temptation, as well as time and flexible routines. As the authors conclude, there is a further need to explore people's experiences with (re-)learning IE [36,37]. The study of the present paper aimed to do both, training people to increase their interoceptive sensitivity (IS) as a prerequisite for IE as well as exploring how such training is experienced.

The immediate social context plays an important role in (re-)learning and changing health-related behaviors, including IE. Evidently, individuals in close (e.g., spousal) relationships influence the IE practices of their significant others [37,38]. More generally, spouses' health-related behaviors have been found to be highly similar, with partner concordance increasing over the course of the relationship [39,40]. This also holds true for dietary practices, i.e., couples tend to synchronize or converge their dietary preferences [41] and food choices [42]. Dietary convergence involves maladaptive eating behavior (e.g., emotional eating [43,44]) as well as favorable [45] dietary styles. However, the extent to which spouses influence each other with regard to IS and IE is still little researched.

Therefore, targeting couples may enhance the effectiveness of health behavior change interventions [37,41]. Previous studies point at the positive effects of couple-based interventions, mostly addressing specific health-related behaviors associated with diet-related illnesses (e.g., diabetes [46]). Yet, the evidence remains largely sparse and inconsistent [46–48]. There is, thus, a need for further studies on couple-based interventions targeting overall health-related behaviors independent from ill-health [47]. By doing so, in-depth knowledge can be gained about the mechanisms influencing the success of such interventions. More specifically, an understanding of how couple dynamics and joint everyday practices affect the implementation of interventions could provide important insights. However, the acceptance of couple-based interventions has not yet been sufficiently researched.

In general, there are ambivalent and inconsistent definitions, conceptualizations, and operationalizations of acceptance within the intervention research field [49]. Against this background, Sekhon et al. [49] stressed the lack of systematic theory-based acceptance analyses in the context of healthcare interventions and developed the Theoretical Framework of Acceptability (TFA), which consists of eight components [50]. The present study was guided by the TFA and, accordingly, refers to the authors' proposed definition of acceptability as "[...] a multi-faceted construct that reflects the extent to which people delivering or receiving a healthcare intervention consider it to be appropriate, based on anticipated or experienced cognitive and emotional responses to the intervention" [49] (p. 4). In this definition, the authors refer to *acceptability*. While acceptability refers to an a priori judgment before exposure to an intervention, the term acceptance describes an a posteriori judgment thereof [51]. In the current study, we analyzed past experiences with the intervention and, hence, unlike Sekhon et al. [50], refer to *acceptance*.

To the authors' knowledge, this is the first mixed-methods acceptance study on a dyadic interoception-based pilot randomized controlled trial (RCT) to increase IS. The major aim of the current study was to analyze participants' overall acceptance of the training, as well as its implementation and (non-)continuation into everyday life [52]. Further aims, specific research questions, and hypotheses of the pilot RCT are described in the study protocol [52]. In the context of the present article, we focus on the following exploratory research questions:

- To what extent do partnered adults aged 50 years and older accept an (couple- vs. single-based) experimental interoception-based training program promoting IS?
- What role does the couple context play in the experience, conduction, and post-intervention continuation of the intervention exercises?

2. Materials and Methods
2.1. Intervention
2.1.1. Intervention Design

The aim of the intervention was to increase IE via training interoceptive sensitivity over 21 days. The training consisted of three interoception-based guided audio exercises. The intervention was a pilot RCT with three measurement points (T0: pre-intervention, training period, T1: post-intervention, and T2: 4-week follow up). We applied a three-arm study design to compare two intervention groups with a control group: *Group 1: Couple-based training* (Index person (G1-I) and partner (G1-P)) vs. *Group 2: Training alone* (Index person (G2-I) and partner (G2-P)) vs. *Group 3: No training* (Index person (G3-I) and partner (G3-P)).

2.1.2. Intervention Description

The training is described in detail in the study protocol [52]. At T0, the participants of G1-I/G1-P and G2-I received a 20-min introductory video about the intervention (study, training, and theoretical background), which they had to watch at home before starting the training. The training consisted of three interoception-based guided audio exercises (Week 1: Body Scan (BS), week 2: hunger (HU) exercise, and week 3: satiety (SA) exercise). The participants had to perform each exercise once a day for 7 days, resulting in a total training period of 21 days. The first exercise was a classic 20-min Body Scan. The exercise was based on a script by Kabat-Zinn and Valentin [53] and was modified according to Fischer and colleagues [54]. The second and third exercises (HU and SA exercises) were based on the IE workbook by Tribole and Resch [55]. In the 8-min HU exercise that was performed before a meal, the participants had to mindfully focus on the perception and quality of hunger signals (e.g., location, intensity, and sensation). In the 9-min SA exercise that was performed after a meal, the participants had to mindfully focus on the perception and quality of satiety signals (location, intensity, and sensation). The aim of the training was to target self-related processes (interoceptive awareness, self-efficacy, self-critical rumination, and self-monitoring), as well as aspects of emotion regulation and attentional control [52,56]. The participants were not instructed to continue to perform the exercises after the 21-day training period.

2.2. Acceptance Study Design

For the purpose of the mixed-methods acceptance study, we utilized a convergent synthesis design to integrate the findings from the quantitative data and qualitative focus groups. The research process followed established criteria for mixed-methods studies [57] and was facilitated by the Pillar Integration Process (PIP) (see Section Mixed-Methods Convergent Synthesis) [58]. The reporting complies with the GRAMMS (Good Reporting of a Mixed-Methods Study) guideline [59].

2.2.1. Operationalization of Intervention Acceptance According to the TFA

To facilitate a comprehensive exploration of the participants' training acceptance, this study and, in particular, the theory-based mixed-methods analysis were oriented towards the TFA [49]. According to this framework, intervention acceptance comprises eight components, which Sekhon et al. [50] operationalized as follows: *Affective Attitudes* address how an individual feels about the intervention, for example, in terms of liking or comfort. *Burden* refers to the amount of effort required to participate in the intervention, including efforts to adhere with the intervention measures. The fit of the intervention with a participant's moral beliefs or ethical value system is another acceptance component referred to as *Ethicality*. *Intervention Coherence* describes the extent to which a participant understands how the intervention works and/or what it aims for. Another central component is called *Perceived Effectiveness*, i.e., an individual's perception of the extent to which the intervention has achieved its intended purpose. *Self-Efficacy* refers to the participant's confidence that they can perform the behavior(s) required to (successfully) participate in the intervention. Another TFA component is called *Opportunity Costs* and refers to the extent to which engaging in the intervention interfered with the participant's other priorities. More specifically, it addresses the benefits, gains, or values potentially relinquished by participating in the intervention. Finally, the TFA suggests an investigation of *General Acceptance*, i.e., an overarching subjective evaluation of the intervention as a whole.

2.2.2. Recruitment and Organization Procedure

QUAN: This pilot RCT is a sub-study of the larger, ongoing, web-based prospective NutriAct Family Study (NFS) that investigates the epidemiological, psychological, and sociological perspectives on food choices in families. For the NFS, we recruited study participants in groups of two or more family members (spouses and siblings) aged 50+. For further information regarding the study design of the NFS, please see [60]. Eligible for participation in the present study were heterosexual cohabiting couples aged 50+. The aim of the intervention recruitment strategy was to identify people with a low level of IE and invite them to take part in the intervention study with their partner. Therefore, we followed a selective prevention approach. Based on the already available data of the NFS, we successively recruited our intervention sample based on the Intuitive Eating Scale-2 (IES-2) [10] rank, starting with those persons who showed the lowest level of IE. First, we contacted these people (index persons) by mail and invited them to take part in our intervention study together with their partners. If an index person and the partner were willing to participate in our intervention study, we clarified the inclusion and exclusion criteria by phone. From November 2020 to September 2021, we recruited the intervention sample.

QUAL: Three months after the intervention was completed, we recruited the qualitative subsample to build four focus groups. Recruitment took place from May to August 2021. Index persons were contacted via phone to ask for their readiness to participate. In the case of agreement, the participants received an email with detailed study information about the content and practical organization of the group discussions, as well as about measures taken to secure data protection. Participation was compensated with an incentive of EUR 20 per person. Initially, we aimed for group sizes between 5 and 8 people. However, due to the COVID-19-pandemic, the group sizes were limited to a maximum of four people. To facilitate comparative analyses, the focus groups were constituted by (1) women only (G1/2-I), (2) men only (G2-I), (3) couples, where both partners had participated in the intervention (G1-I and G1-P), and (4) men and women who had participated in the intervention without their partners (G2-I).

2.2.3. Data Collection

Procedure: Separate, Subsequent Data Collection

QUAN: At each of the three measurement points, we assessed a web-based survey that was filled out by both partners. Furthermore, the pre-assigned index person of each couple was invited to the laboratory and objective variables were assessed. For further evaluation of the acceptance and impact of the training, training evaluation sheets were filled out (paper and pencil) after every week of the training. A detailed flow chart of the intervention design can be found in the study protocol [52]. The trial was registered at the German Clinical Trials Register (DRKS), no. DRKS00024903. The index persons received EUR 10 for each assessment in the laboratory to compensate for travel expenses. For further information regarding the intervention design, please see the study protocol [52].

QUAL: The focus group discussions also took place at the German Institute of Human Nutrition Potsdam-Rehbruecke. Immediately before the discussions, the participants obtained verbal study information, were asked for permission to be audiotaped, and given room for potential open questions. Thereafter, all participants handed in their written informed consent. The recordings were encrypted and stored on a secured institutional drive. The audiotapes were transcribed verbatim and then pseudonymized and anonymized in accordance with the DSGVO (EU 2016/679).

Measures

Data were collected separately for the QUAN and QUAL study parts. In the following section, we will only report those measures that are relevant to our research questions. All further measures included in the RCT are described in the study protocol [52].

QUAN: Intuitive Eating Scale-2 (IES-2)

The German IES-2 [11] was applied to measure the level of IE. The IES-2 was included in the web-based surveys. For the current analysis, assessment of the IES-2 at T0 was used. The IES-2 has 23 items and consists of 4 subscales measuring different facets of IE. The items were answered on a 5-point Likert scale ranging from *strongly disagree* (=1) to *strongly agree* (=5). For the current analysis, only the mean values of the IES-2 were used. Higher mean values on the IES-2 reflect higher levels of IE. Previous validation studies have supported the scale's validity and reliability (e.g., [10,11]). In the current study, Mc Donald's Omega was 0.80.

QUAN: Training Evaluation Sheets (TES)

The participants of G1-I and G2-I completed three training evaluation sheets (one sheet per exercise) after each week of training. The self-constructed items measured how the participants evaluated different aspects of the exercises. For the current analysis, we used the following items: TES_1) *Please evaluate the exercise regarding the following characteristics:* exertion (TES_1_1), easy to follow (TES_1_2), comprehensibility (TES_1_3), pleasantness (TES_1_4), liking (TES_1_5), usefulness for everyday life (TES_1_6), and easy to concentrate on (TES_1_7). The items were rated on a 5-point semantic differential scale, with higher values representing a better evaluation. To assess the overall evaluation of each exercise, we calculated the mean value of acceptance with the 7 items of TES_1 (Mean_TES_1_BS; Mean_TES_1_HU; and Mean_TES_1_SA). TES_2) *Will you continue to perform the exercise in your everyday life after the end of the study?* The answer options were *yes* or *no*.

QUAN: Acceptance-Related Variables (ARVs)

We further assessed ARVs with self-constructed items. For the current analysis, we used the following items at T1 in G1-I, G1-P, and G2-I: ARV_1) *Overall, do you feel that you can better perceive hunger and satiety signals because of the training?* The answer options ranged from 1 (*not at all*) to 6 (*very much*). ARV_2) *Would you recommend the training?* The answer options ranged from 1 (*not at all*) to 6 (*absolutely*). The following item was assessed at T1 only by G1-I and G1-P: ARV_3) *Imagine if you could do the training again: Would you prefer to do the training again with your partner or alone?* The answer options were 1 (*with my partner*) and 2 (*alone*). The following item was assessed at T1 only by G2-I: ARV_4) *Would you have preferred to do the training together with your partner?* The answer options were 1 (*yes*) or 2 (*no*). The following items were assessed at T2 in G1-I, G1-P, and G2-I: ARV_5) *Have you noticed any changes in your everyday life as a result of the exercises after completing the training?* The answer options were *yes* or *no*. If the participants answered *yes*, they were then asked to specify which changes they had noticed. ARV_6) *Have you continued to perform the exercises after the end of the study?* The answer options ranged from 1 (*no*) to 6 (*once a day*).

QUAL: Focus Group Discussions (FG)

A semi-structured guideline was developed to stimulate discussion and support the exchange of experiences among the participants. The guideline development was informed by the tentative descriptive results of the training evaluation sheets (*QUAN: Training Evaluation Sheets (TES)*). The question stimuli focused on the acceptance of the entire intervention, as well as on specific experiences with the three training exercises over time, i.e., both during the intervention period and after the completion of the intervention. Discussions were also stimulated with respect to the couple context, e.g., the influence and support of the partner in carrying out the exercises. To stimulate a conversation dynamic, the introductory stimulus concerned dietary practices in general, irrespective of IE and the intervention. For this purpose, a quote by a previous study participant was shared: "Look, that [(his dietary practice)] can't possibly be healthy. I've had three cups of coffee and so many cigarettes before I even eat anything. That's my weak spot. [. . .] I want to get to the point where I eat at least two pieces of toast and an egg in the morning. I do that occasionally and it even makes me feel better. But I always have to torture myself." The participants were then asked to talk about the extent to which they could identify themselves with this statement and in how far potential attempts to change dietary practices had already succeeded/failed—both as individuals and as a couple.

2.2.4. Data Analysis

The data analysis took place in a two-staged process: First, the quantitative and qualitative data materials were analyzed separately. At the end of this parallel analysis process, several meetings took place between the qualitative and quantitative researchers in order to enable a first overview of the respective findings for triangulation, as well as for validation purposes. In the second step, a mixed-methods data analysis was carried out using a convergent synthesis approach [61].

Separate, Parallel Data Analysis

QUAN: The quantitative data were analyzed in a descriptive manner. Furthermore, to compare which exercise was evaluated best (Mean_TES_1_BS vs. Mean_TES_1_HU vs. Mean_TES_1_SA) and how the specific evaluation aspects (TES_1_1–TES_1_7) differed between the three exercises, we performed Friedman's ANOVA with the data of G1-I and G2-I. To compare the recommendation of the training (ARV_2) between the different groups (G1-I, G1-P, and G2-I), we performed a Kruskal–Wallis test.

QUAL: The qualitative data material was analyzed following the Qualitative Content Analysis by Kuckartz [62] using MAXQDA (version 22.0.1). In an iterative process, categories were inductively and deductively derived by the means of "open coding": in the first step, themes were inductively identified in the transcripts and grouped into so-called "natural categories". These were then reviewed by a second coder and, where necessary, regrouped until consensus was reached. In the second step, these categories were further differentiated into "analytical categories", elaborated upon into sub-categories and revised intersubjectively. The material was subsequently fully re-examined and, where applicable, coded within the established category system. Finally, the category system was adapted according to the given research question. This involved deductive coding, a reduction in the system to the most relevant categories, and a partial rearrangement of (sub-)categories. During the entire analysis process, preliminary findings were continuously discussed within the research team, as well as presented and interpreted (multiple times) in a research colloquium to further ensure inter-coder-reliability.

Mixed-Methods Convergent Synthesis

The mixed-methods approach was informed by the key features put forward by Creamer [61]. In terms of *Priority* (see [61]), we proceeded in an explorative sequential way, whereby qualitative data were analyzed in greater depth and breadth and the survey results were oriented towards the inductively generated qualitative categories (see PIP, Multimedia Supplementary S1). In doing so, the primary aim of the mixed-methods (MM) analysis was to use the qualitative findings to explore and explain the quantitatively assessed outcomes. The *Timing* of the data collection was separate and sequential for the data collection, as well as parallel during the data analysis. To varying degrees, *Integration* took place at each of the six stages of the research process, all of which Creamer proposes as crucial elements of a Fully Integrated MM Design. *Integration* took primarily place on the analysis and interpretation levels, with the latter aiming at drawing so-called meta-inferences [61].

For the synthesis, we utilized the Pillar Integration Process (PIP), which is an analytical technique for systematically integrating qualitative and quantitative results by the means of a joint display [58]. Joint displays provide visual tools to both integrate and represent mixed-methods results to derive meta-inferences [58,63]. Following the PIP, the synthesis was conducted in four subsequent stages: in Stage I (listing of raw data), we listed selective (only those with relevance to the research question) qualitative categories, codes, and respective interview quotes in the joint display. Subsequently, we matched the (Stage II) quantitative results to the qualitative categories. This step first necessitated the "qualitization" (see [61]) of the quantitative numeric data into the qualitative categories. After the initial matching, a second and a third round of matching were conducted, with attributions based on both the QUAN and QUAL results. Each matching round was guided by the constant comparative method, i.e., the focus was on identifying similarities as well as contrasts. If no match was identified, the respective section was left blank.

Stage III involved the checking of the matched results based on the raw data (quantitative and qualitative data material). In doing so, overlaps were identified, categories were renamed and logically rearranged, and the most relevant raw data (numeric and quotes) were selected and harmonized. In Stage IV, the Pillar Building was conducted, whereby themes were derived equally from the quantitative and qualitative results and combined into meta-interferences. This last analytical step did not only involve inductive theme development, but also the deductive derivation of inferences drawing on the TFA. The entire integration process was iteratively conducted by two researchers experienced with qualitative evidence syntheses.

3. Results

3.1. Sample Characteristics

QUAN: We enrolled $n = 71$ heterosexual couples into the study. One couple and one partner dropped out before the groups were allocated and two couples and one partner dropped out before the training started, resulting in $n = 68$ couples and, in total, $N = 134$ participants. The total sample consisted of $n = 68$ women (50.7%). The mean age was $M = 67.4$ years ($SD = 5.6$, range = 53–85 years). Table 1 displays the sample characteristics of the QUAN data separately for each group.

Table 1. QUAN sample characteristics.

	Group 1		Group 2		Group 3	
Couples (n)	24		22		22	
	G1-I	G1-P	G2-I	G2-P	G3-I	G3-P
Group size (n)	24	23	22	22	22	21
Gender						
Women (n)	10	14	10	12	14	8
Men (n)	14	9	12	10	8	13
Age (years)						
M (SD)	66.0 (4.2)	67.2 (6.1)	67.7 (4.9)	67.4 (6.0)	67.8 (6.4)	68.5 (6.2)
Min–Max	56–74	53–82	60–77	56–77	58–85	57–80
BMI (kg/m^2) [1]						
M (SD)	27.8 (4.8)	26.4 (4.9)	27.3 (3.6)	26.0 (3.1)	25.5 (3.1)	23.5 (3.3)
Min–Max	19.0–39.0	20.8–42.2	20.6–35.7	22.2–34.1	20.6–32.5	17.6–28.4

Note. [1] BMI was calculated from height and weight (BMI = weight (kg)/height (m) [64]. BMI values for index persons were based on laboratory measurements of height and weight, while BMI values for partners were based on self-reported height and weight.

QUAL: The final sample for the focus groups consisted of twelve individuals. Among the participants, 50% were women. The mean age of the participants was $M = 65.9$ years ($SD = 4.9$, range = 60–78 years) and the mean BMI was $M = 24.1$ kg/m^2 ($SD = 2.5$, range = 20.3–28.3 kg/m^2).

3.2. Main Results

As a major result of the MM convergent synthesis, a pillar consisting of six overarching themes was developed, which combined the quantitative ("qualitized") and qualitative categories. The QUAN categories primarily concerned aspects of practicability, ease of realization, and the integration into everyday life. Among other things, the QUAL categories provided insights into the participants' lived experiences, attitudes towards the training and the concepts of IE and mindfulness in general, and explained reasons for a perceived (lack of) training effect. The pillar themes reflected six out of the eight TFA components proposed by Sekhon et al. [50], which were empirically derived throughout the synthesis process. Each of these components appeared several times, e.g., for the training exercises. The two TFA components of *Ethicality* and *Opportunity Costs* did not occur in our data. The most significant material, which primarily emerged from the FG, concerned the TFA components of *Perceived Effectiveness* and *Affective Attitude*, indicating their particular importance for the training acceptance.

In Multimedia Supplementary S1, a joint display is depicted showing the results of the Pillar Integration Process (PIP). The joint display provides a detailed overview of the pillar themes, and the inductively generated categories are depicted for the overall intervention, each training exercise, and the couple context. Figure 1 illustrates a condensed overview of the selected results regarding the overall intervention acceptance and the main context factors shaping the participants' acceptance.

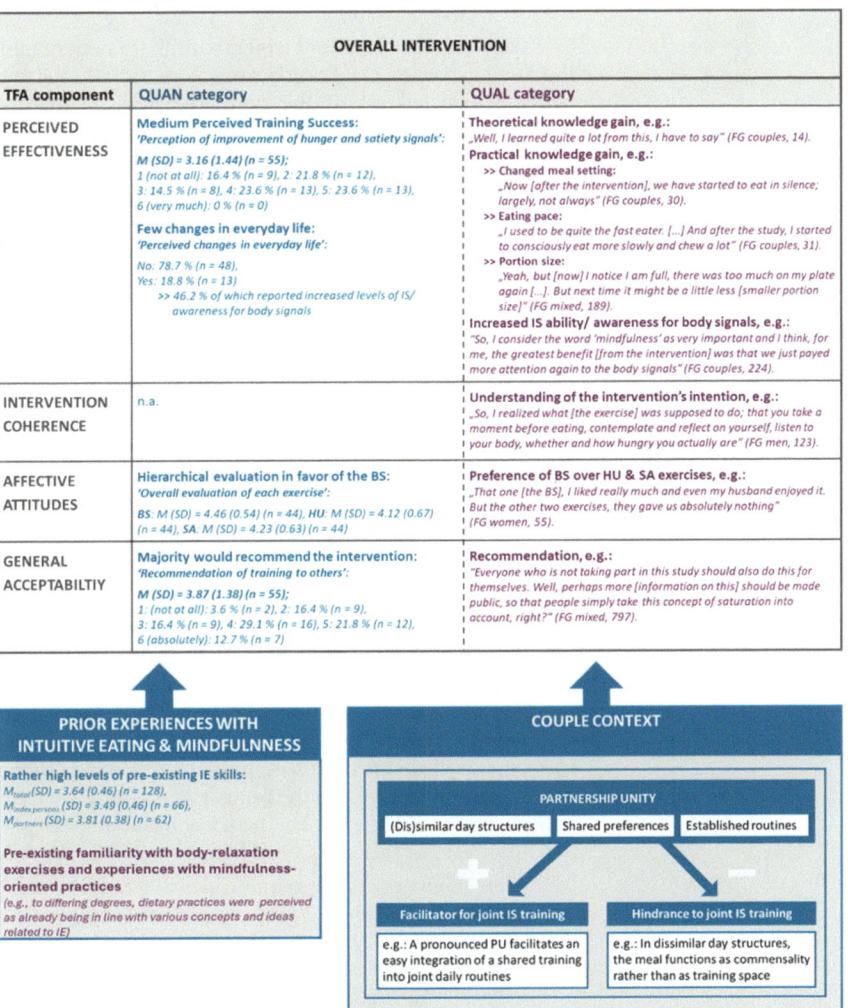

Figure 1. Overview of selected results regarding the overall intervention acceptance and main context factors. Note. QUAN = quantitative, QUAL = qualitative, FG = focus group, M = mean, SD = standard deviation, IE = Intuitive Eating, IS = Interoceptive Sensitivity, BS = Body Scan, HU = hunger exercise,

SA = satiety exercise, and PU = Partnership Unity. This figure contains selected results on the overall intervention acceptance. For more detailed information on the acceptance of the respective exercises and respective TFA components, as well as further primary data (QUAN/QUAL), please see Multimedia Supplementary S1 (PIP).

Subsequently, the results are described for each of the identified TFA components in Section 3.2 (see Sections 3.2.1–3.2.5). In addition, Section 3.3 deals with findings regarding the couple context, which could be reconstructed inductively on the basis of the QUAL FG beyond the TFA-based acceptance analysis. Section 3.3.1 deals with the extent to which the partner and/or a joint participation was perceived as a benefit in carrying out the exercises and achieving the intended training effects. Section 3.3.2 addresses the dynamics of the couples' everyday lives that were identified from the FG, allowing conclusions to be drawn about the barriers and facilitators for joint training execution.

3.2.1. Affective Attitude

Our findings document a hierarchical gradient regarding affective attitudes towards the three exercises: the Body Scan was preferred over the hunger and satiety Exercises, which is reflected in both the qualitative and the quantitative results. The quantitative findings showed relatively high values for pleasantness (BS: M (SD) = 4.56 (0.79), HU: M (SD) = 4.05 (0.91), SA: M (SD) = 4.32 (0.83)) and moderately high values for liking (BS: M (SD) = 4.23 (1.08), HU: M (SD) = 3.61 (1.17), SA: M (SD) = 3.75 (1.28)) for all three exercises. Insights gained from the focus groups allowed us to further understand these outcomes: the participants expressed a relatively pronounced general enjoyability and pleasantness associated with the BS. This also applied to cases where initial skepticism was present, but which gave way to a positive attitude during the course of the training, as one participant described with respect to her husband:

"But [then] he was really pleased by the Body Scan. [...] At the beginning, he said 'that's hocus-pocus' or something like that and I said 'why don't you try it first', yeah? And then [(afterwards)] he said: 'that was really pleasant!' [...] [So,] I really much liked [the BS] and even my husband enjoyed it. But the other two exercises, they gave us absolutely nothing." (FG women, pos. 55/68)

Despite this hierarchical evaluation in favor of the BS, the participants also showed gratitude for the knowledge gain and heightened meal anticipation elicited by the HU exercise:

"At the end [of the HU exercise] I always told myself: 'So, now you can have a delicious dinner'. [...] And then I was really looking forward to eat something and actively went upstairs saying: 'Oh, now you are allowed to eat something really nice!'." (FG mixed, female participant, pos. 445)

Concerning negative attitudes towards the exercises, the qualitative and quantitative findings were somewhat divergent. For instance, while (rather) high levels of pleasantness were reported for the HU, negative affects played a greater role in the group discussions: Here, the participants discussed unpleasant feelings such as annoyance, disappointment, and anger, especially with the hunger and satiety exercises, but also regarding the Body Scan—albeit to a lesser degree. These feelings were often placed in the context of a perceived "needlessness" or "senselessness", as illustrated by the following quote:

"But this hunger exercise and also the satiety exercise, those drove me up the wall, because the questions asked were complete nonsense in my point of view. Like, where do I feel hunger'. [...] I feel it in my stomach and [...] in the digestive tract. And satiety, too. But I don't feel it in my hands and feet—so, these were completely illogical questions [laughs]. Practically every time these questions came—It was over. That's when I got annoyed." (FG men, pos. 92)

3.2.2. Burden and Self-Efficacy

To varying degrees, *Burdens* were identified with respect to each of the three training exercises, whereby this TFA component appeared to largely overlap with aspects related to *Self-Efficacy*. Therefore, both themes were conjointly addressed in the PIP and subsequently. According to both the quantitative and qualitative findings, the BS required low levels of effort (BS: M (SD) = 4.71 (0.70)) and was evaluated as easy to follow (BS: M (SD) = 4.67 (0.64). The associated relatively high degree of perceived self-efficacy may partially be explained by the participants' prior experiences with other kinds of relaxation exercises, such as the regular Qigong practice mentioned by one participant. Regarding the HU and SA exercises, low levels of effort (HU: M (SD) = 4.51 (0.82), SA: M (SD) = 4.70 (0.59)) were reported and the exercises were evaluated as easy to follow (HU: M (SD) = 4.67 (0.56), SA: M (SD) = 4.79 (0.47)), while some burdens and little experiences of self-efficacy were revealed in the group discussions. For example, the participants perceived the exercises as challenging, as they were not used to sensing their hunger and satiety signals: *"[...] It was exhausting because I didn't realize if I was full or not, what is that feeling?"* (FG mixed, male participant, pos. 431). The satiety exercise appeared to be more difficult to perform, partly because the feeling of satiety was reported to be more subtle and, therefore, harder (if at all) to sense as compared to hunger: *„[...] and maybe I had more of a problem with the satiety exercise. So, hunger is easier to identify for me than satiety"* (FG couples, male participant, pos. 288). In spite of these difficulties, however, repeated practice of the exercises seemed to have a positive influence on the level of self-efficacy over time. The participants expressed their experience of a familiarization effect, making the exercises easier as the training progressed, as this quote illustrates: *"Well, you first had to get used to finding a way in, because you—it [the HU exercise] was unfamiliar. But it got better over time [...]"* (FG mixed, pos. 430).

3.2.3. Perceived Effectiveness

In respect to the *Perceived Effectiveness* concerning the overall intervention, the quantitative and qualitative results were inconsistent again. While the quantitative data displayed a relatively low perceived training success (M_{ARV_1} (SD) = 3.16 (1.44)), with more than three-quarters of the participants (78.7% (n = 48)) reporting no associated changes in everyday life, the qualitative results indicated rather positively perceived training effects. In particular, the qualitative analysis revealed two different (but related) types of knowledge gain: on the one hand, the participants shared their perceptions in terms of a theoretical knowledge gain, i.e., of having learnt something new about the concept of mindfulness and/or IE. On the other hand, and seemingly of greater relevance, different types of practical knowledge gains towards more conscious eating practices were discussed in the FGs. These mainly concerned a general greater awareness towards (diet-related) internal body signals. In some cases, this was rather framed as a re-learning or intensifying of already existing skills, rather than establishing new ones:

> *"So, I consider the word 'mindfulness' as very important and I think, for me, the greatest benefit [from the intervention] was that we just paid more attention again to the body signals."* (FG couples, female participant, pos. 224)

Moreover, various changes in mealtime routines and eating habits were mentioned, such as a quieter meal setting, smaller portion sizes, and a slower eating pace, as illustrated by the following quote: *"I used to be quite the fast eater. [...] And after the study, I started to consciously eat more slowly and chew a lot"* (FG couples, male participant, pos. 31). Interestingly, although these changes (e.g., increasing the amount of chewing) were not explicitly addressed as part of the training exercises, they were apparently associated with IE and considered to be integral to the individual intervention success.

In comparison to the other exercises and particularly to the SA exercise, the Body Scan was perceived as the most useful for everyday life. As the FG revealed, its useful benefits included a better ability for interoception, stress reduction, and a general calming and relaxation effect—both physically and mentally—as well as an improvement in sleep quality. One participant recalled his positively experienced effects of the BS exercise as follows:

"It was the first time I consciously felt my body in every corner, right? And then I lay down for another moment and afterwards I got up, let's say, as light as a feather; I was calm, also calm inside, and found it really fascinating what it [the BS exercise] does to your mind." (FG Mixed, male participant, pos. 157)

At the same time, a few participants also criticized a lack of effect and/or were not convinced this exercise could have any kind of influence on their eating practices. While the BS showed a fairly high perceived usefulness for everyday life overall (M (SD) = 3.87 (1.12)), both the HU and SA exercises were perceived as only moderately effective (HU: M (SD) = 3.29 (1.12), SA: M (SD) = 3.09 (1.14)). On the one hand, a large number of participants reported no (lasting) training effects. This may be explained by findings of the participants' pre-existing mindfulness-oriented lifestyle in general, and mindful or IE-related dietary habits in particular. Both of these, as expressed in the FGs, seemed to prevent participants from experiencing training effects:

"I would actually like to emphasize [that] the- the [HU] exercise itself didn't give me anything, because I already live according to this pattern anyway, right?" (FG men, pos. 187)

"So, for us [couple], the meal is a ceremony in a certain sense, right? Not that we make a big fuss about it, but it all happens in a calm manner. We chew thoroughly without counting the amount of chewing actions per bite. But yeah, it all happens in peace." (FG men, pos. 124)

On the other hand, the HU and SA exercises were perceived as being useful due to a gain in knowledge, e.g., the exercises provided new aspects that participants were *"grateful for"* (FG couples, female participant, pos. 89). More strikingly, the participants shared experiences of improved interoception resulting from regular practice of the SA and/or HU exercises. This training effect was not only related to the intervention period, but also to the time afterwards, as this participant remembered:

"[. . .] in retrospect, in the time since [the intervention], I have to say I've become more aware of it. I realize better when I'm hungry and when I'm full. I've become more aware of this feeling. I used to notice it less." (FG mixed, female participant, pos. 178)

With regard to these experiences, however, we found a discrepancy between the objective of IE to improve the sensational attunement to HU/SA signals and the practical realization by the means of "rationality". In this context, one male participant described a heightened reflexive awareness for the concept of satiety, albeit with remaining difficulties with actually sensing this body signal:

"What the study did for me: It raised awareness for the concept of satiety. Because I- even though I don't notice if I am already full at that moment, I might notice it minutes later, but by then, I've already had several other forks or spoons. It [now] has rather become a matter of rationality. The concept of satiety has triggered a bit more reason in me, for now I say: 'No, that's enough. You might not be really full yet, but that's enough, stop it.' Right? That's what my consciousness tells me." (FG mixed, male participant, pos. 797)

Here, the sensation of satiety was perceived as an automatism and an eating practice closely aligned to the principles of IE, which does not (yet) seem possible (merely) by the means of interoception. Instead, the concept of mindfulness is brought into consciousness on a reflexive level, and the habitual eating practice (of overeating) is disrupted through rational action, as in this case through an auto suggestive imperative.

3.2.4. Intervention Coherence

The extent to which the participants understood how the intervention was supposed to improve their interoceptive sensitivity and/or IE skills was not quantitatively assessed. Yet, a few conclusions can be drawn from the qualitative study findings. Albeit in rare cases, the participants seemed to have understood the intended training purpose, as the following quote demonstrates:

> "So, in principle, I realized what it [the HU exercise] was supposed to do; that you take a moment before eating and reflect on yourself, listen to your body and feel how hungry you are." (FG men, pos. 123)

At the same time, ambiguities also became evident, as several questions were raised in the FGs about the intended intervention purpose, for example, why IS was of interest as a research topic. In addition, there appeared uncertainties regarding the concept of interoceptive sensitivity, its specific aims (e.g., as distinct from IE), and its practical implementation by the exercises. Implicitly, this became evident when the participants described IE practices in general, as well as when they put their training experiences in the context of broader mindfulness-oriented lifestyle behaviors and attitudes. While this illustrates a difficulty in separating the overlapping concepts and underlying principles of IS and IE, it may, nevertheless, be an indication of a general understanding of the intervention's associated aims. More explicitly, however, a lack of *Intervention Coherence* was shown when the participants expressed their desire for feedback, both individually on their own performance (e.g., "[...] *some kind of personalized information*" (FG women, pos. 175)), as well as in comparison to the other participants. The following quote shows exemplarily that this desire was associated with the participants' ambition for a correct training execution and an accompanying uncertainty: "*I would be interested in whether all the participants are basically marching in the same direction or if we are generally off the mark*" (FG men, pos. 219). This desire for objectifiable, quantified comparison and external validation implicitly challenges the participants' acceptance in terms of the *Intervention Coherence*.

3.2.5. General Acceptance

General acceptance of the intervention was not directly measured, but could be inferred from several indicators. Foremost, recommendation was used as a proxy, showing that the majority of the participants (n = 35, 63.6%) would have (rather) recommended the training to others. However, a considerable proportion also indicated that they would not at all (n = 2, 3.6%) or rather not (n = 18, 32.8%) have done so. Noteworthy, the recommendation rates were significantly higher among the participants who had completed the training without their partner (G2-I). The qualitative study findings primarily supported a positive view: in the mixed FGs, one participant suggested, "[...] *everyone who is not taking part in this study should also do this for themselves*" (FG mixed, male participant, pos. 787), while another participant emphasized a particular benefit for young people with overweight:

> "[...] *Young people should participate in this kind of dietary study, right? Because I know that currently many, well, let me say overweight people, are really, really young. So that might also be an approach: to invite the younger folks to this kind of intervention to make them realize how important this is, especially for later life. Because if they are already that overdimensioned now, how will this be in old age? That is really important, right?*" (FG mixed, female participant, pos. 36)

This suggestion demonstrates a goal-oriented comprehension of the concept of IE, namely weight reduction. Against this understanding, the participant implicitly positioned herself in contrast to young people with overweight, who she considered to be in particular need of an IE practice, amongst others with respect to healthy ageing. A personal need for IE as an end in itself is, therefore, not considered here. In line with the other participants' statements, this indicates a certain degree of positive self-assessment regarding a healthy, mindful dietary practice. This is reflected in the study sample's IE levels ($M_{\text{index persons}}$ (SD) = 3.49 (0.46); M_{partners} (SD) = 3.81 (0.38)), which are comparable to adults aged 50+ in a German community sample [11]. Moreover, not only was the training itself deemed recommendable, but so was the promotion of the principles associated with IE: "*Well, perhaps more [information on this] should be made public, so that people simply take this concept of saturation into account, right?*" (FG mixed, male participant, pos. 797).

The *General Acceptance* of the training was also reflected in the (partial) continuation of the exercises during the period following the intervention. In the questionnaires, the participants were asked for their intention to continue the training exercises (at T1) and their actual training exercises continuation (at T2). While the HU and SA exercises were not intended to be continued after the intervention by the vast majority (HU: intention yes = 29.5% (n = 13), no = 70.5% (n = 31); SA: intention yes = 36.4% (n = 16), no = 63.6% (n = 28)), the participants seemed to have more positive expectations of the BS. Here, 77.8% (n = 35) indicated they would possibly continue this exercise. However, 22.2% (n = 10) could not imagine themselves doing so.

With respect to the actual training exercises continuation, the quantitative data revealed that approximately half of the participants (54.1%, n = 33) did not continue the training at all, while others indicated they had continued the exercises sporadically (18%, n = 11), regularly (19.7%, n = 12), or in a daily manner (8.2%, n = 5). To further explore which exercises were continued, to what extent, and for what reasons, the qualitative results provide further information:

Congruent with the findings showing a hierarchical exercise evaluation in favor of the BS (also see *Affective Attitudes*, Section 3.2.1), this exercise was continued the most frequently and consistently. At the same time, however, sporadic training exertion was also shared in the FGs: *"Well, I neither do it [the BS exercise] regularly. I somewhat do it as needed"* (FG couples, male participant, pos. 201). Such occasional practice was particularly evident in connection with a purposeful intention set by the participants themselves, such as for improving sleep quality (*"[...] It calms you down, so it's sleep-inducing, if you can't sleep"* (FG couples, female participant, pos. 202)). Thus, the experience of specific needs that were believed to be met by practicing the BS seemed to encourage post-intervention continuation of this exercise. In the case of continuation, the participants reported they did so without listening to the audio instructions.

In the case of the HU exercise, there was some continuation from time to time by a rather small proportion of the participants. Similar to the BS exercise, the HU was then performed without listening to the audio file and only particular parts were selected in response to the individuals' needs and wishes. Moreover, although participants in two FGs reported that aspects of the SA exercise remained "in the back of their minds" (FG couples, female participant, pos. 89), none of the interviewees reported the retention of the SA exercise after the end of the study.

Across all exercises, the reasons for discontinuation included a perceived lack of added value and purpose, which may possibly be related to the level of understanding of the intervention's intended effects (also see *Intervention Coherence*, Section 3.2.4). This was particularly evident for the HU exercise, as the following statement underlines: *"To this day, I still don't really see the (deep) meaning of it [the HU exercise]"* (FG men, pos. 91).

Another reason for discontinuation was that the participants saw no need or little value for themselves due to their already pre-existing mindfulness-related skills: *„I wouldn't say that it didn't give me anything at all, but I was just already eating more consciously before [the training]"* (FG couples, female participant, pos. 284)) (also see *Perceived Effectiveness*, Section 3.2.3). Conversely, there also appeared to be a perceived inability to perform the exercises—especially regarding the HU exercise. Some participants noted that, particularly with increasing age, they either rarely felt hunger (anymore) or did not experience it at all, which rendered the hunger exercise rather pointless to them: *"Well, [...] just like you [(other participants)] don't know the feeling of satiety, I don't really know the feeling of hunger either"* (FG women, pos. 128).

Moreover, the aim of the SA exercise was shown to be in conflict with their own habitual eating practices for some. This was especially the case in connection with certain socialization experiences, whereby socio-culturally shaped normative eating rules played a role: *"I was actually raised to always eat up, you know? [laughs]. That's why I always finish my plate"* (FG mixed, male participant, pos. 204). Here, the norm of eating everything on one's plate seemed to interfere with the principles of IE.

3.3. Couple Context

3.3.1. Intervention Benefit of Partner Participation

Regarding the intervention, the qualitative FGs showed a rather beneficial effect of having the partner involved in the training execution. Only occasionally was the partner perceived as a slight hindrance. On the one hand, this was related to incongruent levels of motivation within the couple, which, in one case, for example, required persuasion on the part of the female participant. On the other hand, a greater distractibility and permission to "cheat" was observed as a barrier when performing the exercises together: *"[laughs] if one cheats, the other one cheats too"* (FG couples, female participant, pos. 100). A much more positive emphasis was placed on the joint participation, whereby motivation also played a decisive role:

"Doing it together always makes it easier.//[male partner:] Exactly. So no, we haven't slowed each other down, you rather motivate each other." (FG couples, female//male participant, pos. 144)

"I didn't need to be motivated by my wife. But it was pleasant to do these two hunger and satiety exercises together with her." (FG mixed, male participant, pos. 417)

As documented in the last quote, there also were participants who explicitly did not need any external motivation from their partner. This may cautiously be explained against the background of the general attitude towards participation in the study: overall, the FGs demonstrated the participants' aspirations of being conscientious and appropriate in the study involvement. For example, one male participant referred to his *"[laughs] Prussian obedience"* (FG male, pos. 89). More importantly, this shows that partner participation was positively associated with an affective component—particularly with feelings of pleasantness and joy. To a certain extent, joint training participation even appeared to have a protective or facilitative effect. As illustrated by the following quote, for instance, the exercise itself was associated with a "struggle", which could be counteracted by the commensal practice and exchange of experience: *"When you do it together it's definitely more fun, obviously, than struggling with it by yourself.//[female partner]: Then you can exchange experiences with one another: 'How was it like for you?'"* (FG couples, male//female participant, pos. 145).

In addition, the partner's influence was also perceived positively when they were not in the training group (G2-P) and did, therefore, not perform the exercises. Here, the partner was perceived as supportive, e.g., by active encouragement of regular practice. Although the partners of training group 2 were not instructed to support their spouses, this encouragement was driven by the positive training effects observed by the partner: *"Even though he didn't participate [...], it was important to him to remind me because he noticed it was good for me."* (FG women, pos. 114).

There was no clear quantitative evidence of a perceived benefit from participation as a couple, which we could only analyze based on a proxy measure: when asked about their preferences for future training participation, the vast majority of participants would not change the way in which they participated. Hence, both those who attended with their partner (G1-I/P: preference with partner: 67.6% (n = 25), without partner: 32.4% (n = 12)) and those who participated alone would like to do so again in the future (G2-I: preference with partner: 38.9% (n = 7), without partner: 61.1% (n = 11)).

3.3.2. Training Intuitive Eating in Everyday Couple Life

The FGs revealed that the couples' everyday lives played a decisive role in the conduction and experience of the training exercises. Some relationship-specific dynamics and routines emerged in this context, allowing conclusions to be drawn about couple-related barriers and—to a greater extent—facilitators. Overall, both couples and individuals in the respective FGs demonstrated the existence of an established *partnership unity* (PU) in terms of their general lifestyle behaviors and shared daily routines. This specifically concerned various diet-related aspects such as meal structures and habits, as well as food preferences and choices. The participants attached a normative, positive meaning to their PU (e.g., by referring to themselves being *"well synchronized"* or *"well attuned"*), indicating an ideal picture of a couple relationship (not only) in the context of food. This became particularly evident in distinction to others, as expressed in this example:

> *"And so, we have—we are both such a, such a unit. And when it comes to cooking and eating habits, we're relatively well-adjusted. [...] Fortunately, I have to say, I know other examples [laughs]..., we are a pretty good unit when it comes to diet and exercise. So that works out quite well."* (FG women, pos. 70)

The perception of a 'good' PU was regarded as an important basis or at least a beneficial starting point for practicing the training exercises as a couple. To differing degrees, this positively perceived PU appeared as a result of (ongoing) negotiation and convergence processes. The following quote illustrates the assumed link between a well-established (diet-related) PU and perceived joint training success:

> *"So, it's not a problem for us, it was already the case that we were largely in alignment when it came to food and nutrition, right? [...] Well, over time, that has also harmonized. [...] In this respect, it wasn't a problem for us to keep it [the intervention] up together."* (FG couple, male participant, pos. 157)

Here, shared dietary practices had been established through mutual negotiations over the course of the relationship. Implicitly, this harmonization process was viewed as a success (or at least the absence of conflict), which the participants relied on as a resource for an unproblematic joint realization of the intervention training program.

As a facilitator or barrier for a positively experienced and successful joint training execution, PU unfolded on several levels, i.e., various aspects of a shared daily life constituted the experience of PU. First, various harmonized diet-related practices such food choices and meal preparation (e.g., also see quote in line 753) appeared in the context of "well-synchronized" PU, which, in turn, was considered to be a constructive pre-condition for joint training success. More specifically, the participants described how their initially (more or less) divergent dietary styles had been subject to a convergence process during the course of their relationship. This concerned ethically and morally motivated dietary styles (e.g., vegetarianism), as well as health-oriented ones (e.g., reduced sugar intake and restricted alcohol consumption). Closely related, some couples also described a gradual alignment in their taste preferences. As an example, in one case, the husband had converged his diet to suit his wife's medical condition. Proceeding from this first step of adaptation, the wife further perceived the development of a harmonized 'PU taste':

> *"[...] Nutrition has always played a bit of a role for me because of my illness [(Diabetes)] and (.) my husband has always supported me in this, in that I've put certain things (2)-less on the table [e.g.,] sweetness has been gradually reduced to the point where we are now and we both like it and I don't have to have a guilty conscience if I bake a cake that isn't as sweet [laughs] as others (.) would perhaps like it to be. [...] [Overall,] we have supported each other well in this respect [(in adjusting dietary preferences)] (.)."* (FG couples, female, pos. 158)

Besides the aforementioned diet-related practices, (in)congruent daily rhythms were discussed as being formative for PU. Primarily, time and setting issues were emphasized, e.g., in relation to working hours and conditions. Spouses' similar everyday structures and shared mealtimes were perceived to have a facilitating effect on the joint training realization. For example, working from home simplified the scheduling of a joint exercise session:

> *"And of course, we have good conditions [(for a proper training realization)]. [...] We are currently working from home, at least I am, due to COVID, and we can really plan our daily routine together now."* (FG couples, male participant, pos. 30)

Mostly, however, couples rarely shared their meals during working weeks, with breakfast being an exception. The training (especially the HU and SA exercises) was then sometimes perceived as being an additional burden interrupting their irregular yet coordinated daily routines. This was also the case among couples in which one spouse only participated in the training. Especially when there was less importance and meaning attached to food as compared to leisure activities, for example, commensal meals were less of a priority and only taken if the schedule allowed so. This consequently impeded regular training realization, as shown in the following:

> "I'd say that we actually make the biggest compromises when it comes to hunger and [as far as hunger is concerned], we had paid the least attention to the study. At the weekends, where we always eat together, there are certain times for us—//male participant: yes//where we have something planned, [such as] doing sports sometimes or I go to church or something. So, [at the weekend] our daily routines are pretty similar. And then it's a compromise as to when the meal fits in. We don't pay that much attention [to hunger]." (FG couples, female participant, pos. 233)

In another way, dissimilar daily "rhythms" appeared as a hindrance, specifically when the meal was one of the few moments of the day that served the purpose of socializing. Here, communicative commensality was prioritized over the training interoception of hunger or satiety signals and other principles related to IE:

> "Well, so far, we haven't managed to concentrate on eating so much, because we don't see each other that much. I work, he doesn't. Erm, and we have more or less the opposite daily rhythm. [laughs] Eh, and for us, mealtimes are more about communication and sharing." (FG couples, female participant, pos. 33)

In contrast, rather than a place of communication, the meal became a place of silence and interoceptive concentration in other couples. Here, achieving a particularly adequate or successful training realization was sought by creating specific facilitation conditions, i.e., the introduction of the rule to eat in silence and/or without speaking:

> "For me, it was like that, [I have learnt]—to eat more consciously or concentrating on eating. [...] This calming down, this relaxing and paying attention to what you eat and how you eat—because we also liked to have the radio on for breakfast and then listen to the news or music, [...]. And we've now abandoned that after the study (.), so to speak. So, we really had breakfast in peace and quiet then." (FG couples, male participant, pos. 21)

> "[...] Well, we have introduced this now [(since the intervention)] as far as possible, not always, that we eat in silence. [...] We have realized that it's good to eat in silence." (FG couples, male participant, pos. 30)

As illustrated by the two above-cited quotes, the training stimulated the impetus to try new and mindful eating practices. Hence, the perceived effectiveness of the intervention training went beyond the intervention's objectives and exercise instructions. While other couples did not establish such new routines or favorable training conditions, these couples identified rather unfavorable settings that hindered them from practicing the exercises. In particular, the restaurant setting and specific temptations due to a larger variety of foods and bigger portion sizes were experienced as impeding the ability to pay attention to one's satiety signals.

Moreover, mindfulness-oriented daily routines some couples had already established prior to the intervention were seen as being a particularly favorable precondition. Specifically, a routinized shared meditation practice facilitated the realization of the training sessions and the understanding of the underlying intervention objectives. The following spouses remembered collectively how they individually had made sense of the more general mindfulness-oriented BS exercise as some kind of preparatory part of the intervention:

> "I found it interesting that this Body Scan was part of it [the diet-focused intervention] [...]. So, that was nothing new to me. Um and, yes, I have already had my thoughts: Yes, as an introduction to a mindfulness exercise, the Body Scan is of course very good, so that you first get to know this kind of approach.//[female partner]: Yes, I also thought that you should first familiarize yourself with your own body and pay attention to body signals. And then I thought to myself: Yes, of course. When it comes to eating, perhaps

that also plays a decisive role (laughs)." (FG couples, male//female participant, pos. 222/223)

Interestingly, this couple further shared that their (mealtime) routines had been subject to a past negotiation process, partly because the wife's diet accorded with principles of intermittent fasting. Among other things, this specific dietary style required finding a compromise regarding the timing of shared meals:

"Well, we have adjusted to each other a bit over the years, and it usually works out well with the mealtimes. [...] We have simply adapted our daily routines over time so that it's okay for both of us. [...] Of course, new aspects were brought in here [(by the training)], but we had already managed it quite well before, I'd say." (FG couples, male participant, pos. 229)

This statement further reflects how the participant viewed the benefits of the training for his and his wife's PU: On the one hand, the training encouraged the integration of "new aspects" into the couple's daily life. On the other hand, however, a (more substantial) change was not considered to be necessary due to a previously negotiated, established PU. Notably, the intended training effect of improving interoceptive sensitivity was not addressed here. Instead, however, the training seemed to be understood more generally and associated with an improvement in their everyday couple life.

4. Discussion

To the authors' knowledge, this is the first mixed-methods acceptance study on a dyadic interoception-based pilot randomized-controlled trial (RCT). The RCT aimed to train interoceptive sensitivity (IS) among couples aged 50+ as a crucial first step towards re-learning intuitive eating (IE). The overarching objective of this study was to analyze the participants' acceptance of the training in general, as well as its practical implementation in everyday life. Two main exploratory research questions were addressed: first, the extent to which partnered adults aged 50+ accepted the (couple- vs. single-based) interoception-based training; and second, the role the couple context played in the experience, conduction, and post-intervention continuation of the training.

While popular as well as scientific research on IE is growing, research on IE and its associated principles—including IS—is still limited to aims that can be achieved by IE (e.g., adaptive eating behavior [22,27,28]) or specific target groups (e.g., individuals with obesity [18,19] or women [30,37,38]). Basic research on the mechanisms involved in practicing IE in general populations is scarce. Against this background, previous work has specifically emphasized the need for qualitative explorations on re-learning IE [37]. Moreover, there is little research on practicing IE that takes the couple context into account, which may, however, decisively shape the ways in which individuals engage in practices of IE [38]. Therefore, our study aimed to investigate a couple- (vs. single-) based intervention. Addressing these research gaps, the present acceptance study provides first insights into the role the couple context plays, e.g., in promoting or inhibiting joint IE training execution.

4.1. Training Acceptance

Overall, our synthesis revealed a fairly moderate *General Acceptance*, whereby the training, in general, was perceived as feasible and associated with a relatively low burden. However, a mixed picture emerged, particularly with respect to the *Perceived Effectiveness* and *Affective Attitudes*. Here, a hierarchization of the more general mindfulness-based Body Scan (BS) over the hunger (HU) and satiety (SA) exercises became evident. Besides a few exceptions, the BS was primarily evaluated as pleasant, enjoyable, and useful for everyday life. The BS was associated with various beneficial effects even apart from eating, such as an improved sleeping quality. Some of these positive experiences associated with the BS in particular were also shown in an earlier study about women who had been practicing IE over a minimum of 1.5 years without an intervention context [37]. For instance, a greater "headspace" and an improved awareness of body signals was described.

As in comparison to the BS, the HU and SA rather evoked negative emotions and were associated with a medium *Perceived Effectiveness*. In addition, the participants expressed some disappointment with the HU and SA training content and reported a lack of training success on various levels. This ranged from mostly slight difficulties with the exercise implementation (both organizationally (e.g., due to the spouses' incongruent daily routines) and in terms of content (e.g., perceived lack of interoceptive ability)) to, in extreme cases, anger about the training content. In these cases, the training experiences, thus, rather fell short of the intended intervention objective.

The hierarchical exercise evaluation may have been related to the participants' pre-existing familiarity with body relaxation exercises and their experiences with mindfulness-oriented practices and lifestyles in general. In contrast, the HU and SA exercises were novel and (mostly) surprising to the participants. Closely related, our findings suggest a partially insufficient understanding of the objectives and intended effects of the HU and SA exercises, resulting in a more negative evaluation compared to the BS. This can be further explained by the quite high popularity of mindfulness-based stress reduction programs that include the Body Scan. The implications of these results are described in Section 4.6.

Compared to German adults aged 50+ [11], our participants showed similar pre-existing levels of IE, which is related to the sampling strategy (see Section 2.2.2). In addition, they demonstrated relatively pronounced mindfulness and health-oriented lifestyles. As an example, they saw their dietary practices as already being in line with various IE ideas to differing degrees, rendering the HU and SA (slightly) obsolete.

Concerning the TFA dimension of *Intervention Coherence*—i.e., the participants' understanding of how the intervention aimed to increase IS—a thin line of conflict between a more reflective awareness and intuitive practices could be observed: for example, for one participant, the training did not lead to an increase in IS, but rather to a stronger pronunciation of rationality regarding the concept of satiety. This style of eating is described as "flexible control" [65]. On the one hand, raising awareness for the concepts of hunger and satiety could be seen as a necessary step or preliminary stage in increasing IS. On the other hand, however, eating guided by control, instead of by one's hunger and satiety sensations, is not in line with the principles of IS.

It appears vital to embed the above-mentioned difficulties with (re-)learning IS and thus IE in a broader societal context: whether for health or ethical reasons, there is a widespread trend of eating according to various kinds of restriction rules. This concerns several types of restrictive dietary practices [66], for instance, regarding specific foods or macronutrients (e.g., low-calorie diet [67] or temporal restrictions (e.g., fasting [68]). Data from a German population-wide consumption study showed that people are dieting more frequently as they age, with around 20% of people over 65 doing so [69]. In light of these trends IE—and more specifically, the training of IS—is facing a challenge. This is also highlighted by a study on IE experiences among British women, where prevailing norms of the diet mentality occurred as barrier for practicing IE [37]. Albeit more implicitly, our findings also suggest a connection of such broader societal norms with the difficulties participants experienced throughout the training. However, there is also an emerging trend towards IE as a counter-movement to the dominant diet culture and related normative discourses [37,70]. It will be the task of future studies to unravel how this affects future cohorts in training IS.

4.2. The Role of the Couple Context

Overall, our synthesis pointed at some conflicting results regarding the wish of spousal training involvement. While the quantitative data rather showed that participants did not want to or could not imagine changing the training mode, the FGs highlighted a beneficial effect of spousal training participation. Since the FGs provided more space and time for reflection and encouraged discussions on these issues, it seems plausible that new stimuli and ideas were triggered here. At the same time, mechanisms related to social desirability may have had a stronger impact here, e.g., with respect to the training staff who had designed a couple-based intervention, or to present themselves as a well-attuned couple to the other participants. Indeed, the qualitative data material on this aspect was particularly rich, underlining its credibility despite the contradictory quantitative results. Moreover, the insights gained regarding the beneficial effects are congruent with prior study findings on general dyadic behavior change interventions [46,47,71].

While in the FGs, the involvement of the spouse in the training was considered to be favorable overall, some results also implied that the partner was experienced as an obstacle to adequately practice IS. As an example, one participant described difficulties in concentrating on her own body signals (e.g., with respect to the portion size) in the presence of her partner, because this might have disrupted the social, communicative function of commensality. This emphasizes a balancing act between eating according to hunger and satiety signals and fulfilling the personal needs of closeness and belonging, as has previously been stressed [72,73].

One of our main findings concerned the Partnership Unity (PU) presented by the couples, which manifested itself on various levels—primarily on the level of diet-related everyday practices and (in)congruent daily rhythms and meal structures. According to a previous study, married couples showed (fairly) higher levels of mindful and IE skills as compared to singles. The authors concluded that this was due to couples having more regular daily routines and eating habits as compared to singles [74]. It is well-established that couples tend to share similar taste preferences and dietary practices habits [75,76]. On the one hand, this can be attributed to the phenomenon of "homogamy", i.e., a similarity in the milieu background and lifestyles from the onset of the relationship [75]. On the other hand, this also results from various negotiation and convergence processes over the course of the relationship [41,75,77].

Two previous studies using data of the NutriAct Family Study (NFS) analyzed such intra-couple dynamics shaping dietary preferences. First, a primarily asymmetrical convergence pattern was found, whereby one partner predominantly adapted the other one's food preferences [41]. Second, the dominant role of women in shaping older-aged couples' dietary habits was shown [41,45]. Such convergence dynamics were also evident in the qualitative FGs of the present study. Generally, however, our couples demonstrated a rather symmetrical, conjointly shaped harmonization, specifically with respect to food choice and mealtime routines.

Focusing on meal practices, prior work on intra-couple dynamics highlights jointly-shaped synchronizations that occurred chronologically across different phases [78]. Thereby, synergetic mealtime practices resulted from the last of three synchronization stages. In this stage, previous individual practices and negotiations thereof are blended or combined, amongst others. Given the emphasized PU, our couples may cautiously be attributed to this stage. Besides such convergence processes, various couple biographical aspects (e.g., relationship length, disruptions, and relationship quality) may have been involved in shaping the spouses' IS- and more general IE-related practices. As previous research suggests, the level of existing IE skills is associated with different relationship types and the perceived relationship quality [38]. Based on our data, we can only assume a relatively high perceived relationship quality, considering how the participants positioned themselves as couples and their PU in the FGs.

4.3. Joint Training Execution within Various Daily Routines

There is ample evidence that biographical transitions shape lifestyle behaviors such as dietary practices [8,79]. For our target group, the retirement transition represents such a critical momentum. There are often asynchronous everyday structures and corresponding meal routines determined by everyday working life, as also shown in our FGs. The retirement transition offers an opportunity to (re-)establish more flexible and shared mealtime routines [80]. In the present study, the retirement status of one or both partners also played a role in the joint participation and the establishment of IS and IE practices, which was mostly related to the (dis)similar daily rhythms of the spouses. At the same time, as some of our FG results indicated, even if both partners are in the same phase of life, they may have different daily mealtime routines and only sometimes share their meals, e.g., because they prioritize other (joint) activities. Therefore, retirement may, to some extent, be a facilitating and inhibiting condition for a joint participation in (dietary) couple interventions. In a broader sense, however, it is the similarity of the life phases in general that appears to be decisive, yet further research is needed here.

Broader societal disruptions, such as the COVID-19 pandemic, also play a role in this respect. Findings of an observational study suggest a positive relationship between the pandemic and its lock-down and pronounced levels of mindful eating and IE skills [74]. Our study took place at the time of the COVID-19 lockdown in Germany. This period entailed changes in (shared) daily structures (e.g., working from home) and mealtime routines for many. As implied by some of our FG findings, it may have, hence, created specific facilitating conditions for the couples' engagement in joint IE practices.

Moreover, the (in)congruent daily rhythms described by our couples can also be framed in terms of broader societal developments. In the context of ongoing individualization processes [81,82], (commensal) traditional day structures are continuously changing. Thus, dietary habits are becoming increasingly flexible, and meals are more frequently eaten alone, rather than in the family context [72,76,83]. In our study, mostly positive meaning and a rather great importance was attached to commensality. However, couples with rather dissimilar daily rhythms described various barriers they faced in the joint training realization. It appears, thus, worthwhile to account for such continually changing everyday realities in future (couple-based) dietary intervention designs. In this way, the practical obstacles to implementing the intervention, as also reported by our couples, could be overcome.

4.4. Overlapping Concepts: Interoceptive Sensitivity, Intuitive Eating and Mindfulness

Looking at the IE construct developed by Tribole and Resch [55], our intervention study primarily focused on the improvement of IS and thus the principles *"Honour your hunger"* and *"Feel your fullness"*. Nevertheless, the participants' discussions also concerned several other principles, such as *"Honour your health-gentle nutrition"*, *"Reject the diet-mentality"*, *"Challenge the food police"* and *"Discover the satisfaction factor"*. Closely related, they also referred to several changes towards more IE-oriented lifestyles and dietary practices as a result of the intervention (e.g., eating in silence and heightened meal anticipation). Such intervention-induced changes were perceived as successful training outcomes, yet went beyond the original objectives of the intervention, and may, thus, be seen as an additional "transfer achievement". At the same time, the participants also found that the training goals were presented too vaguely or abstract and would have liked more detailed information about the conceptual basis and more specific training instructions. In particular, the desire for feedback and comparability with others (e.g., *"whether we are marching in the same direction"*) is notable here, as this demonstrates insecurities with the concepts of IS and IE and stresses their need for more guidance.

Furthermore, the participants associated the interoception-oriented training with more general mindful eating practices [84] (e.g., eating slowly and focusing on the chewing process) or understood IS and mindfulness as being synonymous. The BS is a mindfulness-based exercise that is not directly linked to the specific interoceptive perception of hunger and satiety cues, but rather to a more generic mindfulness towards one's own body. In this respect, the link between mindfulness and IS/IE was already drawn in the context of the intervention. Furthermore, other studies also seem to mix up the concepts of IE and mindfulness, as has been critically remarked by Erhardt (2021) [37]. The question, therefore, arises as to the extent to which a strict separation of these concepts is appropriate and useful for IE interventions. Accordingly, it is also questionable in how far the theoretically defined concepts of IS, IE, and mindfulness are indeed distinguishable and distinctively implementable by laypeople. Our findings emphasize these questions, as our participants' already existing mindfulness orientation seemed to have acted as a facilitator in conducting the training exercises. At the same time, the exercises also stimulated further mindfulness practices, indicating a mixing of the concepts of IS, IE and mindfulness.

4.5. Strengths and Limitations

This is the first acceptance study on a novel couple-based intervention program focusing on the (re-)learning of IS skills without the direct goal of weight loss or health-improvement. Our analysis followed a theoretically oriented iterative approach, drawing on the Theoretical Acceptance Framework by Sekhon et al. [49,50]. So far, there was a lack in consented acceptance definitions and respective theory-driven acceptance analyses on behavioral healthcare interventions [49]. Responding to this gap, the TFA is the first framework providing a definitional and, at the same time, analytical framework [50]. Our study is the first to apply the TFA to an intervention acceptance analysis. Using an explorative qualitative convergent synthesis design involving the Pillar Integration Process (PIP) [58], six out of eight TFA-acceptance components emerged as themes. The benefits of MM in behavioral intervention research, amongst others, for generating a rich and comprehensive understanding has been stressed previously [85]. In our MM design, the explorative-inductive analysis process allowed going beyond the TFA acceptance dimensions and providing in-depth insights into various contextual factors.

Since we conducted a pilot trial, we were not able to recruit a representative sample for German adults aged 50 years and above. Furthermore, although we followed a selective recruitment strategy, the IE levels of our intervention participants were comparable to a German community sample. Especially with regard to the training effects, it should be noted that our participants had previously taken part in the NFS and, therefore, were already experienced with diet-related studies. This might reflect the participants' strong interest and great knowledge about diet-related topics. These aspects might limit the generalizability of our findings. Furthermore, the quantitative measurement of the training evaluation and the intervention acceptance was based on self-constructed items. By the time of the intervention, there was a lack of a validated questionnaires to assess the acceptance of healthcare interventions [50].

With respect to the FGs, there are two major limitations to be addressed: first, cross-case and cross-group comparability was only possible to a limited extent. Due to the COVID-19-restrictions, as well as recruitment problems associated with the pandemic, two of our groups consisted of two people only. Ideally, FGs involve 4-8 individuals, as group sizes may have a crucial effect on interaction dynamics. Moreover, a small group size limits the variety of perspectives, and, at the same time, the discovery of a so-called "collective perspective" [86]. However, our qualitative data material yielded detailed descriptions and showed some contrasting horizons of experiences [87]. Second, specific FG dynamics may occurred due to mechanisms related to social desirability and (self-)positioning as a couple, i.e., the ways in which the individuals and couples portrayed themselves towards the other participants as well as the researcher [88]. In our study, this might have been specifically the case with respect to the couples' representations of their PU, which were emphasized in various ways and to varying degrees. To address the above-mentioned shortcomings, future studies are needed that use qualitative theoretical sampling in further investigating, amongst others, intra-couple dynamics involved in IE-related practices.

4.6. Implications for Future Interventions

Against the background of the intervention acceptance and contextual factors discussed above, several conclusions can be drawn for future interventions. Most importantly, the participants expressed a desire for closer guidance and feedback during the intervention, as well as a personalized evaluation after the study. It seems, hence, vital to promote a better understanding and a more thorough implementation, especially of the HU and SA exercises. First, it might be beneficial to provide more detailed information and conceptual definitions regarding the concepts IS and IE, as well as to explain the intentions of each exercise more explicitly in order to help the participants to monitor their own learning progress.

Second, a regular involvement and (personal or digital) exchange with the study staff and also the opportunity to share experiences with other participants could be fruitful. Here, a(n) (online) group setting (e.g., group videoconferencing) appears to be effective [25,89], which, for example, involves an exchange forum during the respective training weeks.

The participants' wish for interaction may have been related to the web-based study format. Previous studies have challenged web-based behavioral intervention designs and concluded face-to-face-designs to be more effective [25]. This may also be true for our intervention, because older participants might need greater support than younger participants regarding study participation and the conduction of an online training [90]. However, not only during COVID-19 times, web-based interventions may be particularly feasible and practicable, since they are readily available and have rather low access barriers [91,92].

Overall, our findings support benefits of dietary couple-based interventions, which have also been suggested by previous research [47,93]. Regarding the couple-related aspects discussed above, it appears worthwhile for future diet-related interventions to target couples who share similar daily routines or aim to do so. Since different life phases and daily rhythms can hinder a regular joint training participation, the question arises as to in which cases and under which circumstances a couple-based intervention is appropriate and expedient. In a previous intervention combining IE and mindfulness for the treatment of maladaptive eating behaviors, the integration of intervention programs into the workplace or other (institutionalized) settings was emphasized as a successful strategy [94]. How such an approach can be meaningfully applied to the target group of people 50+ and especially to couples is the task of future studies.

Finally, our sample showed IE levels comparable to adults aged 50+ in a German community sample [11] and a general pronounced mindfulness and health orientation. Previous studies have discussed IE as a "privileged approach" [95] and shown "food secure adults" [26] to score higher in IE skills. Hence, future studies on population groups with more diverse and precarious socio-economic backgrounds as well as lower IE skills are needed and a respective tailoring of IS/IE interventions seems essential.

5. Conclusions

Intuitive Eating (IE)—an adaptive eating behavior characterized by an attunement to one's hunger and satiety signals—has gained scientific interest as a critical response to dieting trends. Training interoceptive sensitivity (IS) might be a first step in effectively promoting IE. The couple context plays an important role in (re-)learning and changing dietary practices, including IE. The benefits of couple-based health interventions in general have been demonstrated, but no such studies have yet been conducted in relation to IE. Against this background, a web-based dyadic experimental interoception-based pilot randomized-controlled trial (RCT) was conducted to increase IS—and, thus, IE—among couples aged 50 years and older. The training consisted of three exercises involving a more general mindful-oriented Body Scan (BS) and two exercises specifically concerning IS towards hunger (HU) and satiety (SA).

The present acceptance study was the first to exploratively analyze how couples accept a dyadic interoception-based training program to increase IS and, to explore the role the couple context in the experience and conduct of a joint vs. single training execution. In a mixed-methods convergent synthesis design, findings of a quantitative survey ($n = 68$ couples) and of qualitative focus groups (FGs) ($n = 4$ couples with 12 individuals) were synthesized using the Pillar Integration Process (PIP). The synthesis process was oriented towards the Theoretical Framework of Acceptance (TFA).

Overall, a fairly moderate general acceptance emerged, e.g., with respect to its feasibility and low burden. A hierarchical gradient was shown in favor of the BS, which was associated with benefits beyond the training's intention, such as an improved sleep quality. Amongst others, barriers concerned a perceived lack of the exercises' usefulness and a limited understanding of the training's intended purpose. The participants expressed a wish for regular feedback and exchange with the study stuff and other participants. A rather beneficial effect of having the partner involved in the training execution was demonstrated. Thereby, a jointly established Partnership Unity regarding previously harmonized diet-related practices and shared daily routines (e.g., mealtime structures) appeared as constructive pre-condition for a joint training success.

Our study highlights the potential and implications of a web-based training of IS in a couple context among adults aged 50+. Further studies are needed that address different population groups. Future interventions should take into account the couple context and focus on a regular exchange with other participants and a closer guidance by the study staff to promote a better understanding of the processes and goals of IS and IE.

Supplementary Materials: The following supporting information can be downloaded at: https://www.mdpi.com/article/10.3390/nu16121949/s1. Multimedia Supplementary S1: Synthesis Table according to the Pillar Integration Process.

Author Contributions: Conceptualization: N.-R.B., N.V.G. and U.A.G.; RCT/intervention realization: U.A.G., H.R.W. and P.W.; QUAN methods: H.R.W. and U.A.G.; QUAL methods: N.-R.B. and N.V.G.; mixed methods: N.-R.B. and N.V.G.; software: N.-R.B., N.V.G., H.R.W. and U.A.G.; resources: L.S. and P.W.; data curation: N.-R.B., N.V.G., H.R.W. and U.A.G.; writing—original draft preparation: N.-R.B., N.V.G. and U.A.G.; writing—review and editing: all authors; project administration: H.R.W.; funding acquisition: L.S. and P.W. All authors have read and agreed to the published version of the manuscript.

Funding: This research was funded by the Federal Ministry of Education and Research (FKZ: 01EA1806B). The funding resource has no role in the design of the study, the collection, analysis, and interpretation of data, and in writing the manuscript.

Institutional Review Board Statement: The study was conducted in accordance with the Ethikkommission Landesärztekammer Brandenburg(läkB) (E38933). Approval date: 7 September 2019.

Informed Consent Statement: Informed consent was obtained from all subjects involved in the study.

Data Availability Statement: As this study is part of the ongoing NutriAct Family Study, access to data will be arranged on a reasonable request and with the permission of all collaboration partners.

Acknowledgments: First of all, the authors would like to thank the study participants. Moreover, we thank Manuela Bergmann, Ulrich Harttig, Julia Luff-Heinke, Jule Burblies, Shirley Ohme, Afifah Pribadi, Anastasia Krasnikova, Birgit Czullay, Juliane Wakim, Nadine Bespalenko, Bianca Weigel, Tabea Albroscheit, Malina Pyttlik, and Ellen Schöley-Pohl for support in conducting the study.

Conflicts of Interest: The authors declare no conflicts of interest.

References

1. Chen, P.-J.; Antonelli, M. Conceptual Models of Food Choice: Influential Factors Related to Foods, Individual Differences, and Society. *Foods* **2020**, *9*, 1898. [CrossRef]
2. Zorbas, C.; Palermo, C.; Chung, A.; Iguacel, I.; Peeters, A.; Bennett, R.; Backholer, K. Factors perceived to influence healthy eating: A systematic review and meta-ethnographic synthesis of the literature. *Nutr. Rev.* **2018**, *76*, 861–874. [CrossRef]
3. Keller, C.; Siegrist, M. Does personality influence eating styles and food choices? Direct and indirect effects. *Appetite* **2015**, *84*, 128–138. [CrossRef]
4. Larson, N.; Story, M. A Review of Environmental Influences on Food Choices. *Ann. Behav. Med.* **2009**, *38* (Suppl. S1), s56–s73. [CrossRef]
5. Constantinides, S.V.; Turner, C.; Frongillo, E.A.; Bhandari, S.; Reyes, L.I.; Blake, C.E. Using a global food environment framework to understand relationships with food choice in diverse low- and middle-income countries. *Glob. Food Secur.* **2021**, *29*, 100511. [CrossRef]
6. Mustajoki, P. Obesogenic food environment explains most of the obesity epidemic. *Duodecim Laaketieteellinen Aikakauskirja* **2015**, *131*, 1345–1352.
7. Caspi, C.E.; Sorensen, G.; Subramanian, S.V.; Kawachi, I. The local food environment and diet: A systematic review. *Health Place* **2012**, *18*, 1172–1187. [CrossRef]
8. Devine, C.M. A Life Course Perspective: Understanding Food Choices in Time, Social Location, and History. *J. Nutr. Educ. Behav.* **2005**, *37*, 121–128. [CrossRef]
9. Vesnaver, E.; Keller, H.H. Social influences and eating behavior in later life: A review. *J. Nutr. Gerontol. Geriatr.* **2011**, *30*, 2–23. [CrossRef]

10. Tylka, T.L.; Kroon Van Diest, A.M. The Intuitive Eating Scale–2: Item refinement and psychometric evaluation with college women and men. *J. Couns. Psychol.* **2013**, *60*, 137–153. [CrossRef]
11. Ruzanska, U.A.; Warschburger, P. Psychometric evaluation of the German version of the Intuitive Eating Scale-2 in a community sample. *Appetite* **2017**, *117*, 126–134. [CrossRef]
12. Robinson, E.; Blissett, J.; Higgs, S. Social influences on eating: Implications for nutritional interventions. *Nutr. Res. Rev.* **2013**, *26*, 166–176. [CrossRef]
13. Craig, A.D. Interoception: The sense of the physiological condition of the body. *Curr. Opin. Neurobiol.* **2003**, *13*, 500–505. [CrossRef]
14. Cameron, O.G. *Visceral Sensory Neuroscience: Interoception*; Oxford University Press: Oxford, UK, 2001; ISBN 0198031106.
15. Herbert, B.M.; Blechert, J.; Hautzinger, M.; Matthias, E.; Herbert, C. Intuitive eating is associated with interoceptive sensitivity. Effects on body mass index. *Appetite* **2013**, *70*, 22–30. [CrossRef]
16. Richard, A.; Meule, A.; Georgii, C.; Voderholzer, U.; Cuntz, U.; Wilhelm, F.H.; Blechert, J. Associations between interoceptive sensitivity, intuitive eating, and body mass index in patients with anorexia nervosa and normal-weight controls. *Eur. Eat. Disord. Rev.* **2019**, *27*, 571–577. [CrossRef]
17. Stevenson, R.J.; Mahmut, M.; Rooney, K. Individual differences in the interoceptive states of hunger, fullness and thirst. *Appetite* **2015**, *95*, 44–57. [CrossRef]
18. Willem, C.; Gandolphe, M.-C.; Roussel, M.; Verkindt, H.; Pattou, F.; Nandrino, J.-L. Difficulties in emotion regulation and deficits in interoceptive awareness in moderate and severe obesity. *Eat. Weight. Disord.-Stud. Anorex. Bulim. Obes.* **2019**, *24*, 633–644. [CrossRef]
19. Robinson, E.; Foote, G.; Smith, J.; Higgs, S.; Jones, A. Interoception and obesity: A systematic review and meta-analysis of the relationship between interoception and BMI. *Int. J. Obes.* **2021**, *45*, 2515–2526. [CrossRef]
20. Murphy, J.; Geary, H.; Millgate, E.; Catmur, C.; Bird, G. Direct and indirect effects of age on interoceptive accuracy and awareness across the adult lifespan. *Psychon. Bull. Rev.* **2018**, *25*, 1193–1202. [CrossRef]
21. Linardon, J.; Tylka, T.L.; Fuller-Tyszkiewicz, M. Intuitive eating and its psychological correlates: A meta-analysis. *Int. J. Eat. Disord.* **2021**, *54*, 1073–1098. [CrossRef]
22. Ruzanska, U.A.; Warschburger, P. Intuitive eating mediates the relationship between self-regulation and BMI—Results from a cross-sectional study in a community sample. *Eat. Behav.* **2019**, *33*, 23–29. [CrossRef]
23. Carrard, I.; Rothen, S.; Rodgers, R.F. Body image concerns and intuitive eating in older women. *Appetite* **2021**, *164*, 105275. [CrossRef]
24. Babbott, K.M.; Cavadino, A.; Brenton-Peters, J.; Consedine, N.S.; Roberts, M. Outcomes of intuitive eating interventions: A systematic review and meta-analysis. *Eat. Disord.* **2023**, *31*, 33–63. [CrossRef]
25. Hensley-Hackett, K.; Bosker, J.; Keefe, A.; Reidlinger, D.; Warner, M.; D'arcy, A.; Utter, J. Intuitive Eating Intervention and Diet Quality in Adults: A Systematic Literature Review. *J. Nutr. Educ. Behav.* **2022**, *54*, 1099–1115. [CrossRef]
26. Jackson, A.; Sano, Y.; Parker, L.; Cox, A.E.; Lanigan, J. Intuitive eating and dietary intake. *Eat. Behav.* **2022**, *45*, 101606. [CrossRef]
27. Warren, J.M.; Smith, N.; Ashwell, M. A structured literature review on the role of mindfulness, mindful eating and intuitive eating in changing eating behaviours: Effectiveness and associated potential mechanisms. *Nutr. Res. Rev.* **2017**, *30*, 272–283. [CrossRef]
28. Hazzard, V.M.; Telke, S.E.; Simone, M.; Anderson, L.M.; Larson, N.I.; Neumark-Sztainer, D. Intuitive eating longitudinally predicts better psychological health and lower use of disordered eating behaviors: Findings from EAT 2010–2018. *Eat. Weight Disord.-Stud. Anorexia Bulim. Obes.* **2021**, *26*, 287–294. [CrossRef]
29. Grider, H.S.; Douglas, S.M.; Raynor, H.A. The Influence of Mindful Eating and/or Intuitive Eating Approaches on Dietary Intake: A Systematic Review. *J. Acad. Nutr. Diet.* **2021**, *121*, 709–727.e1. [CrossRef]
30. Belon, K.E.; Serier, K.N.; VanderJagt, H.; Smith, J.E. What Is Healthy Eating? Exploring Profiles of Intuitive Eating and Nutritionally Healthy Eating in College Women. *Am. J. Health Promot.* **2022**, *36*, 823–833. [CrossRef]
31. Kerin, J.L.; Webb, H.J.; Zimmer-Gembeck, M.J. Intuitive, mindful, emotional, external and regulatory eating behaviours and beliefs: An investigation of the core components. *Appetite* **2019**, *132*, 139–146. [CrossRef]
32. Healy, N.; Joram, E.; Matvienko, O.; Woolf, S.; Knesting, K. Impact of an intuitive eating education program on high school students' eating attitudes. *Health Educ.* **2015**, *115*, 214–228. [CrossRef]
33. Schaefer, J.T.; Magnuson, A.B. A Review of Interventions that Promote Eating by Internal Cues. *J. Acad. Nutr. Diet.* **2014**, *114*, 734–760. [CrossRef]
34. Van Dyke, N.; Drinkwater, E.J. Review Article Relationships between intuitive eating and health indicators: Literature review. *Public Health Nutr.* **2014**, *17*, 1757–1766. [CrossRef]
35. Bacon, L.; Stern, J.S.; Van Loan, M.D.; Keim, N.L. Size Acceptance and Intuitive Eating Improve Health for Obese, Female Chronic Dieters. *J. Am. Diet. Assoc.* **2005**, *105*, 929–936. [CrossRef]
36. Van Dyke, N.; Murphy, M.; Drinkwater, E.J. What do people think of intuitive eating? A qualitative exploration with rural Australians. *PLoS ONE* **2023**, *18*, e0278979. [CrossRef]
37. Erhardt, G.A. Intuitive eating as a counter-cultural process towards self-actualisation: An interpretative phenomenological analysis of experiences of learning to eat intuitively. *Health Psychol. Open* **2021**, *8*, 20551029211000957. [CrossRef]

38. Carbonneau, N.; Carbonneau, E.; Cantin, M.; Gagnon-Girouard, M.-P. Examining women's perceptions of their mother's and romantic partner's interpersonal styles for a better understanding of their eating regulation and intuitive eating. *Appetite* **2015**, *92*, 156–166. [CrossRef]
39. Skoyen, J.A.; Blank, E.; Corkery, S.A.; Butler, E.A. The interplay of partner influence and individual values predicts daily fluctuations in eating and physical activity. *J. Soc. Pers. Relatsh.* **2013**, *30*, 1000–1019. [CrossRef]
40. Brazeau, H.; Lewis, N. Within-couple health behavior trajectories: The role of spousal support and strain. *Health Psychol.* **2021**, *40*, 125–134. [CrossRef]
41. Baer, N.; Zoellick, J.C.; Deutschbein, J.; Anton, V.; Bergmann, M.; Schenk, L. Dietary Preferences in the Context of Intra-Couple Dynamics: Relationship Types within the German NutriAct Family Cohort. *Appetite* **2021**, *167*, 105625. [CrossRef]
42. Bove, C.; Sobal, J.; Rauschenbach, B. Food choices among newly married couples: Convergence, conflict, individualism, and projects. *Appetite* **2003**, *40*, 25–41. [CrossRef]
43. Bartel, S.J.; Sherry, S.B.; Molnar, D.S.; Mushquash, A.R.; Leonard, K.E.; Flett, G.L.; Stewart, S.H. Do romantic partners influence each other's heavy episodic drinking? Support for the partner influence hypothesis in a three-year longitudinal study. *Addict. Behav.* **2017**, *69*, 55–58. [CrossRef]
44. Mason, T.B.; Dayag, R.; Dolgon-Krutolow, A.; Lam, K.; Zhang, D. A systematic review of maladaptive interpersonal behaviors and eating disorder psychopathology. *Eat. Behav.* **2022**, *45*, 101601. [CrossRef]
45. Wortmann, H.R.; Gisch, U.A.; Jannasch, F.; Knüppel, S.; Bergmann, M.M.; Warschburger, P. Dyadic analysis of the relationship between food neophilia and dietary quality among older heterosexual couples: Findings from the NutriAct Family Study. *Food Qual. Prefer.* **2023**, *110*, 104952. [CrossRef]
46. Trief, P.M.; Fisher, L.; Sandberg, J.; Hessler, D.M.; Cibula, D.A.; Weinstock, R.S. Two for one? Effects of a couples intervention on partners of persons with Type 2 diabetes: A randomized controlled trial. *Diabet. Med.* **2019**, *36*, 473–481. [CrossRef]
47. Arden-Close, E.; McGrath, N. Health behaviour change interventions for couples: A systematic review. *Br. J. Health Psychol.* **2017**, *22*, 215–237. [CrossRef]
48. Albanese, A.M.; Huffman, J.C.; Celano, C.M.; Malloy, L.M.; Wexler, D.J.; Freedman, M.E.; Millstein, R.A. The role of spousal support for dietary adherence among type 2 diabetes patients: A narrative review. *Soc. Work. Health Care* **2019**, *58*, 304–323. [CrossRef]
49. Sekhon, M.; Cartwright, M.; Francis, J.J. Acceptability of healthcare interventions: An overview of reviews and development of a theoretical framework. *BMC Health Serv. Res.* **2017**, *17*, 88. [CrossRef]
50. Sekhon, M.; Cartwright, M.; Francis, J.J. Development of a theory-informed questionnaire to assess the acceptability of healthcare interventions. *BMC Health Serv. Res.* **2022**, *22*, 279. [CrossRef]
51. Février, F. Vers un Modèle Intégrateur "Expérience-Acceptation": Rôle des Affects et de Caractéristiques Personnelles et Contextuelles dans la Détermination des Intentions D'usage d'un Environnement Numérique de Travail. 2011. Université Rennes 2, Université Européenne de Bretagne. Available online: https://theses.hal.science/tel-00608335 (accessed on 10 June 2024).
52. Warschburger, P.; Wortmann, H.R.; Gisch, U.A.; Baer, N.-R.; Schenk, L.; Anton, V.; Bergmann, M.M. An experimental approach to training interoceptive sensitivity: Study protocol for a pilot randomized controlled trial. *Nutr. J.* **2022**, *21*, 74. [CrossRef]
53. Kabat-Zinn, J.; Valentin, L. *Stressbewältigung Durch Die Praxis der Achtsamkeit*; Arbor: Freiburg im Breisgau, Germany, 2014; ISBN 9783867811217.
54. Fischer, D.; Messner, M.; Pollatos, O. Improvement of Interoceptive Processes after an 8-Week Body Scan Intervention. *Front. Hum. Neurosci.* **2017**, *11*, 452. [CrossRef]
55. Tribole, E.; Resch, E. *The Intuitive Eating Workbook*; New Harbinger Publications: Oakland, CA, USA, 2017; ISBN 978-1-62625-622-4.
56. Schuman-Olivier, Z.; Trombka, M.; Lovas, D.A.; Brewer, J.A.; Vago, D.R.; Gawande, R.; Dunne, J.P.; Lazar, S.W.; Loucks, E.B.; Fulwiler, C. Mindfulness and Behavior Change. *Harv. Rev. Psychiatry* **2020**, *28*, 371–394. [CrossRef]
57. Döring, N.; Bortz, J. *Forschungsmethoden und Evaluation in den Sozial- und Humanwissenschaften*, 5th ed.; Springer: Berlin/Heidelberg, Germany, 2016; pp. 185–544, ISBN 978-3-642-41088-8.
58. Johnson, R.; Grove, A.; Clarke, A. Pillar Integration Process: A Joint Display Technique to Integrate Data in Mixed Methods Research. *J. Mix. Methods Res.* **2017**, *13*, 301–320. [CrossRef]
59. O'Cathain, A.; Murphy, E.; Nicholl, J. The quality of mixed methods studies in health services research. *J. Health Serv. Res. Policy* **2008**, *13*, 92–98. [CrossRef]
60. Schwingshackl, L.; Ruzanska, U.; Anton, V.; Wallroth, R.; Ohla, K.; Knüppel, S.; Schulze, M.B.; Pischon, T.; Deutschbein, J.; Schenk, L.; et al. The NutriAct Family Study: A web-based prospective study on the epidemiological, psychological and sociological basis of food choice. *BMC Public Health* **2018**, *18*, 963. [CrossRef]
61. Creamer, E. *An Introduction to Fully Integrated Mixed Methods Research*; SAGE Publications: Thousand Oaks, CA, USA, 2018; ISBN 9781483350936.
62. Kuckartz, U. Qualitative Inhaltsanalyse. In *Methoden, Praxis, Computerunterstützung*; Beltz Juventa, Auflage: Weinheim, Germany, 2018; Volume 4.
63. Guetterman, T.C.; Fetters, M.D.; Creswell, J.W. Integrating Quantitative and Qualitative Results in Health Science Mixed Methods Research Through Joint Displays. *Ann. Fam. Med.* **2015**, *13*, 554–561. [CrossRef]
64. WHO. Obesity: Preventing and Managing the Global Epidemic: Report of a WHO Consultation. 2000. Available online: https://iris.who.int/handle/10665/42330 (accessed on 10 June 2024).

65. Tylka, T.L.; Calogero, R.M.; Daníelsdóttir, S. Is intuitive eating the same as flexible dietary control? Their links to each other and well-being could provide an answer. *Appetite* **2015**, *95*, 166–175. [CrossRef]
66. Bandelin-Franke, L.; Schenk, L.; Baer, N.R. To Eat or Not to Eat—A Qualitative Exploration and Typology of Restrictive Dietary Practices among Middle-Aged and Older Adults. *Nutrients* **2023**, *15*, 2466. [CrossRef]
67. BMEL. Deutschland, Wie es Isst. Der BMEL-Ernährungsreport 2023. Bundesministerium für Ernährung und Landwirtschaft. Available online: https://www.bmel.de/SharedDocs/Downloads/DE/Broschueren/ernaehrungsreport-2023.pdf?__blob=publicationFile&v=4 (accessed on 10 June 2024).
68. DAK-Gesundheit. Fasten Bleibt 2022 Trotz Pandemie Weiter im Trend. 2022. Hamburg. Available online: https://www.dak.de/dak/bundesthemen/fasten-bleibt-2022-trotz-pandemie-weiter-im-trend-2533580.html#/ (accessed on 10 June 2024).
69. BMEL. *Nationale Verzehrsstudie II*; Bundesministerium für Ernährung, Landwirtschaft und Verbraucherschutz: Berlin, Germany, 2008.
70. Kilger, M.; Pérez Aronsson, F. "You were born into this world an intuitive eater": Healthism and self-transformative practices on social media. *Food Foodways* **2024**, *32*, 35–55. [CrossRef]
71. Voils, C.I.; Coffman, C.J.; Yancy, W.S.; Weinberger, M.; Jeffreys, A.S.; Datta, S.; Kovac, S.; McKenzie, J.; Smith, R.; Bosworth, H.B. A randomized controlled trial to evaluate the effectiveness of CouPLES: A spouse-assisted lifestyle change intervention to improve low-density lipoprotein cholesterol. *Prev. Med.* **2013**, *56*, 46–52. [CrossRef]
72. Rückert-John, J.; Reis, S. Zur Reproduktion der sozialen Sinnform "Mahlzeit" in Zeiten des globalisierten Lebensmittelmarkts. In *Waren–Wissen–Raum: Interdependenz von Produktion, Markt und Konsum in Lebensmittelwarenketten*; Baur, N., Fülling, J., Hering, L., Kulke, E., Eds.; Springer: Wiesbaden, Germany, 2020; pp. 401–419, ISBN 978-3-658-30719-6.
73. Fischler, C. Commensality, society and culture. *Soc. Sci. Inf.* **2011**, *50*, 528–548. [CrossRef]
74. Sanlier, N.; Kocabas, Ş.; Ulusoy, H.G.; Celik, B. The Relationship between Adults' Perceptions, Attitudes of COVID-19, Intuitive Eating, and Mindful Eating Behaviors. *Ecol. Food Nutr.* **2021**, *61*, 90–109. [CrossRef]
75. Burkart, G. Soziologie der Paarbeziehung. In *Eine Einführung. Studientexte zur Soziologie*; Funcke, D., Hillebrandt, F., Vormbusch, U., Wilz, S., Eds.; Springer: Wiesbaden, Germany, 2018.
76. Barlösius, E. *Soziologie des Essens*; Juventa: München, Germany, 2011; ISBN 3779914891.
77. Caso, G.; Vecchio, R. Factors influencing independent older adults (un)healthy food choices: A systematic review and research agenda. *Food Res. Int.* **2022**, *158*, 111476. [CrossRef]
78. Khanijou, R.; Cappellini, B.; Hosany, S. Meal for two: A typology of co-performed practices. *J. Bus. Res.* **2021**, *134*, 675–688. [CrossRef]
79. Wethington, E.; Johnson-Askew, W.L. Contributions of the Life Course Perspective to research on food decision making. *Ann. Behav. Med.* **2009**, *38* (Suppl. S1), s74–s80. [CrossRef]
80. Baer, N.; Deutschbein, J.; Schenk, L. Potential for, and readiness to, dietary-style changes during the retirement status passage: A systematic mixed-studies review. *Nutr. Rev.* **2020**, *78*, 969–988. [CrossRef]
81. Beck, U.; Giddens, A.; Lash, S. *Reflexive Modernization: Politics, Tradition and Aesthetics in the Modern Social Order*; Stanford University Press: Redwood, CA, USA, 1994; ISBN 0804724725.
82. Reckwitz, A. *Die Gesellschaft der Singularitäten: Zum Strukturwandel der Moderne*; Suhrkamp: Berlin, Germayn, 2017; ISBN 3-518-58706-4.
83. Yates, L.; Warde, A. Eating together and eating alone: Meal arrangements in British households. *Br. J. Sociol.* **2017**, *68*, 97–118. [CrossRef]
84. Peitz, D.; Schulze, J.; Warschburger, P. Getting a deeper understanding of mindfulness in the context of eating behavior: Development and validation of the Mindful Eating Inventory. *Appetite* **2021**, *159*, 105039. [CrossRef]
85. Gallo, J.J.; Lee, S.Y. Mixed Methods in Behavioral Intervention Research. In *Behavioral Intervention Research—Designing, Evaluating, and Implementing*; Gitlin, L.N., Czaja, S.J., Eds.; Springer: New York, NY, USA, 2016.
86. Bohnsack, R.; Nentwig-Gesemann, I.; Nohl, A.-M. *Die Dokumentarische Methode und ihre Forschungspraxis: Grundlagen Qualitativer Sozialforschung*; Springer: Berlin/Heidelberg, Germany, 2013; ISBN 3531198955.
87. Przyborski, A.; Wohlrab-Sahr, M. *Qualitative Sozialforschung: Ein Arbeitsbuch*; Ouldenbourg: München, Germany, 2013; Volume 4, ISBN 3486719556.
88. Wimbauer, C.; Motakef, M. Das Paarinterview. In *Methodologie-Methode-Methodenpraxis*; Springer: Wiesbaden, Germany, 2017; ISBN 978-3-658-17977-9.
89. Banbury, A.; Nancarrow, S.; Dart, J.; Gray, L.; Parkinson, L. Telehealth Interventions Delivering Home-based Support Group Videoconferencing: Systematic Review. *J. Med. Internet Res.* **2018**, *20*, e25. [CrossRef]
90. Nahm, E.-S.; Bausell, B.; Resnick, B.; Covington, B.; Brennan, P.F.; Mathews, R.; Park, J.H. Online research in older adults: Lessons learned from conducting an online randomized controlled trial. *Appl. Nurs. Res.* **2011**, *24*, 269–275. [CrossRef]
91. Al-Dhahir, I.; Reijnders, T.; Faber, J.S.; van den Berg-Emons, R.J.; Janssen, V.R.; Kraaijenhagen, R.A.; Visch, V.T.; Chavannes, N.H.; Evers, A.W.M. The Barriers and Facilitators of eHealth-Based Lifestyle Intervention Programs for People with a Low Socioeconomic Status: Scoping Review. *J. Med. Internet Res.* **2022**, *24*, e34229. [CrossRef]
92. Wilson, J.; Heinsch, M.; Betts, D.; Booth, D.; Kay-Lambkin, F. Barriers and facilitators to the use of e-health by older adults: A scoping review. *BMC Public Health* **2021**, *21*, 1556. [CrossRef]

93. Burke, T.J.; Segrin, C. Examining Diet- and Exercise-Related Communication in Romantic Relationships: Associations With Health Behaviors. *Health Commun.* **2014**, *29*, 877–887. [CrossRef]
94. Bush, H.E.; Rossy, L.; Mintz, L.B.; Schopp, L. Eat for Life: A Work Site Feasibility Study of a Novel Mindfulness-Based Intuitive Eating Intervention. *Am. J. Health Promot.* **2014**, *28*, 380–388. [CrossRef]
95. Burnette, C.B.; Hazzard, V.M.; Larson, N.; Hahn, S.A.; Eisenberg, M.E.; Neumark-Sztainer, D. Is intuitive eating a privileged approach? Cross-sectional and longitudinal associations between food insecurity and intuitive eating. *Public Health Nutr.* **2023**, *26*, 1358–1367. [CrossRef]

Disclaimer/Publisher's Note: The statements, opinions and data contained in all publications are solely those of the individual author(s) and contributor(s) and not of MDPI and/or the editor(s). MDPI and/or the editor(s) disclaim responsibility for any injury to people or property resulting from any ideas, methods, instructions or products referred to in the content.

MDPI AG
Grosspeteranlage 5
4052 Basel
Switzerland
Tel.: +41 61 683 77 34

Nutrients Editorial Office
E-mail: nutrients@mdpi.com
www.mdpi.com/journal/nutrients

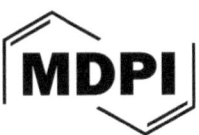

Disclaimer/Publisher's Note: The title and front matter of this reprint are at the discretion of the Guest Editors. The publisher is not responsible for their content or any associated concerns. The statements, opinions and data contained in all individual articles are solely those of the individual Editors and contributors and not of MDPI. MDPI disclaims responsibility for any injury to people or property resulting from any ideas, methods, instructions or products referred to in the content.

www.ingramcontent.com/pod-product-compliance
Lightning Source LLC
LaVergne TN
LVHW072359090526
838202LV00019B/2583